I0464386

# Hyperbaric Oxygen, Hypoxia, Hyperoxia & EMODs (ROS):

## SEPARATING FACT FROM FACTITIOUS

BY

### Prof Randolph M. Howes MD,PhD
**Physician, Surgeon, Scientist (Biochemist)**
**Prolific Author and Academic Scholar**

## A CRITIQUE & SELECTIVE REVIEW

# Hyperbaric Oxygen, Hypoxia, Hyperoxia & EMODs (ROS):

## SEPARATING FACT FROM FACTITIOUS

BY

### Prof Randolph M. Howes MD,PhD
Physician, Surgeon, Scientist (Biochemist),
Prolific Author and Academic Scholar

Adjunct Assistant Professor of Plastic Surgery, (RET.)
The Johns Hopkins Hospital, Baltimore, MD USA

Espaldon Professor of Plastic and Reconstructive Surgery,
University of Santo Tomas, Manila, Philippines

Adjunct Professor of Biological Sciences,
Southeastern Louisiana University

Founder, Director and Chairman of the Scientific Advisory
Board;
U.S. Medical Scientific Research Foundation, Inc.

**Copyright © 2015**
**Free Radical Publishing Co.**
**ISBN-13: 9781515207962**

**ISBN-10: 151520796X**

**By Dr. Randolph "HealR" Howes The "PHENOM"**
Copyright © 2015
**Free Radical Publishing Co.**
**27439 Hwy 441**
**Kentwood, Louisiana 70444**

Address for communication: 27439 Highway 441, Kentwood, Louisiana 70444-8152, USA. Email: rhowesmd@hughes.net

# DISCLOSURE AND DISCLAIMER

It is understood that medicine is an ever-changing science. As new research and clinical experience broaden our knowledge, changes in treatment and drug therapy are required. The author and the publisher of this work have checked with sources believed to be reliable in their efforts to provide information that is complete and generally in accord with the standards accepted at the time of publication. However, in view of the possibility of human error or changes in the medical sciences, neither the authors nor the publisher nor any other party who has been involved in the preparation of publication of this work warrants that the information contained herein is in every respect accurate or complete, and they disclaim all responsibility to any errors or omissions or for the results obtained from use of the information contained in the work. Readers should confirm the information contained herein with other sources. For example and in particular, readers are advised to check the product information sheets (or labels) included in the package of each drug they plan to administer to be certain that the information contained in this work is accurate and that changes have not been made in the recommended dose or in the contraindications for administration. This recommendation is of particular importance in connection with new or infrequently used drugs, additives or supplements.

**Disclaimers**: Please note: only your personal physician or other health professional you consult can best advise you on matters of your health based on your medical history, your family medical history, your medication history, and how information from any of these databases may apply to you. Neither Dr. Howes nor any party involved in creating, producing or delivering this web site shall be liable for any damages arising out of access to or use of this material or web site, or any errors or omissions in the content thereof.

The information given herein is not intended as medical advice. Always consult with your doctor for underlying illness. Before beginning dietary investigation, consult a dietician or a physician with an interest in nutrition. Information is drawn from the scientific literature, web research, and personal enquiry; while all care is taken, information is not warranted as accurate and the author cannot be held liable for any errors and omissions.

The information contained herein is not intended to replace a one-on-one relationship with a qualified health care professional and is not intended as medical advice. It is intended as a sharing of knowledge and information from the research of Dr. Howes. Dr. Howes encourages you to make your own health care decisions based upon your research and the advice of a qualified health care professional.

Financial disclosure: **Dr. Howes has no financial conflicts of interest and is not involved in the sale of dietary supplements or fitness equipment. The author holds no stocks or interests in companies in the food additive or antioxidant supplement business.**

# ACKNOWLEDGEMENTS

Special thanks Don Neale Piatt, Sr. for proof reading. Also, special thanks to Michael R. Root, M.S. for his unwavering encouragement.

Truth be told,

I can scarcely begin to explain

the overwhelming, biochemical complexity

of a singular living, breathing critter.

In truth, it approximates

being utterly ineffable,

all the while, reflecting the

stunning beauty of Creation.

R. M. Howes, M.D., Ph.D.

2/2/15

# DEDICATION

To my mentors Dr. Richard H. Steele, Dr. Alan White,
Dr. C.T. Su, Dr. George Zuidema, Dr. John Cameron, Dr. Vincent Gott,
Dr. John Hoopes and Dr. Andrew Schally

Oxygen is not optional.

It is essential for creating and

perpetuating aerobic life and for

sustaining homeostatic health,

especially in man.

R. M. Howes, M.D., Ph.D.

4/2/15

Radically increase your chances

for establishing long term homeostatic health

by increasing your oxidative capacity,

- your oxidative bliss.

R. M. Howes, M.D., Ph.D.

4/3/15

**Breathing –**
**a significantly under-appreciated activity**
**Oxygen –**
**a significantly under-valued element**
**Free Radical Theory –**
**a significantly over used, flawed notion**
**Oxidative Stress –**
**a significant misinterpretation of facts**
**Antioxidant –**
**a significant misuse of words**
**EMODs –**
**a significant correction of terms**
**UTOPIA Theory –**
**a significant contribution to redox biochemistry**
**ROSI Theory of Howes –**
**a significant new, unique concept of disease coexistence**

R.M. Howes, M.D., Ph.D.
7/5/15

**EMODs** (electronically modified oxygen derivatives, previously called reactive oxygen species, ROS); **ROSI theory**, ROS Insufficiency theory, reactive oxygen species insufficiency theory; **UTOPIA theory**, Unified theory of oxygen participation in aerobiosis

# Hyperbaric Oxygen, Hypoxia, Hyperoxia & EMODs (ROS):

## SEPARATING FACT FROM FACTITIOUS

# TABLE OF CONTENTS:

# SECTION SEVEN
## HBOT AND CANCER.................................................227

# NOTICE:

Throughout this book, I have placed significant hyperbaric oxygen positive effects in **arial black print**

---

**Abbreviations**: Hyperbaric oxygen, HBO or $HBO_2$; hyperbaric oxygen therapy (treatment), HBOT; electronically modified oxygen derivatives, EMODs; reactive oxygen species, ROS; reactive nitrogen species, RNS; nitric oxide (NO); stem/progenitor cells, SPCs; hypoxia inducible factors, HIF; basic fibroblast growth factor (bFGF); platelet derived growth factor (PDGF); Vascular endothelial growth factor (VEGF); tumor necrosis factor (TNF); interleukin (IL); insulin-like growth factor I (IGF-1); central nervous system (CNS); UTOPIA (Unified Theory Of Oxygen Participation In Aerobiosis); ROSI syndrome theory of Howes (Reactive Oxygen Species Insufficiency); reactive oxygen intermediates, ROIs; peripheral blood mononuclear cells (PBMCs); mitogen-activated protein kinases (MAPKs); metalloproteinase (MMP); diabetic foot ulcers (DFU); age-related macular degeneration (AMD); delayed onset muscle soreness (DOMS); anterior cruciate ligament (ACL); low-level laser therapy (LLLT); low-intensity laser irradiation (LILI) or phototherapy; adenosine triphosphate (ATP); H.Ep.2 cells (laryngeal carcinoma cells); MTT (thiazolyl blue tetrazolium bromide); murine melanoma (B16F10) cells; intracellular calcium ($ICa^{2+}$); a photosensitizer (PS); photodynamic therapy (PDT); photodynamic reaction (PDR)

# PREFACE

As an intro, and since oxygen and its electronically modified oxygen derivatives (EMODs) are at the center of the mechanisms of hyperbaric oxygen therapy, I will include this little "scientific teaser", which I composed in 2006, as follows:

## THE FABLE OF
## "CLOTHES are KILLERS"
(a free radical/antioxidant parody)

Once upon a half a century ago, investigators studied a group of cancer patients and found that all had worn clothing. It was impossible to deny this obvious and direct association and they questioned why others hadn't made this apparent connection before.

It had been known for many years that articles of clothing could be destructive and harmful by getting caught in machinery, producing dismemberment, holding hot liquids and/or strangulating blood supply to various body parts.

Scientists set out and verified in the laboratory that clothes could strangle, maim, mutilate, dismember and harm people. Thus, under *in vitro* laboratory conditions, clothes could destroy the underlying biochemicals of life, i.e., proteins, lipids, and even DNA culminating in the death of the individual. The potential of this horrific scene had been skillfully and boldly scrawled in crayon on the nonscience/nonsense canvas of pseudoscience.

Medical researchers obtained grants to study the extent of the clothing menace. They studied a group of patients with atherosclerosis and they had similar findings of a direct relationship between the wearing of clothes and the occurrence of vascular plaques.

Diabetes showed the same thing as did arthritis, Alzheimer's, obesity and cataracts. In fact, all of these diseased patients had worn clothes. The more sick patients they studied, the more they found that all had worn clothing. This was a revelation akin to the discovery of the atom or the circulation of blood.

Additional studies verified a straight line relationship between over 100 pathophysiologies and the wearing of clothing. Study after study demonstrated the same deleterious effect of clothes. The conclusions were undeniable and obvious, i.e., clothes are damaging, toxic, pernicious, deleterious and harmful, even though they may by needed for survival at times.

This conclusion was becoming an established and well accepted fact.

However, some scientists were puzzled by the fact that not all of those who wore clothes actually developed any of these diseases. Consequently, this unsettling observation was immediately dubbed a "paradox" and was shrugged off and swept under the scientific rug of academic cover up. After all, the data was so strong for a direct relationship between the donning of clothes and the occurrence of a vast array of diseases that it had to be a scientifically accurate observation.

They had discovered causality of disease.

These deep thinkers found that if they further segmentalized the diseased patients into categories according to the type of fabric, predominant color of their ensemble, mixing of colors, exposure of the individual and the clothing to sunlight or UV, associated smoking, diesel fumes, sex, race, creed or fondness for pets and Twinkies, they could on occasion find statistically significant subgroups for specific diseases.

By running the data through the statistical pseudo-scientific meat grinder, they could produce a confusing, "virtual sausage" of association, which no one would question. This was especially true if they kept the groups small, observational and non-randomized.

This mathematically proven revelation inspired the **"clothes cause disease theory."** Thence arose the powerful movement of the very vocal "clothes phobes."

For the next fifty years, the "clothes phobes" continued to dismiss the fact that many bearers of clothing did not become ill at all and that they, in fact, lived normal, healthy long lives. They repeatedly made the point that a paradox here or a paradox there does not dismiss or falsify the fact that all of the studied sick people had, in actuality, been wearing clothes on a regular basis and that association was indisputable.

Paper after paper seemingly confirmed their apparent assertion, built peer momentum and over rode common sense observations.

Moreover, it had become increasingly clear that the longer the people had worn clothes, the more likely it was that they were going to develop illness and undergo aging.

Further, it was reasoned that the mere condition of wearing clothes must be producing accumulating stressful and disease causing conditions.

It became obvious to them that the random summation of the clothes-wearing-condition was responsible for the onset of diseases and it, evidently, promoted aging. Thus, was born the **"clothing stress and aging theory."**

Of particular note, one celebrated West Coast biochemist was quoted as saying, "The things which protect our bodies the most, i.e., clothes, are the very things that are killing us." Other respected chemists published "**The Clothes Paradox.**"

The clothes phobes widely and emphatically disseminated their message to the extent that anyone doubting their claims of clothing toxicity would be snubbed by the "clothes phobe clique" and labeled a crack pot.

Forthrightly, they were boldly quoted as saying, "Even Forrest Gump could see that all sick people had worn clothes and that the longer any of them wore clothes, the older they became." Their conclusions were as clear as the nose on your face...or the clothes on your back.

However, it had been pointed out that some infants were born ill and the clothes phobes explained this anomaly by the fact that the sperm donor was probably a wearer of clothes and such was likely the case for the mother. The unspecified clothing toxic factor was likely passed on to the fetus.

Shockingly, it had also been pointed out by some renegades that there were occasions whereby clothes were beneficial and good. Conflicting observations and conclusions were surfacing.

In addition, one study found that the wearing of clothes in polar climates could be life saving and thus, the confusion grew.

But alas, the clothes phobic scientists reasoned that if clothing was the culprit, then illness, disease and aging could be prevented, stopped and/or reversed by not wearing clothes (nudity or an "anti-clothes condition"). Thus, they had millions remove their clothes, followed their clinical course but they unexpectedly observed many contrary and conflicted results which they dismissed as being disturbingly "disappointing."

It appeared that there were just as many sick nude people as there were in people who were wearing clothes. In fact, removal of clothing, which could result in parasite attacks, malaria, yellow fever, frost bite, freezing, extreme sunburns, animal bites and general trauma, could result in an overall increase in disease and mortality.

These observations shook the **"clothes cause disease and aging theory"** to its core. All of the clothes phobe grants were put in jeopardy.

However, the clothes phobes struck back with full, vitriolic, venomous force. With the injudicious use of statistical smoke and mathematical mirrors, they could still show that clothes and disease and aging were directly related.

They repeated the fact that in the lab, items of clothing could readily be made to produce or be associated with harm to the body and if this was the case, "What could be more clear?"

The clothes must go. **"Loathe the clothes"** was their mantra.

They hastily formed the Committee for Dreaming Up Excuses to refute the ineffectiveness of nudity in prevention or reversal of disease and aging. The Excuse Committee published prolifically and clever marketers rushed in to sell "virtual see-through clothes" with the implication that this could supplement the nude state.

Yet, they were still getting disappointing results. The Excuse Committee produced a litany of pretexts and alibis to negate the failed studies but it wasn't enough.

Clear thinking and common sense ultimately prevailed and ushered in the rise and fall of the **"clothes cause disease and aging theory."**

Respectfully (with tongue in cheek) submitted,

Randolph M. Howes, M.D., Ph.D.

p.s. I could have sworn that I had heard something like this before concerning oxygen free radicals and antioxidants, but no one could have been that stupid....or could they?

Oxygen made a good target because of its crucial role in the metabolism of all aerobic cells. Thus, it could be linked to almost anything the cell was doing but the proposal that happenstance associations were "cause and effect" was the main factor which led so many down the "corridor of confusion."

**"Relative to oxygen metabolism,
the most damaging chain reaction that occurs,
is the uncontrolled dispersal of misinformation and
the perpetuation of erroneous conclusions."**
R. M. Howes, M.D., Ph.D.
8/21/04

---

Hyperbaric oxygen, Hypoxia, Hyperoxia & EMODs (ROS) is the scientific companion book to backup the clinical application and use of hyperbaric oxygen therapy.

After reviewing the past and current hyperbaric oxygen (HBO) literature, I have been impressed by two things. Hyperbaric oxygen therapy (HBOT) has been used to varying degrees of effectiveness to treat a wide spectrum of diseases but HBOT has not established itself as a popular mainstay in overall medical practice.

The number of randomized controlled trials on HBO is limited but there is ample additional data to glean an opinion as regards the usefulness of hyperbaric oxygen therapy (HBOT).

HBOT has definitely evolved past the experimental stage and should be recognized as part of the armamentarium of established medical science. And, the experimental field is open to exciting and widespread investigations.

There are a large number of in vitro experiments and animal models which suggest a positive role for HBOT in clinical practice.

Of particular interest to me, is the fact that electronically modified oxygen derivatives (EMODs, formerly incorrectly called reactive oxygen species, ROS) are front and center in the biochemical mechanisms involving HBOT. This dovetails with other treatment modalities such as phototherapy, photodynamic therapy (PDT), sonodynamic therapy, the Howes tumoricidal system, chemotherapy and radiation therapy.

EMOD involvement also has a commonality with the benefits seen with exercise and in the highly oxidatively stressed metabolism of the naked mole rat. Of all voluntary human activities, the one proven most important to prevent disease, and promote and maintain health is exercise.

No doubt, EMOD-induced apoptosis (cellular suicide) is a key factor in holding cancer at bay and in killing cancerous cells.

Additionally, EMODs are essential for the killing of pathogens, such as bacteria, fungi, protozoans and viruses, in particular, viruses that have a lipid coating. I believe that this explains many of the healing and preventative aspects of HBOT.

HBOT has proven to be a safe, non-invasive and a welcomed addition to other common forms of medical care.

Now, let's take a serious look at oxygen, hyperbaric oxygen and its relationship to EMODs.

How important is oxygen to the existence and perpetuation of life in carbon based aerobic life forms....in particular, man?

The nearly unbelievable role of oxygen in sustaining aerobic life is illustrated by the frequently overlooked fact that a constant and invariant supply of $O_2$ is essential to maintain the life force.

**Blood, if oxygenated, carries the life force within its bio-fluid; whereas, un-oxygenated blood is just bio-fluid. HBOT endeavors to increase the oxygen carrying capacity of blood plasma and increase its amount at the cellular and subcellular levels.**

In man, this requires that the body circulate its entire volume of blood every minute of our lives, or 1,440 times/day, or 525,600 times/year or 36,792,000 times for a 70 year old man...at rest!

The human heart beats over 2.5 billion times and pumps 5 million gallons of blood in the average lifetime.

This illustrates the amazing capability of **"specialized flesh", all the while on auto pilot.**

All of this work and energy is expended primarily to remove $O_2$ from the air and to transport it to all of our cells, for the perpetuation of life as we know it. **To me, it is incomprehensible that nature would work so very hard to actively bring an alleged "killer substance, a toxin, a poison, e.g., ($O_2$)" into its midst but it**

**would logically do so to sustain itself with the life rendering energy potential possessed by oxygen.**

**With billions of years to perfect aerobic metabolism, I remain highly circumspect that the generation of superoxide or hydrogen peroxide from one of every 20 processed oxygen molecules, which passes through the electron transport chain en route to oxidative phosphorylation, is the result of a "leak" or a colossal design flaw. A glaring mistake of this magnitude is implausible, since it had billions upon billions of years to get it right.**

**Obviously, we have been looking at the situation from the wrong perspective. Any evolving system, possessing the ingenuity to create beautifully complex molecules, such as the $O_2$-binding heme proteins, surely would have corrected a "lethal leak" occurring directly in the midst of its most vital chemical pathway.**

**There is a general failure to appreciate the imposing biochemical grandeur encased within the living/breathing cell and its inter-connectedness to the whole organism.**

Basic energy-producing metabolism for aerobic organisms starts with $O_2$ (di-radical, ground state oxygen) and ends with $H_2O$ (water). At first glance, that appears ever so simple but that is far from the actual case.

$O_2$ plus direct electron reductions and hydrogen abstractions lead to **$2H_2O$ plus energy production.**

Studies are further complicated by combining all of EMODs under one incorrect "radical" heading and by not recognizing their individual re-activities or chemical properties. It is inexcusable that these known inaccuracies are perpetuated.

The situation only worsens when one reviews the literature on "anti-oxidants and antioxidant enzymes."

**Sweeping erroneous generalities are everywhere and appear to be readily accepted** but the true biochemical facts must be applied to make interpretation of the data as accurate as possible. For example:

- It is rarely pointed out that many of the standard antioxidants can serve equally well as reductants or that pro-oxidants can also serve as antioxidants.
- The idea that any free radical or oxidant is merely present to kill us or to make us ill, is a blatant distortion of biochemical facts.

Tragically, the erroneous concept that EMODs are only agents of destruction and harm has been indelibly etched into the medical, scientific and lay psyche.

- It is rarely pointed out that free radicals and oxidants play an ever-increasing role in indispensable and crucial cellular signaling functions and they are operative at many metabolic levels.
- It is rarely mentioned that either standard or large excessive doses of antioxidants can be harmful or even deadly.
- It is even more rarely mentioned that normal steady state levels of EMODs are necessary to maintain cellular homeostasis and to fend off infections and cancer via their **bactericidal, fungicidal, parasiticidal, virucidal and tumoricidal activity**.
- Antioxidant enzymes can also generate free radicals and oxidants, further confusing the unknowing reader of the literature, and antioxidant enzymes are frequently inhibited or inactivated by various EMOD species.
- Rarely mentioned is the possible reaction of hydrogen peroxide with transition metals which produces the superoxide anion, not the hydroxyl radical.
- EMODs, including singlet oxygen, did not come on the scene for just the past 100 years, when cancer, heart disease and CNS disease rates started to soar or for just the past ½ century, since the free radical theory was introduced. They have been around since aerobic life evolved on Earth, which was approximately 2.3-2.5 billion years before these diseases became a cause celebre. Actually, they have been around since light (photons) first reacted to excite a pigment, in the presence of oxygen. During the intervening eon, these alleged killers of aerobic life (EMODs) should surely have destroyed aerobic life, according to the predictions of the free radical theory, but they did not. In fact, EMODs sustained aerobic life and accompanied the evolutionary process. Consequently, Dr. Harman, and the oxy-moronic sycophants, did not release EMODs upon helpless and vulnerable aerobic life forms. They just mistakenly attributed all disease states and aging to them.
- Evolutionary history has proven the predictors of doom and gloom to be wrong, as it relates to EMODs and aerobic cellular interactions.
- The probable interaction of EMODs with themselves or feed back/self-control of EMODs is rarely mentioned. Control of EMOD levels does not necessarily require antioxidants, either endogenous or exogenous, once one understands the myriad of inter-actions possible with EMODs and redox chemistry. I believe that complex EMODs interactions may be, in a large part, self-regulating.

**Medical and scientific literature concerning oxidative metabolism is loaded with confusing, conflicting, contradictory and controversial data.** Nothing is more disturbing than the claims by thousands of researchers that **O$_2$ is a toxic killer**, contrasted with the claims of thousands of alternative practitioners that **O$_2$ therapy is a cure**.

On the one hand, O$_2$ and its products are blamed for causing over 100 human diseases; whereas, on the other hand, O$_2$ therapy is touted as the cure for these very same diseases.

Thus, we must continue to look for "patterns of predictability" to lead to a greater understanding of the unbelievable complexities of the living/breathing cell.

**I have become increasingly skeptical and weary of overly exaggerated interpretations of in vitro studies and at epidemiological associations which are presented and touted as cause and effect relationships. Remember, by definition, a cause invariably leads to its effect.**

**The introduction of biometry, which is the application of statistics to biology and medicine, has been a double edged microtome. Causality may be unrelated to correlations.**

**One good clinical study is worth countless expert opinions.**

## UTOPIA CONNECTIONS AND CONVERGENCE

My studies of the biochemical intricacies connecting reactive oxygen radicals and excited states has led me to the following unifying concepts:

- EMODs, including excited states, have levels or ranges, which I prefer to call zones, which determine certain biological outcomes, relative to the appearance of cancer and infection. Zones of EMODs and excited states appear to be multi-phasic and at least triphasic. In general, these zones refer to the whole organism but due to the heterogeneity of tissue and/or organs necessitates that they be considered on an individual basis at times.

- **Howes' TRIPHASIC ZONES OF EMODs & EXCITED STATES**

- **Apoptosis Zone** - the **highest zone (hyper-zone, levels of EMODs above normal homeostatic levels)** of EMODs and excited states (EMODs). Based on the results of thousands and thousands of papers, it is well established that very high levels of EMODs and excited states which can be produced by PDT, many chemotherapeutic drugs, radiation, HBOT and the Howes Singlet Oxygen delivery system, **will kill cancer**. Also, a hyper-stimulated immune system, such as is seen in spontaneous regression of cancer, **kills cancer**.

- **Abeyance Zone** - the **middle zone (mid-zone, adequate homeostatic EMOD levels)** of EMODs, including excited states. Based on the fact that millions and millions of people go through life without the manifestation of cancer is evidence, par excellence, for the existence of this mid zone of EMODs and excited states, which **hold cancer cell development in abeyance**. It is an accepted scientific fact that all aerobic cells undergo exponential numbers of potentially mutagenic oxidative damaging events on a continual basis yet, **millions do not manifest or develop continual infections or tumors in a life time.** This is the zone of **homeostasis**.

- **Allowance Zone** - the **lowest zone (hypo-zone, a deficiency or insufficiency)** of EMODs, including excited states. This zone is based on the millions of cases of patients with immunosuppression (acquired or innate) and on genetic diseases such as chronic granulomatous disease, obesity and diabetes. We know that low levels of EMODs, including excited states **allow the development of cancer**.

**"Aerobic life is choreographed by its oxygen instructor to perform the dance of the electron."**
R. M. Howes, M.D., Ph.D.
2/25/04

Overall, I have found sound biochemical rationale for the use of HBOT in pathogen protection, increased wound healing and cancer prevention and potential cure.

I have included in this book both the pros and cons as regards HBOT in treating chronic wounds and a wide spectrum of diseases. I have arduously summarized the studies and provided a condensed listing of the conditions that have been successfully treated with HBOT.

As with all medical science topics, experiments range from low quality to those that are conducted carefully for wound healing, wounds in diabetics, radiation tissue injury, multiple sclerosis, autism, Crohn's disease, cancer, Alzheimer's disease, etc. One has to try to assimilate the data and arrive at a reasonable substantiated conclusion as regards the risk/benefit ratio for HBOT. Fortunately, for HBOT, the benefits far outweigh the risks.

Perhaps one of the most reliable sources of studies is the Cochrane Collaboration and I have tried to include their work where possible.

Overall, HBOT is considered safe but I have included possible adverse effects where ever data was available. In 2008, the Department of DefenseWhite Paper report stated: "side effects are uncommon and severe or permanent complications are rare..."

Serious side effects, such as seizures, temporary visual disturbances and oxygen toxicity are rare but some lesser adverse effects, such as discomfort during decompression, claustrophobia, abdominal pain and ear pain are more common and are mild and self limiting.

It must be mentioned that there has been some risk associated with the use of the hyperbaric equipment itself, but it is also rare.

In short, I feel that HBOT has a promising future. I can only hope that it will make deeper inroads into common medical practice and that patients can avail themselves to its benefits. I am also hopeful that research on HBOT will move forward at an accelerated pace for the prevention of pain and suffering.

I find it particularly exciting that another prooxidant therapy, HBOT, has established itself in the general arena of medical science.

**"The raw materials needed to construct a man are worth less than**
**five dollars of basic chemical components.**
**Yet, when properly oxygenated, hydrated, nourished and assembled,**
**they form entities of value beyond estimation,**
**which we love and call**
**'self**
**and**
**our fellow man'."**
R. M. Howes, M.D., Ph.D.
7/11/04

Undoubtedly, my book may spark some controversy, but I sincerely hope that it may, in some way, stimulate discoveries in this most exciting area of medical science and thus, bring cures to the patient's bedside and lessen pain and suffering for mankind.

### First, Do No Harm. ("Primum non nocere")

The **"dogma de jour"** (**dogma of the day),** can hold medical advances at a virtual standstill.

**The mere fact that a procedure is called a "therapy" or that a drug is called a "medicine" does not guarantee you that it is good for you or that it will not cause you serious harm. In fact, it may kill you.**

Big Pharma certainly follows the Golden Rule, in that "He, who has the gold, makes the rules." They market and promote **"pharmaceuticide."**

The mantra of Big Pharma seems to be **"profit, profit and more profit".**

**The definition of successful research programs has been narrowed to those most likely to yield a marketable product, rather than to those that generate new knowledge.**

**The work that is being done, and that is ultimately published, tends to favor the interest of those who fund the research.**

For scientific work to maintain quality and reliability, it must adhere to the principles of the scientific method.

**Following a lifetime of research, I have arrived at an overall conclusion regarding disease allowance, disease coexistence and aging as follows: as age increases, oxygen availability to the cell and its intracellular organelles decrease, and an EMOD insufficiency results, which "allows" diseases and the signs of aging to become manifest realities. Sustaining sufficient oxygen, and its EMOD progeny levels, maintains homeostasis and an increased healthspan and lifespan. RMH 8-7-15**

# SECTION ONE

## CRUCIAL OXYGEN

### The Self-evident Importance of Oxygen

Oxygen is ubiquitous and omnipresent on the Earth's surface and throughout our bodies. As we breathe it in, plants breathe it out.

In our cells, mitochondria "breathe" $O_2$ and pyruvic acid into the Kreb's cycle to produce ATP. When a mitochondrion "breathes out" it releases ATP, $H_2O$, and $CO_2$.

Oxygen is the subject of immense chemical, physiological, and clinical literature.

The energy for life derives from the large free energy difference between hydrogen and oxygen. The energy of radiation from the sun is used in the photosynthetic processes of plants to separate water into oxygen and hydrogen.

The oxygen in the atmosphere is believed to represent but 0.1 % of the oxygen content of the Earth. The greatest store of oxygen remains combined with minerals in the solid earthen crust and in water.

The relative amounts of oxygen consumed by the tissues of an adult human male are directly related to the content and capacity of the mitochondrial respiratory chain. (Tyler, 1992)

**Oxygen's history stems from the original observations of Lavoisier, Priestley, and Scheele.** (Lavoisier, 1777) (Priestley, 1775) (Scheele, 1777)

In the beginning, there was no free $O_2$ in the atmosphere. The subsequent outgassing of the outer layers of the Earth then contributed to the atmosphere **the small amount of oxygen required for initiating life processes** in which oxygen combined with carbon to form $CO_2$, with N2, formed the next stage of our atmosphere. (Herbig, 1981)

The linkage to the development of life, as we understand it, in particular the key role played by oxygen, remains a challenge for scientific investigation. Life presumably developed in **the original reducing atmosphere using oxidation-reduction reactions dependent on such elements as sulfur and iron**; but at some point photosynthesis developed and reactions were established for the dissociation of water, thereby markedly increasing the availability of oxygen for chemical and biological reactions. (Kamen, 1963)

Oxygen in the atmosphere is continually being replenished by photosynthesis but consumed by oxidation of organic compounds, including respiration by living organisms including the small plants that produce it, in the sea as well as on land, at a rate of about 0.04% per year.

As life forms evolved into multicellular organisms with convective systems that in effect surround each cell with an oxygen-containing environment, they were able to grow in size. **Claude Bernard immortalized this concept in his "milieu interieur".** (Bernard, 1878)

**Pasteur noted that lack of $O_2$ produced changes in the structure of yeast, and he concluded that $O_2$ was the key to differentiation.** (Pasteur, 1861)

**Warburg later extended this principle, believing that the lack of $O_2$ caused cells to de-differentiate.** (Warburg, Geissler, Lorenz, 1968)

The physical properties of oxygen, combined with its thermodynamic and kinetic properties, **place oxygen in a unique position so "that no other element could effectively replace it."** (Hamilton, 1990)

Central to this theme is the large free energy release available in discrete increments that occurs during the reduction of oxygen to water. **The four one-electron equivalent stepwise reduction of molecular oxygen to water results in a great variety of chemical species as intermediates.** (Koppenol, 1988)

In biological systems the one-electron reduction of oxygen results in **(a)** the formation of the **free radical superoxide anion**. For example, during the reaction of some flavoproteins or hemoproteins with oxygen or during the redox cycling of quinones, significant amounts of superoxide are formed. The microbicidal role of superoxide formed during the "oxygen burst" of phagocytosis is an essential component of the response to inflammation and the killing of pathogens.

**The protonated form of the superoxide anion, the perhydoxy radical, is the dominant form at neutral pH** and is more invidious (undesirable) because of its increased lipid solubility.

**(b) The two-electron reduction state of molecular oxygen is hydrogen peroxide.** This compound is generally formed by a dismutation of the perhydroxy radical in a reaction catalyzed by the enzyme superoxide dismutase (a prooxidant enzyme). Hydrogen peroxide can dissociate (in the presence of a suitable metal) to form an electrophilic oxene intermediate together with water. Of course, this highly reactive form of oxygen can also arise from the heterolytic cleavage of molecular oxygen.

**(c)** Most reactive of the reduction intermediates of molecular oxygen is the strongly oxidizing **hydroxyl radical, HO** ; i.e. the three-electron reduced state of molecular oxygen. Classic Fenton reaction chemistry or the metal (iron) catalyzed Haber-Weiss reaction leads to this species of oxygen.

Lastly, **(d)** the four-electron reduced form of molecular oxygen is **water**.

The reactivity and alleged toxicity of the reactive oxygen species (EMODs) formed during the reduction of oxygen have been proposed to be major contributors to the pathogenesis of many chronic degenerative diseases and aging. **However, I take strong objection to this position.**

Although molecular oxygen is used by higher animals in the synthesis of a great variety of important chemical compounds that serve as constituents and regulators of cellular metabolism, **the amount of oxygen used for these reactions is minor compared to that consumed for energy production.**

A specified amount of $O_2$ is required for all energy needs by all aerobes. $O_2$ delivery must be adjusted within seconds for any changes in metabolic rate in order to maintain cell $pO_2$ and avoid cell death.

Some of the following material was adapted from: (Forster, Estabrook, 1993)

The $pO_2$ in blood entering the cellular capillary bed is normally 100 mm Hg while the $pO_2$ at the mitochondria is certainly less than 15 mm Hg. (Coburn, Marers, 1974)

This drop of $pO_2$ of some 85 mm Hg within the cells is the largest decline in the entire path from ambient air to the mitochondrial cytochrome c oxidase.

The minimal $pO_2$ at which a mitochondrion will continue to reduce $O_2$ is thought to be low, possibly less than 1 mm Hg, but this value is in dispute.

The $O_2$-carrying capacity of the blood can be regulated by altering the concentration of erythrocytes.

Peripheral skeletal muscles have extremely low resting capillary blood flow, but with exercise and the associated metabolic demands the blood flow increases enormously. (Grieb et al, 19985)

Athletic training increases muscle capacity for work by increasing the number of mitochondria and, of necessity, the capillary bed to supply them.

**The relative amounts of oxygen consumed by the tissues of an adult human male are directly related to the content and capacity of the mitochondrial respiratory chain.** (Tyler, 1992)

Skeletal muscle, which makes up about 42% of body weight, uses about 30% of oxygen consumed at rest, and over 86% of oxygen consumed during heavy work. The abdominal organs use 25% and the brain uses 20% of the oxygen consumed at rest. Their relative contributions proportionately decrease during heavy work.

The human brain and heart can survive for only brief intervals of $O_2$ deprivation without sustaining irreversible damage or cell death.

A cell may die from lack of oxygen long before it can starve because of a failure of nutrient transport. For example, the normal arterial concentration of glucose is 5.5 mM and the normal arterial $pO_2$ is 100 mm Hg, equivalent to 0.12 mM $O_2$.

In addition, 6 molecules of $O_2$ are required to oxidize 1 molecule of glucose so that from the viewpoint of supplying metabolic needs, the concentration of glucose is 275 times greater than that of $O_2$ in the extracellular fluid at the surface of the cell. Thus, oxygen turnover is the highest among essential nutrients.

If one looks at **levels of consciousness**, decreasing levels of $O_2$ results directly in decreased levels of consciousness. Pilots or those exploring high altitudes, experience confusion, and dizziness up to the point of total loss of consciousness, with progressively decreasing levels of $O_2$.

Conditions such as ischemic encephalopathy, present with decreased brain oxygen levels and with the attendant mental confusion pattern. **If the $O_2$ levels are stopped for just a few minutes, one can experience death of brain neurons**, in an irreversible fashion and brain function ceases. Again, this is analogous to pulling the plug on a computer, thereby stopping or interrupting its power supply.

One can see that a situation can exist whereby the brain still has an $O_2$ supply but does not function properly, such as in traumatic unconsciousness or coma. This would be analogous to traumatizing a computer, whereby it is still plugged into a power supply but does not function.

Thus, it appears to me that at least one fundamental requirement for consciousness is the presence and flow of a constant supply of electrons via oxygen.

Furthermore, **I believe, as do others, that the reactivity of ground state oxygen is far too slow to participate in usual brain function (thinking, thought storage and retrieval) and that speeds of electromagnetic phenomena can be achieved primarily by oxygen radicals and electronic excitation states.**

Howard Mason (personal communication to Foster and Estabrook) has cataloged over 350 different classes of enzymes in biology that react with oxygen. Of these about 150 different types may be present in mammals, although many are shared with lower forms of life. This calculation does not include the large number of isoforms (isoenzymes) that subdivide a specific class of oxygen-reacting enzyme.

These enzymes include oxidases, oxygenases, hydroxylases, and peroxidases. They consist of hemoproteins, flavoproteins, copper proteins, and proteins containing metals such as molybdenum, manganese, cobalt, vanadium, etc. Clearly, Nature has devised many different approaches to capture the potential energy present in oxygen.

Another class of hemoproteins present in many cells is the cytochrome P450 super family. These hemoproteins catalyze an oxygenase reaction for the incorporation of molecular oxygen into a wide spectrum of organic chemicals. Most interesting is the diversity of oxygen-dependent reactions catalyzed by different P450s. These reactions touch nearly every aspect of biology and medicine.

In the 1970s, Dr. Richard H. Steele and I were to first to show the involvement of EMODs in lipid peroxidation and aryl hydroxylations in P450 hepatic systems. (Howes, Steele, 1971) (Howes, Steele, 1972)

Oxygen radicals are generated during the reintroduction of oxygen to a tissue, such as the reperfusion of the ischemic myocardium. (Kato, 1987)

As a result, a peroxidation of cellular lipids may modify the properties of cellular membranes or an oxidation of key cellular proteins may produce conformational change or denaturation with a concomitant loss of enzymatic activity. The result of these irreversible injuries to the cell is necrosis.

**The $O_2$ transport system regulates the delivery of $O_2$ to peripheral cells to maintain $pO_2$ within a narrow range, from about 1 mm Hg to about 15 mm Hg.** (Coburn et al, 1986)

Older literature states that if a healthy adult breathes essentially pure $O_2$ at sea level, his lungs become irritated; a rat exposed in the same way will die in a matter of hours; newborn humans will develop retrolental fibrodysplasia. Chronic exposure of rats to high oxygen can diminish or destroy the ability of the carotid bodies to monitor low arterial blood $pO_2$. These are but a few examples of the deleterious effects of inspiring higher than normal $0_2$ concentrations.

Some believe the rather absurd notion that $O_2$ is both an absolute requirement for life and at the same time, a toxin, giving rise to the **"oxygen paradox."**

> **I lived another day.**
> **I breathed another day.**
> **I shared another wondrous day of living**
> **with my beautiful chemical cohort,**
> **oxygen.**
> R. M. Howes, M.D., Ph.D.
> 2/22/11

**Ames & Gold estimate that "the DNA hits per cell per day from endogenous oxidants are normally in the $10^5$ rat and $10^4$ in humans.** (Ames, Gold, 1991)

"Oxygen radicals are thought to account for the major share of agents causing disease and aging damage. Thus, there is a paradox. Oxygen is essential to life, yet we must balance this positive effect with the recognition that oxygen may also limit life processes.

The misleading term "oxygen (or oxidative) stress" has been coined to encompass the physiological and pathological situations that result from increased cellular loads of oxygen radicals. (Sies, 1991)

The critical balance of an "oxygen limited" cellular metabolism places oxygen at the fulcrum point for dictating the energy charge required for homeostasis.

In individuals who expire calmly, the life force leaves them concurrent or simultaneous with the cessation of breathing. **In other words, when the constant and invariant supply of oxygen is gone, so is life, as we know it.**

Not only is oxygen directly tied or linked to consciousness but it is also directly linked to the life process itself. At times, it appears that some scientists have overlooked these most basic of observations.

There is a plethora of comments condemning $O_2$ and its modifications, which tend to overlook its beneficence.

I can only feel that conditions such as dementia and Alzheimer's disease are related at least in part, to lowering of oxygen levels and EMODs in the brain.

Investigators utilizing **hyperbaric oxygen** treatments have made interesting contributing studies to these areas but **it has received little attention or mention. Studies show that, although the brain is only 2% of the total body weight, it requires 20-25% of the body's consumed oxygen.**

Additionally, **brains shrink at the rate of 20-30 grams per decade until the age of 60, and 30-40 grams thereafter.** The average male brain weighs 1,350 grams, that of females 1,200grams; but females have a slightly higher proportion of brain to body. Brain size is roughly proportional to body size.

The heart and the brain have the highest requirements for oxygen than any other organ or tissue in the body. Additionally, heart and brain cells have low levels of superoxide dismutase and catalase, again indicating that these tissues have a need for higher levels of reactive oxygen products and peroxide and excited states.

Just as with the living/breathing cell, the complexities of the human brain should not be underestimated. By way of illustration, **the National Academy of Sciences estimates that, "a single human brain has a greater number of possible connections among its nerve cells than the total number of atomic particles in the universe." RMH Note: somehow I doubt the accuracy of this statement by the National Academy of Sciences, since each of the brain's interconnections are established via atoms.**

Studies on the toxicity of massive doses of hydrogen peroxide, given intravenously to laboratory animals, show that it selectively injures the lungs, thymus, liver and kidneys.

I believe that **this indicates that both the heart and the brain can "handle or tolerate" excessively high levels of peroxide and oxygen.**

In fact, it appears that these two tissues require higher levels of peroxides and oxygen.

Also, I feel that non-polar oxygen species such as hydrogen peroxide, singlet oxygen or hypochlorite, may be the way to treat certain ischemia or $O_2$ deficiency conditions, since these species can readily cross cell membranes.

Additionally, peroxide would be more stable but it could be rapidly decomposed by catalase, while in the blood stream.

Further, if one were to attempt to administer $^1O_{2*}$ or $^1O_{2*}$ generating reagents, one would have to consider the short life time of singlet oxygen as 3-4 $ms$ and short diffusion distance, such that it would have to be generated at or near the target site. Still, singlet oxygen can serve as a signaling agent and have extended biochemical effects for days or even months, as seen with photodynamic therapy.

This could, however, give concerns for air embolism in the small arterioles of the brain, which could be lethal but this could theoretically be overcome by decreasing concentrations of reagents or decreasing the flow rates of reagents, as was done using $H_2O_2$ in the 1960s by Urschal's group at Baylor.

Hypochlorite could break down to chlorides or chloramines and be harmful in that form. Thus, perhaps a better route would be to try to increase levels of ground state triplet oxygen. This can be done by either increasing the concentration of inspired $O_2$, increasing the $O_2$ carrying capacity of hemoglobin, by a hyperbaric oxygen chamber or by a combination of all of these modes.

**Of interest is the fact that the Baylor group found that intra-arterial administration of $H_2O_2$ had the same physiological effect on $O_2$ saturation as did hyperbaric $O_2$ administration.**

The main effect of stroke or heart attack is that they interrupt or stop the flow of oxygen to either the heart or the brain. **Nearly 90% of all strokes result from clots that block the brain's arteries, cutting off circulation and starving the brain cells of oxygen**.

In surgery, we can tourniquet off the blood supply to the arm or hand for up to 2 hours before irreversible damage occurs. Yet, the heart or the brain can only tolerate oxygen stoppage for a few minutes, as is evidenced with angina, myocardial infarction or stroke. Oxygen is, indeed, magical or an essential to these vital organs in sustaining life as we know it.

Many investigators have shown that **calcium is essential for production of EMODs** and believe that elevated calcium levels are responsible for activation of EMOD-generating enzymes and formation of free radicals by the mitochondrial respiratory chain. Conversely, **an increase in intracellular calcium concentration may be stimulated by EMODs** and $H_2O_2$ has been recently shown to accelerate the overall channel opening process in voltage-dependent calcium channels in plant and animal cells.

Data support the speculation that **$Ca^{2+}$ and EMODs are two cross-talking messengers in various cellular processes.** (Gordeeva et al, 2003)

Please keep in mind that many investigators believe that $Ca^{2+}$ overload is considered to be the final pathway leading to cell death under pathological conditions. I believe that this is related to **EMOD** induced apoptosis.

In an interview with Franklin Cameron, Dr. Harman stated that, "I knew when Mother Nature finds something that works, she uses it over and over, like variations of a theme. **I approached the problem with the idea that there is a single cause of aging.** This cause would be responsible for the aging and death of everything, modified by genetics and environment."

**Harman concluded that free radicals of oxygen were the source of basically all human disease and aging**.

I submit that he so biased his initial approach, that it forever forced him to try to knowingly manipulate the data to fit the biased concept. The acceptance of this apocryphal concept has led generations of oxymorons to follow in lock step.

Based on decades of evaluation, **I believe that his conclusion that there is a singular cause for all human disease and aging is, at best, naive and at worst, just plain wrong.**

I am reminded of the words of the Irish author, Elizabeth Bowen, who said, "One can live in the shadow of an idea without grasping it."

## "The R. M. Howes, M.D., Ph.D. Tribute to the Living/Breathing Cell."

**The living /breathing cell is a heterogeneous isothermal conglomerate, containing a dynamic commingled biochemical infrastructure, held rather precariously, yet intentionally, in a most meaningful spatial conformation by lipid interlinks utilizing weak non-covalent and covalent forces, and capable of assimilating nutrients and processing data during energy production. Stretching the laws of thermodynamics, it maintains steady states of oxygen free radicals and electronic excitation states far from equilibrium.**

**With an uncanny degree of self awareness, the living/breathing cell is :**

**Self-sustaining**
**Self-contained**
**Self-adjusting**
**Self-assembling**
**Self-medicating**
**Self-healing**
**Self-replicating**
**Self-mutilating**
**Self-mutating**
**Self-terminating**

**It is an anti-chaotic/anti-entropic living unit, one hundred trillionth of the whole man, which carries on light speed to-and-fro cross talk within itself and throughout the whole, all for the sake of self-survival. As I grapple with its spiritual overtones, I am awe-struck by its biochemical beauty, mystified by its ability to pass on the self-replication dictum and inspired by its will to live and thus, to win.**

**The living /breathing cell is home to the savant of living matter and to the pundit of protoplasm.**

After a selective review of the world's literature, I have found that others are also beginning to **seriously question and reject the hallowed free radical theory**. Research by University College of London, published in Nature in February 2004, states that the theory may be incorrect and flawed.

Dr. Tony Segal said, **"Many patients might be using expensive antioxidant drugs based upon completely invalid theories."**

Since the 1970s, pharmaceutical companies have developed and flooded the market with drugs, including vitamins and dietary supplements, designed to mop up or inactivate the production of damaging free radicals, which are produced during normal metabolism of oxygen. Tons of vitamins A, C and E are consumed on a daily basis and are regarded as healthy because they allegedly "attack" free radicals.

This is being done and perpetuated, even though **the data relating to it is contradictory and at times indicates considerable potential harm or even death from many of these antioxidants**. The power of the lay press, the media and the pharmaceutical industry is enormous. Unfortunately, their bottom line is profit and not the well being of our citizenry.

Dr. Segal further states, **"Our work shows that the basic theory underlying the toxicity of oxygen radicals is flawed."** Segal's group discovered that production of lytic enzymes, which are triggered by potassium flow, are responsible for digestion of foreign invaders and that free radicals are by no means the toxic particles they had been accused of being.

Segal said, **"Pharmaceutical companies have spent millions on what effectively amounted to a red herring. All the theories relating to the free radical causation of disease and the therapeutic value of antioxidants, at the very least, must be re-evaluated."**

I feel that an entire multi-billion dollar industry, including lecturers, publishers, health gurus, antiaging clinics, drug manufacturers, etc., is likely based on the extremely shaky ground of speculation and not the terra firma of scientific experimentation.

After cataloging numerous DNA mutations that are associated with cellular progression from normalcy to malignancy, it is becoming obvious **that events in the tissues surrounding cancer cells play a major formative role**.

Some researchers have shown that a cancer cell's so-called microenvironment can determine its tumorigenic potential. Lisa Coussens, Ph. D. of the University of California, San Francisco, says, "You can't proliferate as a cancer cell all by yourself unless you can orchestrate that microenvironment to allow you to proliferate."

It is becoming increasingly clear that **only certain tissues permit cancer growth with particular DNA mutations.**

Mina Bissell, Ph.D. of the Lawrence Berkeley National Lab, has shown that the abnormal behavior of cancer cells is due not only to mutations from within but also to influences from without. (Fredrich, 2003)

**I believe that the micro-oxygen environment is a major player in the "allowance" of either primary, secondary or metastatic tumor growth. I am referring to the EMOD micro-environment and not to just ground state oxygen, as was proposed by Otto Warburg.**

Throughout my writings I have argued against the use of the term "inducer" (when applied to hypoxia) and have insisted on the use of the term "allowed." I believe that, in many instances, **it is the absence of EMODs which "allows" cancer to develop; whereas, in other circumstances, EMOD levels either hold cancer cells in abeyance or if EMOD levels are high enough, they cause death of the cancer cells by induction of apoptosis.**

> **"Medicine's history and its practice teaches us that physicians and scientists alike, can be blinded by obviousness and entrapped by ignorance."**
> R. M. Howes, M.D., Ph.D.
> 5/2/04

"To be possessed with the gift to see the unseen or
to know the unknown, even for a fleeting second,
can be an unparalleled blessing,
rife with reward or
a daunting flash of peril,
the immediate result of which will be determined, not by ultimate truth, but by the amplitude of reactionaries."
R. M. Howes, M.D., Ph.D.
5/25/04

## Hyperoxia and hyperbaric oxygen

Hyperoxia and hyperbaric oxygen enhance hydrogen peroxide
generation at the subcellular and cellular levels at different
extents (60 to 200%). All mitochondria exhibit lower (or negligible) rates of hydrogen peroxide production in State 3 (active
ATP production), whereas, it is maximum in State 4 (resting,
nonphosphorylating mitochondria).

Hyperbaric oxygen and hyperoxia exposure results in a marked increase in hydrogen peroxide production by isolated heart and liver mitochondria. (Forman et al, 2003)

In hyperbaric oxygen, tissue levels may approach 1200 mmHg,
in which increased production of superoxide, peroxide and
other oxygen radicals occurs. However, some organisms adapt by
producing increased levels of superoxide dismutase. There is no direct
antibacterial effect of enhanced oxygen on aerobic organisms.

Indirect antibactericidal effects are related to improved PMN function
in killing bacteria. Results with hyperbaric oxygen are similar to
that obtained by the Baylor investigators using intra-arterial
$H_2O_2$.

Aminoglycosides such as gentamicin, tobramycin, alizarin and
netilmicin are oxygen dependent for their antimicrobial activity. Vancomycin is another antibiotic that does not kill microorganisms
well under low oxygen tensions.

Sulfonamides antimicrobial effect is potentiated in hyperbaric
oxygen. Similarly, many of the chemotherapeutic drugs are
oxygen dependent.

**Chronic wounds have been studied with implanted polygraph-ic oxygen electrodes and found to be hypoxic with levels of 5 to 20 mmHg compared to control values of 30 to 50 mmHg. This is a very important point.**

**The Free Radi-Crap theory states that chronic wounds induce cancer by the over-production of EMODs, whereas in reality, these chromic wounds have an oxygen deficiency state and the body could likely kill the infecting pathogen if adequate levels of oxygen were available and it would also kill pro-neo-plastic cells.**

**In situations where oxygen delivery is impaired, chronic non-healing wounds may develop.**

In summary, oxygen is essential for maintaining cellular integrity, func-tion and repair when tissues are injured. Oxygen not only plays an important role in energy metabolism, but also is very important in poly-morphonuclear cell function, neovascularization, fibroblast proliferation and collagen deposition.

**I point out that oxygen is not our enemy but is our greatest ally.**

Supplemental oxygen has been shown to enhance healing dependent on dose and frequency, however, excessive or continuous oxygen may impair the normal healing process. Some period hypoxia in conjunction with other stimuli (including lactate and other intermediates) is neces-sary to promote the healing process.

In a normal host, despite a large wound with definite hypoxia, healing will occur as long as factors such as nutrients, blood flow and immune function remain adequate to allow regeneration of capillaries and res-toration of nutrient delivery.

A delicate balance exists between one of the major stimuli to heal-ing hypoxia and the **paradoxical** need for oxygen for wound repair. **In situations where oxygen delivery is impaired chronic non-healing wounds may develop.**

**It has been shown in numerous studies that the degree of polymorphonuclear cell function in killing of bacteria is directly dependent on oxygen tension.** (DeChatelet, 1975) (Hohn, 1977)

**Hyperbaric oxygen has been shown to be a beneficial adjunct to therapy in Bacteroides fragilis, Fusobacterium infections and nonclostridial anaerobic infections.** (Schreiner, 1974)

**Both NAD- and FAD-linked substrates support rates of hydrogen peroxide production (0.2-0.8 nmol hydrogen peroxide/min mg protein) modulated by various metabolic states.** (Boveris, Chance, 1973) (Loschen et al, 1973)

## Head and Neck Squamous Cell Carcinoma

Head and neck squamous cell carcinomas (HNSCC) is the fifth most common malignancy worldwide. These tumors arise from diverse anatomical locations, including oral cavity, or pharynx, larynx and hypo pharynx, but have common epithelial origin and etiological association with tobacco and alcohol exposure.

Despite modern intervention, the five year survival rate for this disease has improved only marginally over the past decade. (Greenlee et al, 2001), and recurrent disease is observed in ~50% of the patients.

## Hypoxia

In a recent study on HNSCC, **the median tumor $pO_2$ was consistently lower than that of normal squamous cell tissues from the same patient, for all patients.** (Le et al, 2003)

The impact of hypoxia in increasing radiation resistance to a variety of biologic end points has been known for almost 70 years. It was demonstrated 35 years ago that **hypoxia limited the radio-curability of murine tumors. That hypoxia exists in human tumors was demonstrated 45 years ago by Thomlinson.**

This diffusion-limited hypoxia was felt to be an important reason for the inability of radiation therapy to achieve local tumor control, and consequently, an extensive laboratory and clinical effort was undertaken to overcome this effect starting with the use of hyperbaric oxygen in the mid-1960s.

It must kept in mind that molecules other than oxygen are also abnormally distributed within tumor cells, when compared to normal cells. In general, there are two types of hypoxia: 1) chronic or diffusion-limited hypoxia, where tumor cells are too far from a functional vessel and 2) acute/intermittent or perfusion-limited hypoxia, where there is abnormal periodic flow within a tumor vessel.

Overall, hypoxia relates to molecular biology, biochemistry, physiology, angiogenesis and imaging. **Hypoxic cells are radio-resistant, requiring two or three times the radiation dose to kill them compared to the same cells in a eu-oxic (normal oxygen) state.**

Hypoxia can be of two types: 1) chronic hypoxia, which is diffusion limited and 2) acute hypoxia, which is perfusion limited.

**Tumor oxygen status is a reliable prognostic marker that impacts malignant progression and outcome of tumor therapy.** However, tumor oxygenation is heterogeneous and cannot be sufficiently described by a single parameter. It is influenced by several factors including microvessel density (MVD), blood flow (BF), blood volume (BV), blood oxygen saturation, tissue $pO_2$, oxygen consumption rate, and hypoxic faction.

Hypoxia-inducible factor-1 (HIF-1) is a transcription factor that plays a critical role in tumor growth by increasing resistance to apoptosis and the production of angiogenic factors such as vascular endothelial growth factor (VEGF). (Welsh et al, 2003)

**Hypoxia is a feature inherent in solid tumors as is increased energy demand and diminished vascular supply.** Tissue hypoxia is a characteristic property of cervical cancers that **makes tumors resistant to chemo- and radiation therapy.**

Erythropoietin (Epo) is a hypoxia-inducible stimulator of erythropoiesis. Acting via its receptor (EpoR), Epo up regulates bcl-2 and inhibits apoptosis of erythroid cells and rescues neurons from hypoxic damage.

In addition to human papillomavirus infection, increased bcl-2 expression and decreased apoptosis are thought to play a role in the progression of cervical neoplasia. (Acs et al, 2003)

The present understanding of the changes in cellular function during hypoxia are rather complex. **The hypoxia-inducible factors (HIF-1$\alpha$ and HIF-2$\alpha$)** dimerize with the constitutively expressed HIF-1$\beta$ subunit to bind to a hypoxia-responsive element to **activate a wide array of genes, including those involved in anaerobic**

**metabolism, cell cycle arrest, differentiation, stress adaptation, angiogenesis and others**. (Semenza, 2000)

These can result in profound alterations on tumor and cellular phenotype, including an obvious role in angiogenesis by upregulation of angiogenic factors such as vascular endothelial growth factor.

**Hypoxia, with or without reoxygenation, is a mediator of malignant progression**, with mechanisms that include selection pressure, genomic instability, genomic heterogeneity, decreasing apoptotic potential, increasing angiogenesis, and a chaotic microcirculation. Radioresistance of hypoxic cells is well established.

Clinically, **hypoxic tumors tend to do worse in terms of both local recurrence and distant metastases**. (Fyles et al, 2002)

This has been reported after surgical resection as well as after radiation therapy. (Nordsmark, Overgaard, 2000)

Hypoxia may also adversely effect chemotherapy response. (Telcher, 2001)

**Biochemical and Clinical Aspects**

**Tumor hypoxia**

**Materials in the following section have been excerpted from and based upon the following paper**: (Hockel, Vaupel, 2001)

Hypoxia in tumors is primarily a pathophysiologic consequence of structurally and functionally disturbed microcirculation and the deterioration of diffusion conditions. **Tumor hypoxia appears to be strongly associated with tumor propagation, malignant progression and resistance to therapy**, and it has thus become a central issue in tumor physiology and cancer treatment.

Biochemists define it as $O_2$-limited electron transport and physiologists and clinicians define it as a state of reduced $O_2$ availability of decreased $O_2$ partial pressure that restricts or even abolishes functions of organs, tissues or cells.

For the purposes of applications to my **Unified Theory**, I am ultimately concerned with the levels of EMODs that are generated intracellularly, thus, I must consider all factors that can affect these levels.

Traditionally, **tumor hypoxia has been considered a potential therapeutic problem because it renders solid tumors more resistant to sparsely ionizing radiation.** (Hall, 1994)

More recent experimental and clinical studies, suggest that **intratumoral oxygen levels may influence a series of biologic parameters that also affect the malignant potential of a neoplasm.** (Vaupel, Kelleher, 1999)

**Sustained hypoxia in a growing tumor may cause cellular changes that can result in a more clinically aggressive phenotype.** (Hockel et al, 1996)

**During the process of hypoxia-driven malignant progression, tumors may develop an increased potential for local invasive growth, perifocal tumor cell spreading, and regional and distant tumor cell spreading.** (Hockel et al, 1999)

Likewise, hypoxia may cause intrinsic resistance to radiation and other cancer treatments may be affected. (Sethi et al, 1999)

Hypoxia-induced or hypoxia-mediated changes of 1) the **proteome (i.e., the complete set of proteins within a cell at a given time)** of the neoplastic and stroma cells and 2) the genome of the genetically unstable neoplastic cells may explain the fact that tumor oxygenation is associated with disease progression, a link that has been demonstrated for a variety of human malignant tumor types.

With hypoxia and because of finely tuned regulatory processes, increases in tissue $O_2$ consumption are generally matched by an increase in blood flow and, therefore, do not usually lead to hypoxia unless the system regulating blood flow fails to meet the increased $O_2$ demand of the tissue in question.

**In solid tumors, oxygen delivery to the respiring neoplastic and stroma cells is frequently reduced or even abolished by a deteriorating diffusion geometry, severe structural abnormalities of tumor microvessel, and disturbed microcirculation.** (Vaupel et al, 1987)

## Solid Tumor Hypoxia

**When an unrestricted supply of oxygen is available, for most tumors, the rate of $O_2$ consumption (respiration rate) and adenosine triphosphate (ATP) production is comparable to that found in the corresponding normal tissue,** despite the deregulated organization of cells in malignant tumors. To maintain a sufficient energy supply for membrane transport systems and synthesis of chemical compounds, an adequate supply of $O_2$ is required.

In hypoxia, **the mitochondrial $O_2$ consumption rate and ATP production are reduced,** which hinders inter alia active transport in tumor cells. Specifically, major effects of the reduced production of ATP are 1) collapse of Na+ and K+ gradients, 2) depolarizaiton of membranes, 3) cellular uptake of Cl-, 4) cell swelling, 5) increased cytosolic Ca2+ concentration, and finally, 6) decreased cytosolic pH, resulting in intracellular acidosis in tumor cells.

## Hypoxia (Oxygen) Threshold Levels

On the basis of experimental results from isolated engrafted human breast cancer tissue, **tumor tissue hypoxia with reduced $O_2$ consumption rates is expected when the $O_2$ partial pressure in the blood at the venous end of the capillaries (end-capillary blood) falls below 45-50 mmHg.**

**Mitochondrial oxidative phosphorylation is limited at $O_2$ partial pressures of less than approximately 0.5 mmHg. Above this threshold, mitochondria should function physiologically.**

In general, a number of key findings have been described as follows: 1) **Most tumors have lower median $O_2$ partial pressures than their tissue of origin;** 2) many solid tumors contain areas of low $O_2$ partial pressure than cannot be predicted by clinical size, stage, grade, histology and site; 3) tumor-to-tumor variability in oxygenation is usually greater than intratumoral variability in oxygenation; and 4) **recurring tumors have a poorer oxygenation status than the corresponding primary tumors.**

Anoxia/hypoxia-induced proteome changes in neoplastic and stroma cells may lead to the arrest or impairment of neoplastic growth through molecular mechanisms, resulting in cellular quiescence, differentiation, apoptosis and necrosis.

**Cells exposed to hypoxia are generally arrested at the G1/S-phase boundary.** (Giaccia, 1996)

**Under anoxia, most cells are arrested immediately, regardless of their position in the cell cycle.**

**Hypoxia can induce programmed (apoptotic) cell death in normal and neoplastic cells.** The level of p53 in cells increases under hypoxic conditions, and **the increased level of p53 induces apoptosis by a pathway involving Apaf-1 and caspase-9 as downstream effectors.** (Soengas et al, 1999)

However, hypoxia also initiates p53-dependent apoptosis pathways involving hypoxia-inducible factor-1 (HIF-1), genes of the BCL-2 family, and other unidentified genes. (Shimizu et al, 1995)

**Below a critical energy state, hypoxia/anoxia may result in necrotic cell death, a phenomenon seen in many human tumors** and experimental systems.

**Hypoxia stimulates the transcription of glycolytic enzymes, glucose transporters (GLUT1 and GLUT3), angiogenic molecules, survival and growth factors (e.g. vascular endothelial growth factor [VEGF], angiogenin, platelet-derived growth factor-B, transforming growth factor-B, and insulin-like growth factor-II), enzymes, proteins involved in tumor invasiveness (e.g., urokinases-type plasminogen activator), chaperones, and other resistance-related proteins.**

At the same time, hypoxia-induced inhibition of gene expression has been demonstrated for cell-surface integrins facilitating tumor cell detachment.

Again, **I take issue with the term "stimulates" in that the best term here should be "allows". If something isn't there (oxygen), then it can not induce something else since it is not there but its absence can "allow" for subsequent events.**

Hypoxia-mediated clonal expansion of tumor cells with diminished apoptotic potential has been shown both experimentally and clinically, such as occurs in hypoxic surgical scars as a major pathogenetic event for local recurrences, despite cell free margins on complete surgical excisions.

In general, hypoxia-induced changes are detectable at an $O_2$ partial pressure of less than 1 mmHg, which is one order of magnitude below the $O_2$ partial pressures associated with proteome changes.

**RMH Note: It is stated that hypoxia "induces" an increased mutation rate; however, I feel that induction requires the presence of an inducing factor (not its absence) and hence, I feel that hypoxia "allows" for genomic changes instead of inducing them.**

Hypoxic oxygen levels limits the cells ability to produce adequate amounts of reactive oxygen species and electronic excitation states (EMODs) to keep newly developed cancer cells in abeyance.

My **Unified Theory** approach assumes that the intracellular metabolic machinery of the electron transport system is functioning properly.

### Hypoxic Tumor Resistance

Hypoxic $O_2$ partial pressures in a tumor present a severe problem for X and Gamma radiation because the presence of ground state $O_2$ increases DNA damage with "an oxygen enhancement effect." **It requires 3 times more radiation to kill cancer cells in the absence of $O_2$ than it does in the presence of normal levels of $O_2$.**

Hypoxia-associated resistance to photon radiotherapy is multifactorial. The presence of molecular oxygen increased DNA damage through the formation of oxygen free radicals, which occurs primarily after the interaction of radiation with intracellular water.

**Oxygen dependence has also been established for a number of chemotherapeutic agents such as cyclophosphamide, carboplatin, doxorubicin,** etc. and levels are different for each agent.

Hypoxia can impart resistance to many chemotherapeutic agents. (Teicher et al, 1990)

Tissue **acidosis is frequently found in hypoxic tumors with a high glycolytic rate.** (Wike-Hooley et al, 1984)

Photodynamic Therapy-mediated tumor cell death also requires the presence of oxygen and **cells are not killed under anoxic conditions**.

The critical threshold below which progressively reduced cell death was observed varied from 15 to 35 mmHg, probably **because of the reduced production of singlet oxygen ($^1O_2$)** species and different sensitivities to the treatment in different cell lines. (Henderson, Fingar, 1987) (Chapman et al, 1991)

This means that because of the utilization of oxygen by PDT, it is a self-limiting process. In contrast, the **Howes Singlet Oxygen Delivery System** brings its own oxygen supply with it and is, therefore, not self-limiting. (Howes, 2005) (Howes, Farber, 2005)

PDT prodrugs, such as ALA, may be further limited because conversion of the prodrug to the active photosensitizer appears to be less effective under hypoxic conditions.

Additionally, **tumor hypoxia can dramatically effect cytokines (interferon gamma and tumor necrosis factor-*a*) and alter Interleukins 2-induced activation of lymphokine-activated killer cells**.

**Tumor oxygenation is the strongest independent prognostic factor**, followed by FIGO stage and the disadvantage in outcome for patients with hypoxic tumors was independent of the mode of primary treatment (radiation therapy or radical surgery).

Critical oxygen or $O_2$ levels that characterize the upper limit of the hypoxic range (below which activities or specific functions of tumor cells progressively change) are as follows:

Immunotherapies, PDT, X and gamma radiation requires 25-30 mmHg $O_2$.

Binding of hypoxic markers, cellular ATP synthesis and cellular $O_2$ consumption rate is about 10-15 mmHg $O_2$.

Mechanisms at the subcellular and molecular levels such as, gene amplification, genomic instability and loss of apoptotic potential occurs at less than 20 mmHg $O_2$.

Mitochondrial $O_2$ consumption requires about 1 mmHg $O_2$ and oxidation of the cytochromes requires about 0.05 mmHg $O_2$.

## Hypoxia Miscellaneous Facts

-Hypoxia has been seen in cervical cancer, squamous cell cancer of the head and neck, melanoma, breast, sarcoma and recently in prostate cancer.

-Hypoxia promotes angiogenesis, metastasis and selection of cells with a more malignant phenotype.

**RMH Note: According to my Unified Theory, lower levels of oxygen lead to deficiency levels of EMODs, which "allows" the development or progression of cancer.**

-Another $O_2$ **Paradox**: $O_2$ contributes significantly to initial mutations through oxidative damage, but lack of $O_2$ promotes metastasis, angiogenesis and selection of cells with a more malignant phenotype.

-Hb concentration is directly related to outcome of radiotherapy of cancer. **RMH Note: This would be predicted. $O_2$ (EMODs) are needed to kill cancer.**

-Carbogen (95% $O_2$ and 5% $CO_2$) and nicotinamide reduce hypoxia and increases radiotherapy effects.

-Hypoxia sensitizers to improve radiotherapy (i.e., nimorazole, a widespread antimicrobial) and is used in Denmark to treat head and neck cancer.

-Another $O_2$ paradox: cancer is mainly initiated by mutations due to oxidative damage but radiotherapy can cure cancer by producing DNA damage with oxidative free radical damage.

**RMH Note: There is no paradox, ROS (EMODs) and $^1O_2$ do not cause cancer. Their absence "allows" cancer to develop.**

-Erythropoietin (EPO), is a glycoprotein hormone produced by the kidney in response to hypoxia to stimulate RBC production in bone marrow.

-Bioreductive drugs (take advantage of hypoxia, i.e, TPZ tirapazamine) forms a radical to produce DNA damage and kills regardless of p53 status. When $O_2$ is restored, the TPZ radical is oxidized back to less toxic form.

-Another **$O_2$ paradox:** hypoxia increases malignancy of tumors and increases treatment resistance, but induction of severe, acute hypoxia (anoxia) also has a therapeutic effect.

**RMH Note: Since these cells still require some $O_2$ or they die, hypoxia is better than no "oxia" at all.**

-In hypoxia, the $O_2$ sensor, is a prolyl hydroxylase.

-HIF-1, induces expression of more than 30 known genes, including EPO, VEGF, NOS2, Flt-1, GIUT-1 & 3, PK-M and IGF-2.

-Tumor hypoxia stimulates expressing of vascular endothelial growth factor (VEGF) and hypoxia-inducible factor-1$a$ (HIF-1$a$).

-Interleukin-8 (IL-8) is a member of the C$a$C chemokines and originally it was called, "neutrophil-activating peptide," but is also activates lymphocytes and monocytes and angiogenesis factor. It is inducible in tumors by hypoxia.

**RMH Note: I believe that hypoxia induces the release of $H_2O_2$ to compensate for low $O_2$ levels, for an effect similar to that seen by dripping $H_2O_2$ to maintain viability of heart cells by the Baylor Research Group.**

**-HIF-1$a$ is regulated by a proline hydroxylase.**

**Like a mystical present,<br>
I've been shaking the "box of life",<br>
trying to ascertain what are<br>
the wondrous things hidden inside it.<br>
At this point,<br>
I believe it is a box crammed full of EMODs.**<br>
R.M. Howes, M.D., Ph.D.<br>
4/12/15

# SECTION TWO

## RADICALS AND EMODS

### The Free Radical Theory

The realization that energy consumption by mitochondria may result in $O_2^- \cdot$ production linked the free radical theory and the rate of living theory irrevocably: a faster rate of respiration, associated with a greater generation of oxygen radicals, allegedly hastened aging.

Now, the two concepts have essentially merged. However, **data on birds, bats and the naked mole-rat counter the association of EMODs and aging in these theories.**

### Origins of the free radical theory: a brief review

In 1956, Denham Harman suggested that free radicals produced during aerobic respiration cause cumulative oxidative damage, resulting in aging and death. He noted parallels between the effects of aging and of ionizing radiation, including mutagenesis, cancer, and gross cellular damage. (Harman, 1956)

At the time, it had recently been discovered that radiolysis of water generates hydroxyl radical ($\cdot$OH), and early experiments using paramagnetic resonance spectroscopy had identified the presence of $\cdot$OH in living matter.

Harman therefore hypothesized that endogenous oxygen radical generation occurs in vivo, as a by-product of enzymatic redox chemistry. He ventured that the enzymes involved would be those "involved in the direct utilization of molecular oxygen, particularly those containing iron."

Finally, he hypothesized that traces of iron and other metals would catalyze oxidative reactions in vivo and that peroxidative chain reactions were possible, by analogy to the principles of in vitro polymer chemistry.

**However, Harman has been repeatedly wrong over the last sixty plus years**. (Howes, 2006)

**Knowing the truth
beats living in blissful ignorance
every time.**
R. M. Howes, M.D., Ph.D.
4/10/07

The realization that energy consumption by mitochondria may result in $O_2^-\cdot$ production linked the free radical theory and the rate of living theory irrevocably: a faster rate of respiration, associated with a greater generation of oxygen radicals, allegedly hastened aging. By now, the two concepts have essentially merged. **Data on birds, bats and the naked mole-rat counter the association of EMODs and aging in these theories. Basically, 100 exceptions to the FRTA are listed in the beginning section of one of my books and another 150 exceptions are mentioned in my book on Cancer and Longevity Answers.**

### Sources of oxidants (EMODs)

Ground-state diatomic oxygen ($^3\Sigma g^- O_2$ or more commonly, $O_2$), **despite being a radical species and the most important oxidant in aerobic organisms, is only sparingly reactive itself** due to the fact that its two unpaired electrons are located in different molecular orbitals and possess "parallel spins."

**This flies in the face of the axiom that all radicals are highly reactive species, which they are not.** As a consequence, if $O_2$ is simultaneously to accept two electrons, these must both possess antiparallel spins relative to the unpaired electrons in $O_2$, a criterion which is not satisfied by a typical pair of electrons in atomic or molecular orbitals (which have opposite spins according to the Pauli exclusion principle).

As a result, **$O_2$ preferentially accepts electrons one at a time from other radicals** (such as transition metals in certain valences).

Thus, in vivo, typical two- or four-electron reduction of $O_2$ relies on coordinated, serial, enzyme-catalyzed one-electron reductions, and the enzymes that carry these out typically possess active-site radical species such as iron. One- and two-electron reduction of $O_2$ generates $O_2^-\cdot$ and hydrogen peroxide ($H_2O_2$), respectively, both of which are generated by numerous routes in vivo.

In the presence of free transition metals (in particular iron and copper), $O_2^-\cdot$ and $H_2O_2$ together generate the extremely reactive hydroxyl radical ($\cdot OH$).

Ultimately, $\cdot OH$ is *assumed* to be the species responsible for initiating the oxidative destruction of biomolecules. In addition to $O_2^-\cdot$, $H_2O_2$, and $\cdot OH$, two energetically excited species of $O_2$ termed "singlet oxygens" can result from the absorption of energy (for instance, from ultraviolet light).

Designated by the formulas $^1\Delta g O_2$ and $^1\Sigma g^+ O_2$, both of these species differ from the triplet ground state ($^3\Sigma g\ O_2$) in having their two unpaired electrons in opposite spins, thereby eliminating the spin restriction of ground-state $O_2$ and enabling greater reactivity.

**Both ground state oxygen and superoxide are only minimally reactive and superoxide is a better reductant at physiological pH than it is an oxidant.**

It is now beyond doubt that oxidants (EMODs) are generated in vivo and can allegedly cause significant harm and **Beckman and Ames have overlooked the numerous beneficial and crucial actions of EMODs.**

Because all of these species ($O_2^-\cdot$; $H_2O_2$, $\cdot OH$, $^1\Delta g O_2$, and $^1\Sigma g^+ O_2$), by different routes, may be involved in oxygen's alleged toxicity, **Beckman and Ames** collectively and erroneously refer to them as "oxidants."

There are numerous sites of oxidant generation, four of which have attracted much attention: mitochondrial electron transport, peroxisomal fatty acid metabolism, cytochrome P-450 reactions, and phagocytic cells (the "respiratory burst").

It appears **mitochondrial electron transport is imperfect**, and one-electron reduction of $O_2$ to form $O_2^-\cdot$ occurs. The spontaneous and enzymatic dismutation of $O_2^-$· yields $H_2O_2$, so a significant by-product of the actual sequence of oxidation-reduction reactions may be the generation of $O_2^-$· and $H_2O_2$.

Measurements of $H_2O_2$ generation by isolated mitochondria indicated that it is maximal when ADP is limiting and the electron carriers are consequently reduced ("state 4" respiration). (Boveris, Chance, 1973)

**I believe that this so-called "leak" is not a mistake** and I believe that it represents a unique path for the formation of essential EMODs (RSVP pathway of Howes). (Howes, 2004, UTOPIA) (Howes, 2005)

Estimates of state 4 $H_2O_2$ generation by pigeon and rat mitochondrial preparations amounted to 1-2% of total electron flow. When $H_2O_2$ is measured with more physiological concentrations, the flux is ~10-fold lower. (Hansford et al. 1997), and experiments using subcellular fractions of SOD-deficient *Escherichia coli* suggest in vivo leakage of 0.1% from the respiratory chain. (Imlay, Fricovich, 1991)

Because two $O_2^-$· molecules dismutate (either spontaneously or with the help of mSOD) to form one molecule of $H_2O_2$, such results suggest that **virtually all mitochondrial $H_2O_2$ may originate as $O_2^-$·** (Boveris et al, 1972) But, **this is incorrect.**

Moreover, because most cellular $H_2O_2$ originates from mitochondria, $O_2^-$· from the ETC may be a cell's most significant source of oxidants. (Chance et al, 1979

**This is also controversial, depending upon the investigators cited.**

**Some investigators** suggest that the actual role of mSOD in vivo may be to increase $H_2O_2$ generation (with $O_2^-$· as a rapidly consumed intermediate). (Forman, Azzi, 1997)

Beckman and Ames state that there remains a good deal of uncertainty surrounding the mechanisms, quantity, and meaning of mitochondrial $O_2^-$· generation in vivo. (Nohl et al, 1996)

A second source of oxygen radicals is peroxisomal beta-oxidation of fatty acids, which generates $H_2O_2$ as a by-product. **Peroxisomes possess high concentrations of catalase**, so it is unclear whether or not leakage of $H_2O_2$ from peroxisomes contributes significantly to cytosolic oxidative stress under normal circumstances.

However, a class of nonmutagenic carcinogens, the peroxisome prolif- erators, which increase the number of hepatocellular peroxisomes and result in liver cancer in rodents, also cause oxidative stress and damage. Interestingly, **during the regeneration of the liver after partial hepatectomy, there exist peroxisomes that do not stain for catalase activity,** hinting that during rapid cell proliferation, oxidant leakage from peroxisomes may be enhanced.

**Again, I believe that this emphasizes the importance of EMODs for self-healing.**

Microsomal cytochrome $P$-450 enzymes metabolize xenobiotic com- pounds, usually of plant origin, by catalyzing their univalent oxidation or reduction. Although these reactions typically involve NADPH and an organic substrate, some of the numerous cytochrome $P$-450 isozymes directly reduce $O_2$ to $O_2^-\cdot$ and may cause so-called oxidative stress.

An alternative route for cytochrome $P$-450-mediated oxidation involves redox cycling, in which substrates accept single electrons from cyto- chrome $P$-450 and transfer them to oxygen. This generates $O_2^-\cdot$ and simultaneously regenerates the substrate, allowing subsequent rounds of $O_2^-\cdot$ generation.

Finally, phagocytic cells attack pathogens with a mixture of oxidants and free radicals, including $O_2^-\cdot$, $H_2O_2$, NO $\cdot$, and hypochlorite. **(RMH Note: This is normal and essential for pathogen protection.)**

In addition to these four sources of oxidants, there exist numerous other enzymes capable of generating oxidants under normal or patho- logical conditions, often in a tissue-specific manner. As originally articu- lated by Harman. (Harman, 1956), the free radical theory of aging did not distinguish between these different sources of oxidants.

**I have studied this aspect of oxygen metabolism in depth.**
(Howes et al, 1977)
(Howes, Steele, 1976) (Howes et al, 1976) (Howes, Steele, 1972)
(Howes, Steele, 1971)
(Howes, 2006, H2O2) (Howes, 2006, AOX A,C,E) (Howes, 2006, CVD)
(Howes, 2006, Diabetes) (Howes, 2008, ROSI)

## Targets of oxidants

The three main classes of biological macromolecules (lipids, nucleic acids, and proteins) are susceptible to free radical attack but that does not mean that this occurs normally in the living/breathing cell.

In the context of aging, a particularly relevant aspect of oxygen's alleged toxicity is its promotion by some metals and by elevated $O_2$ partial pressure. Iron and copper catalyze the homolytic cleavage of ROOH (the Fenton reaction), leading to the generation of $\cdot OH$. In humans, **the body's content of iron increases with age (in men throughout their lives, and in women after menopause**), and it has been suggested that this accumulation may increase the risk of oxidative damage with age.

Finally, **oxidative stress in vivo is aggravated by increasing $O_2$ partial pressure, due to a more pronounced flux of mitochondrial $O_2^-$**: (Chance et al, 1979)

However, this is proving to be a good thing, as with hyperbaric oxygen therapy.

## Antioxidant defenses

Cells are equipped with an impressive repertoire of antioxidant enzymes, as well as small antioxidant molecules mostly derived from dietary fruits and vegetables.

These include *1*) enzymatic scavengers such as SOD, which hastens the dismutation of $O_2^- \cdot$ to $H_2O_2$, and catalase and glutathione peroxidase (GPx), which convert $H_2O_2$ to water; 2) hydrophilic radical scavengers such as ascorbate, urate, and glutathione (GSH); 3) lipophilic radical scavengers such as tocopherols, flavonoids, carotenoids, and ubiquinol; 4) enzymes involved in the reduction of oxidized forms of small molecular antioxidants (GSH reductase, dehydroascorbate reductase) or responsible for the maintenance of protein thiols (thioredoxin reductase); and 5) the cellular machinery that maintains a reducing environment (e.g., glucose-6-phosphate dehydrogenase, which regenerates NADPH).

The complement of defenses deployed differs not only between organisms or tissues, but even between cellular compartments. For instance,

**GPx plays an important role in mammals but is absent from flies and nematodes,** and there exist in humans three forms of SOD (cytosolic Cu, Zn-SOD, mitochondrial Mn-SOD, and extracellular SOD), encoded and regulated independently.

Clearly, an indifference to oxygen free radicals is allegedly inconsistent with life, underlining the supposed centrality of oxidative damage. Moreover, **the fact that antioxidant defenses are not uniform** has been incorporated into the free radical theory; differences in antioxidant defenses between species have been put forth to explain differences in life span.

Although **there are two different interpretations of the data, they are not inconsistent.** Whereas aerobic life requires organisms to cope with oxidation to some extent, different evolutionary pressures appear to have selected for more or less investment in these defenses.

Measurements of individual antioxidant activities do not have great relevance. In fact, as is discussed below, measurements of age-related changes in individual antioxidants have led to conflicting results. (Sohal, 1993)

For this reason, aggregate assays have been devised, such as the susceptibility of crude cellular homogenates to in vitro oxidation by ionizing radiation. Although **these assays do not provide any information about the specific mechanisms of defense**, they allegedly may measure overall effectiveness.

## Oxidants and evolutionary theories of aging

The intracellular generation of oxidants capable of limiting life span appears **paradoxical.** It seems reasonable to expect that natural selection might have devised aerobic cells that do not leak toxic by-products. Evolutionary biologists have contributed to the free radical theory by suggesting why physiologically harmful generation of oxygen radicals occurs.

They have argued that natural selection favors genes that act early in life and increase reproduction, rather than genes that act to preserve non-germ cells (the "disposable soma"), a principle called "antagonistic pleiotropy". **This is another SWAG. It is counterintuitive that nature would evolve such a destructive EMOD "leak" if it endeavors to improve its chances of survival.**

## Accumulation of oxidative end products

The gradual and steady accumulation of intracellular yellow-brown fluorescent pigments, referred to as lipofuscin, occurs in numerous phyla. **In 2015, we do not know the significance of lipofuscin presence or of any possible role for it.** Even Beckman and Ames admit that despite extensive in vitro experiments, it is not known with certainty.

Results suggest that **the evolution of longevity has not been associated with a clear-cut increase in antioxidant capacity**, at least across the broad sweep of evolution. In any case, what emerged from the comparative biochemistry of free radical defenses is a fascinating **paradox:** birds, which typically have much longer long life spans than rodents, have **lower activities of antioxidants and higher metabolic rates**.

This paradox has inspired the interspecies comparisons of mitochondrial oxidant generation.

**In my opinion, this is only a paradox because they are applying a flawed theory.**

The rate of living hypothesis identified an inverse correlation between metabolic rate and life span, and the free radical theory supplied a convenient mechanistic link: the mitochondrial generation of oxidants.

Appealing as this theory is, one of the problems with the rate of living hypothesis is the conspicuous lack of fit of a few groups, notably birds and primates. **Both of these groups live longer than their specific metabolic rate would predict.**

**Yet, Beckman and Ames conclude** that taken together, interspecies comparisons of oxidative EMOD damage, antioxidant defenses, and oxidant generation provide some of the **most compelling evidence that oxidants are one of the most significant determinants of life span.**

**I believe that lack of convincing evidence effectively undermines the free radical theory of aging.**

**It is said** that a humming bird eats 2X its body weight each day and that the shrew eats 3X its body weight per day. The humming bird eats the equivalent of 200,000 cal/d or 170# of hamburger. **Both animals are only 2 hours away from starvation.**

According to the rate of living theory of aging, these animals are doomed from day one.....but in actuality, they are not.

As one of the most intuitive approaches to testing the free radical theory, nutritional supplementation has been attempted with numerous species and compounds, with the result that mean life span has been extended in some instances. (Harman, 1981)

Negative results from the feeding of antioxidants have been rationalized by arguing that many of the antioxidants fed to mammals interfere with mitochondrial respiration, and so the failure of antioxidant trials to extend MLSP may have been due to their toxicity. (Harman, 1987)

No large-scale human nutritional intervention trials have been aimed specifically at the study of aging.

In spite of overwhelming data to show the unpredictability of dietary antioxidants, Beckman and Ames concluded, "**These negative results, as well as negative results described above using laboratory rodents, should not be taken as evidence that the free radical theory of aging is flawed.**

In fact, they prove merely that a complex organism like a human or rodent is unlikely to respond predictably to crude manipulations such as supplementation with one or a small number of compounds, as well as that a single end point (such as lung cancer) is not equivalent to aging. Since the time when the results of these human trials were announced, a number of explanations have been forwarded to explain the paradoxical promotion of cancer by beta-carotene." "....until the biochemistry of dietary and cellular antioxidants is better understood, dietary trials in laboratory animals or humans will remain unreliable tests of the free radical theory; molecular gerontology should focus on more instructive experiments."

**In essence, Beckman and Ames turn a blind eye to negative studies with antioxidants and ignore the lack of predictability. It is just this type of approach that misled us from the beginning.**

### Harman....again

Dr. Denham Harman, the "father" of the free radical theory of aging, has defined "aging" as the increased probability of death as the age of an organism increases, and diverse adverse physiologic changes accumulate. Thus, aging can be defined as a progressive functional decline and increasing mortality with time. (Harman, 1956)

Briefly, the theory states that the aging process results from the **"stochastic"** (random) accumulated damage caused by reactive oxygen species (ROS), reactive molecules that, among other sources, are normal by-products of cellular metabolism. (Harman, 1981) (Beckman, Ames, 1998) (Finkel, Holbrook, 2000) (Balaban et al, 2005)

In their 1998 review, Beckman and Ames concluded that, "The free radical theory of aging is not just one of the oldest and still current theories of aging - it is one of the best proven. Any serious long-term anti-aging program must be based upon practical knowledge of, and disciplined use of various techniques and supplements to cope with, the reality of free radicals. And even if an antioxidant/ anti-free radical program doesn't ultimately lengthen one's life, it should still seriously reduce the risk of heart attacks, strokes, cancer, Alzheimer's disease, and many other of the "plagues" of the modern world."

**Yet, Beckman and Ames have repeatedly been proven wrong**. (Howes, 2011, Anti-aging)

In fact, contrary to their theory, **the most reliable current scientific studies have shown that the antioxidant vitamins A, C and E increase the risk of cancer, strokes, heart attacks and overall mortality**. (Howes, 2007, #75) (Howes, 2004, UTOPIA) (Howes, 2005, Med Sci) (Howes, 2006, H2O2) (Howes, 2006, CVD) (Howes, 2006, Diabetes) (Howes, 2006, fantasy)

Although estimates vary, it is commonly accepted that, **under normal physiological conditions, between 0.1 and 3% of the oxygen utilized by mitochondria is diverted to the generation of $O_2^{\cdot-}$**. (Chance et al, 1979) (Fridovich, 2004). **RMH Note: figures vary from 0.1% up to 5%.**

# SECTION THREE

## RADICAL IDEAS

### Hyperthermia

**Hyperthermia can also effect tumor cell survival** and cell lines vary considerably in their intrinsic heat sensitivity. In addition, cell cycle position, intracellular pH, nutrient deprivation, and ATP depletion can affect cell survival after a heat treatment. (Vaupel, Kellecher, 1995)

At 43°C hyperthermia, hypoxia per se may not cause cell death as long as concomitant changes in the nutritional and/or bioenergetic status of the cells do not occur. (Gerweck, Richards, Jennings, 1981)

Recent studies show clear evidence that **hypoxia (defined as the fraction of measured $O_2$ partial pressures of <5 mmHg) is a statistically significant adverse prognostic factor of disease-free survival.**

Similarly, poor outcomes have been shown to be associated with low oxygen tensions in advanced squamous cell carcinomas of the uterine cervix. Also, **tumor hypoxia appears to adversely effect the prognosis of patients with primary and metastatic squamous cell carcinomas of the head and neck** (HNSCC).

In summary, there is a wide range of hypoxia in malignant tumors, but they all appear to have hypoxic thresholds, below which, activities and functions become progressively restricted. These $O_2$ levels can encompass $O_2$ partial pressures from 35 mmHg (start of reduced cell death in conventional photodynamic therapy or restricted efficacy of some immunotherapy) to 0.02 mmHg (below this level, cytochromes aa3 and c are no longer fully oxidized) with all other critical $O_2$ levels for specific cellular functions or activities distributed in between.

Considerable data indicates that low $O_2$ in tumor cells is an adverse prognostic sign and this would be in direct contradiction to the Free Radi-Crap theory of aging and oxidative stress. Low tumor $O_2$ is associated with:

increased aggressiveness of primary cancerous lesions
their ability to metastasize
and an increased resistance to treatments with:
> irradiation,
> chemotherapeutics,
> surgery

The lowered $O_2$ levels generate lowered levels of EMODs, which "allows" the cancer to grow and metastasize; whereas, high levels of EMODs from PDT, irradiation, chemotherapeutics or the Howes Singlet Oxygen Delivery System, kill the cancerous cells.

**Get it?....high levels of EMODs kills cancer and low levels "allow" cancers to grow.**

This directly supports my Unified Theory. Also, remember the above work of Reynolds, who showed that low levels of $O_2$ resulted in a 3.4 fold **increase of mutations,** which again supports my Unified Theory and is contradictory to the Free Radi-Crap theory.

## Oxygen Facts

Normally, oxygen exists as a bound pair of atoms or a diradical.

Unbound oxygen is referred to as a **"singlet of oxygen,"** which is **to distinguish atomic or elemental oxygen from electronically excited molecular metastable singlet oxygen (singlet oxygen).**

It is the bound gas which is an essential for human life, although it is reported that some small amounts of "singlets of oxygen" are also produced during normal metabolism.

Please keep in mind the fact that ground state oxygen is relatively stable and unreactive and it is only when electrons are exchanged or have their spin or orbitals altered do we see the phenomenon of life manifested. Basically, stable atoms and molecules are not participating in life rendering energetics and atoms and molecules of non-change (stable) are more associated with conditions characteristic of "dead" or inanimate objects.

**I see living/breathing entities are products of "change", i.e., changing energy potentials, changing electronic configurations, changing membrane potentials, changes in proton osmosis, changing gene regulators, changing intra- and inter-cellular signaling, changing electron orbitals and changing numbers of valence electrons.**

It is these changes which burn the organic fuels to provide the energy of life.

**I submit that these changes sustain the life forces and these are the changes that are associated with EMODs ( free radicals, reactive oxygen species, active oxygen species, reactive oxygen metabolites, active oxygen intermediates and electronic excitation states).**

**Stable and non-changing electrons, atoms and molecules are the hallmark of states of death or of inanimate objects. Life is a state of change.**

Free radicals are defined as any species capable of independent existence (hence the term "free") that contains one or more unpaired electrons. **These highly maligned species are the ones that make life, as we know it, possible.** Yet, current literature is obsessed with the idea that, specifically, oxygen free radicals are the harbingers of all death and disease.

Quite to the contrary, the **oxygen free radicals (EMODs) give us life**.

In fact, reactive oxygen species are now being found to be produced in many cells of the body on an ongoing basis, at rates which were previously unappreciated. These **oxygen modifications (EMODs) are responsible for ever-increasing important cellular regulatory and signaling processes of normal metabolism and for controlling the cellular life cycle.**

Thus, **free radical "leaks" seems naïve, at best and at worst, the oxidative stress theory of Sies appears out and out wrong.**

At the Nov. 21, 2003 meeting of the Society of Free Radical Biology and Medicine, Dr. Irwin Fridovich presented a glimpse into the evolution of the free radical hypothesis of chronic disease and aging (which I now, tongue and cheek, refer to as the free radi-crap theory of aging and oxidative stress).

However, his prior graduate student, **Dr. Joe McCord,** (Webb-Warring Institute, University of Colorado), **discussed the shift in paradigm from viewing reactive oxygen species as cytotoxic species to their more subtle roles as second messengers or modulators of metabolic pathways.** He proposed that a physiological role of superoxide may be for the modulation of lipid peroxidation.

### Oxygen Miscellaneous Facts
### (Referenced and unreferenced)

-Lungs have 300 million alveolar sacs.

**-90% of cellular oxygen is consumed by the mitochondrial electron transport system.**

-We consume approximately each day: 3.5 kg of oxygen,
of which, 2.8% (2-5%) forms free radicals

**RMH Note: figures vary as to the % of free radical formation.**

-It is like being irradiated at low levels all the time.

-Free radicals in vivo are in the pico molar range $10^{-12}$ (Lam).

-An adult uses the equivalent of 250 ml of pure $O_2$/min
15,000 ml/hr
**360,000 ml/day or 360 liters of pure $O_2$/day**
131,400,000/yr

-Only 1.5% $O_2$ is dissolved in plasma.

-Paramagnetic - unpaired electronic spins; $O_2$ has 2 unpaired electrons and they have the same spin state (direction) and is a (thermodynamic) barrier to insertion of a pair of electrons. Therefore, $O_2$ has to have electrons added one at a time.

-Exercise increase $O_2$ consumption 10-20 fold to 35-70 ml/kg/min of which 2.5% forms free radicals, or 0.6 to 3.5 ml/kg/min free radicals produced in exercise.

-The electrons seem to escape at the ubiquinone-cytochrome c level (Sjodin, 1990).

-We breathe 10-20 liters/min of $O_2$ (air), 21% $O_2$.

- ATP anaerobic production requires almost 20-fold increases in glucose utilization compared to aerobic ATP production.

- **Numerous studies have shown that the degree of PMN bactericidal function is directly dependent on oxygen tensions (and EMOD generation).**

- Oxygen independent killing can occur with lysosomes, acidic vacuoles and lactoferrin, but they are less efficient and vary according to the organism.

- Aminoglycosides such as gentamicin, tobramycin, amikacin and netilmicin are **oxygen dependent** for antimicrobial activity. Sulfonamides antimicrobial effect is **potentiated by hyperbaric oxygen.**

- There is no direct antimicrobial effect of enhanced $O_2$ on aerobic organisms. Indirect antimicrobial effects are related to improved PMN function in killing bacteria.

**RMH Note: It is not ground state $O_2$, but rather EMODs which do the killing.**

- Each cell contains hundreds of mitochondria, each contains mtDNA in the cytoplasm and is maternally inherited.

- Mitochondrial diseases commonly involve tissue with high energy requirements: heart, muscle, renal and endocrine systems.

**-Lung capacity decreases 5% with every decade of life.**

-At sea level, each breath is about 500 ml and contains about 21% $O_2$.

-Pressure at sea level is 760 mm Hg for air and partial pressure at sea level of $O_2$ is 160 mm Hg.

-Partial pressure of alveolar air is 100 mm Hg.

-Partial pressure of pulmonary arteries is 40 mm Hg.

-Thus, oxygen diffuses into venous blood to red cells and hemoglobin.

-Hgb leaving the lung is 98% saturated with $O_2$.

-Hgb in one liter of blood is about 200 ml, of which 50 ml (25%) is extracted each pass through the capillaries.

-A 60 kg man requires 200-250 ml of pure $O_2$ per minute.

-Human suffocation occurs at around 7% $O_2$.

-Johnson found in rabbits, that 0.01 volume of 0.12% $H_2O_2$ caused gas embolism and completely shut down capillary blood flow.

-100 ml of plasma at 100 mm Hg can hold only 0.3 ml of $O_2$.

**-Thus, a 60 kg adult has about 20 ml $O_2$ in their plasma.**

-Our body is at least 80% $H_2O$ which is 8/9 oxygen. Thus, we are composed of over 2/3 oxygen, twice as much as everything else in us combined.

**- $O_2$ is the most common free radical, having 2 unpaired electrons.**

- Oxygenation refers to increasing $O_2$ content and $O_2$ supply refers to the $O_2$ available.

-Oxygen and nitrous oxide are the only important biological molecules that exist in a triplet ground state.

**-$O_2$ concentration is 0.07 mM in living tissue.**

-A few puffs on a cigarette will reduce your oxygen absorbing capability by about 25%.

**RMH Note: I believe that, in smokers, this oxygen reduction "allows" for development of a wide variety of diseases and cancer.**

**-A mitochondrion "breathes in," $O_2$ and pyruvic acid into the Kreb's cycle to produce ATP. When a mitochondrion "breathes**

out" it releases ATP, $H_2O$, and $CO_2$ into the cytoplasm. ATP is especially important to neurons because in a resting human about 40% of total energy consumption is used to operate the "pumps" that keep certain ions (e.g., $Na^+$, $K^+$), either inside or outside of the neurons to regulate their excitability. This is why the brain is so sensitive to damage by $O_2$ deprivation or reduction in ATP.

-The brain has about 100 billion cells (neurons), each connected to about 1,000 other cells (this is probably a low estimate).

**RMH Note: In the brain, $O_2$ is the energy source that produces and promotes consciousness. The brain is a "heavy breather" using 20% of the body's total $O_2$ intake.**

I believe that the above fact "that the antioxidant enzymes in the brain do not completely deplete $H_2O_2$ levels" is again evidence of the need for these EMODs for normal brain function.

According to the Free Radi-Crap theory, leaving steady state levels of $H_2O_2$ and extremely dangerous EMODs would have disastrous consequences, especially a chain reaction involving lipid peroxidation, but ....under normal physiological conditions, that does not happen!

-Normal tissue $O_2$ gradient is from 2-5% across a 400 μm distance from a blood supply. Tumor cells are hypoxic with cells adjacent to capillaries with an $O_2$ gradient of 2% and with cells located 200 μm from the nearest capillary have a mean $O_2$ concentration of 0.2%. Thus, tumors have increased lactic acid and other acids and it is an acidic environment.

-$O_2$ concentration is of the order of 0.07 mM in living tissue (Johan Moan, 2001).

| | |
|---|---|
| -Mitochondrial $O_2$ partial pressure | 0.5 mm Hg |
| -Tissue levels with hyperbaric $O_2$ | 1200 mm Hg |
| -Rabbit ear capillaries range | 3-30 mm Hg |
| -Wounds range | 30-50 mm Hg |
| -Chronic wounds range | 5-20 mm Hg |

**RMH Note: My Unified Theory (UTOPIA) is supported by the fact that chronic wounds are associated with cancer. This is because the chronic wound does not have enough $O_2$ to kill bacteria or form collagen and it certainly does not have enough $O_2$ with EMODs to kill cancer cells.** (Howes, 2004, UTOPIA)

Prof Randolph M. Howes MD, PhD

**-Molecular $O_2$ is the only homonuclear diatomic that has triplet spin multiplicity in its ground state ($^3\Sigma_y^-$).**

- Oxygenation is usually exothermic and hence, can thermodynamically occur in every place on this planet. This means that **organisms live under an oxidative environment.**

- Aerobic respiration produces **686 kcal** by complete oxidation of 1 mole glucose to $CO_2$ and $H_2O$; while fermentation releases only 47 kcal for conversion of 1 mole of glucose to lactate.

- $O_2$ is an absolute requirement for differentiation and it is more than an essential cofactor for aerobic metabolism.

-1 in $10^4$ electrons (1:10,000) in respiratory transport chain is caught and produces $O_2^-$. However, other say that as many as one in every twenty oxygen molecules is converted into the superoxide anion as leak from the electron transport chain.

**-$10^{12}$ $O_2$ molecules are consumed everyday.**

-Skeletal muscle accounts for 20-30% of the total resting oxygen uptake and the brain takes 20%.

**RMH Note: The incidence of skeletal muscle and brain cancer should therefore total 40% of the body cancer rate....but it does not.**

-Oxygen can be "our dangerous friend" (Passwater interview).

**RMH Note: So could countless other compounds in deficiency or excessive levels.**

> **"The cell's intracellular cytoplasmic sea is an ocean of symphonic motion awash with incomprehensible complexity."**
> R. M. Howes, M.D., Ph.D.
> 1/24/04

---

I have included this article because EMODs are right in the heart of HBOT and an understanding of this general background information is crucial.

The following article was adapted from: (Turrens, 2003)

## Mitochondrial formation of reactive oxygen species (ROS, EMODs)

(Turrens, 2003)

The reduction of oxygen to water proceeds via one electron at a time. In the mitochondrial respiratory chain, Complex IV (cytochrome oxidase) retains all partially reduced intermediates until full reduction is achieved. Other redox centers in the electron transport chain, however, may leak electrons to oxygen, partially reducing this molecule to superoxide anion ($O_2^-\bullet$).

**Even though $O_2^-\bullet$ is not a strong oxidant**, it is a precursor of most other reactive oxygen species, and it also becomes involved in the propagation of oxidative chain reactions. Despite the presence of various antioxidant defenses, the mitochondrion appears to be the main intracellular source of these oxidants, although this is controversial.

Reactive oxygen species (ROS) is a phrase used to describe a variety of molecules and free radicals (chemical species with one unpaired electron) derived from molecular oxygen.

Molecular oxygen in the ground state is a bi-radical, containing two unpaired electrons in the outer shell (also known as a triplet state).

Since the two single electrons have the same spin, oxygen can only react with one electron at a time and **therefore it is not very reactive** with the two electrons in a chemical bond. On the other hand, if one of the two unpaired electrons is excited and changes its spin, the resulting species (known as singlet oxygen) becomes a powerful oxidant as the two electrons with opposing spins can quickly react with other pairs of electrons, especially double bonds (unsaturated lipids, fats).

**The reduction of oxygen by one electron at a time produces relatively stable intermediates.** Superoxide anion ($O_2^-\bullet$), the product of a one-electron reduction of oxygen, is the precursor of most EMODs and a mediator in oxidative chain reactions.

Dismutation of $O_2^-\bullet$ (either spontaneously or through a reaction catalysed by superoxide dismutases) produces hydrogen peroxide ($H_2O_2$), which in turn may be fully reduced to water or partially reduced to hydroxyl radical ($OH\bullet$), one of the strongest oxidants in nature.

In addition, $O_2^-$• may react with other radicals including nitric oxide (NO•) in a reaction controlled by the rate of diffusion of both radicals. The product, peroxynitrite, is also a very powerful oxidant. (Beckman & Koppenol, 1996) (Radi et al, 2002b)

The oxidants derived from NO• have been called reactive nitrogen species (RNS).

So-called 'oxidative stress' is an expression used to describe alleged various deleterious processes resulting from an imbalance between the excessive formation of EMODs and/or RNS and limited antioxidant defenses. (Sies, 1991)

In vivo, $O_2^-$• is produced both enzymatically and non-enzymatically. Enzymatic sources include NADPH oxidases located on the cell membrane of polymorphonuclear cells, macrophages and endothelial cells and cytochrome $P_{450}$-dependent oxygenases. The proteolytic conversion of xanthine dehydrogenase to xanthine oxidase provides another enzymatic source of both $O_2^-$• and $H_2O_2$.

The non-enzymatic production of $O_2^-$• occurs when a single electron is directly transferred to oxygen by reduced coenzymes or prosthetic groups (for example, flavins or iron sulfur clusters) or by xenobiotics previously reduced by certain enzymes (for example, the anticancer agent adriamycin or the herbicide paraquat).

The mitochondrial electron transport chain contains several redox centers that may leak electrons to oxygen, constituting the primary source of $O_2^-$• in most tissues.

The standard reduction potential for the conversion of molecular oxygen to $O_2^-$• is -0.160V. The respiratory chain includes a variety of redox centers with standard reduction potentials between -0.32 V (NAD(P)H) and +0.39 V (cytochrome $a_3$ in Complex IV).

Given the highly reducing intramitochondrial environment, various respiratory components, including flavoproteins, iron-sulfur clusters and ubisemiquinone, are thermodynamically capable of transferring one electron to oxygen.

Moreover, most steps in the respiratory chain involve single-electron reactions, further favoring the monovalent reduction of oxygen.

On the other hand, the mitochondrion possesses various antioxidant defenses designed to eliminate both $O_2^-$• and $H_2O_2$. As a result, **the steady state concentrations of $O_2^-$• and $H_2O_2$ have been**

**estimated to be around $10^{-10}$ M and $5 \times 10^{-9}$ M, respectively.** (Cadenas & Davies, 2000)

Over the past 35 years several laboratories have identified a variety of mitochondrial sources of $O_2^-\bullet$ including several respiratory complexes and individual enzymes.

Superoxide formation occurs on the outer mitochondrial membrane, in the matrix and on both sides of the inner mitochondrial membrane. Whilst the $O_2^-\bullet$ generated in the matrix is eliminated in that compartment, part of the $O_2^-\bullet$ produced in the intermembrane space may be carried to the cytoplasm via voltage-dependent anion channels.

The relative contribution of every site to the overall $O_2^-\bullet$ production varies from organ to organ and also depends on whether mitochondria are actively respiring (State 3) or the respiratory chain is highly reduced (State 4).

Although Complex III appears to be responsible for most of the $O_2^-\bullet$ produced in heart and lung mitochondria, $O_2^-\bullet$ formation by **Complex I appears to be the primary source of $O_2^-\bullet$ in the brain under normal conditions.**

Moreover, Complex I is allegedly the primary source of EMODs in a variety of pathological scenarios ranging from aging to Parkinson's disease.

**The rate of $O_2^-\bullet$ formation by the respiratory chain is controlled primarily by mass action, increasing both when electron flow slows down** (increasing the concentration of electron donors, R•) **and when the concentration of oxygen increases.** (Turrens et al, 1982)

The energy released as electrons flow through the respiratory chain is converted into a $H^+$ gradient through the inner mitochondrial membrane. (Mitchell, 1977)

This gradient, in turn, dissipates through the ATP synthase complex (Complex V) and is responsible for the turning of a rotor-like protein complex required for ATP synthesis.

**In the absence of ADP**, the movement of $H^+$ through ATP synthase ceases and the $H^+$ gradient builds up **causing electron flow to slow down** and the respiratory chain to become more reduced (State IV respiration). As a result, **the physiological steady state concentration of $O_2^-\bullet$ formation increases.**

**The formation of $O_2^-\bullet$ may be further increased in the presence of certain inhibitors (for example rotenone, which inhibits Complex I, or antimycin, an inhibitor of Complex III),** which cause those carriers upstream from the site of inhibition to become fully reduced. In Complex I, the primary source of $O_2^-\bullet$ appears to be one of the iron-sulfur clusters

The simultaneous formation of $O_2^-\bullet$ and nitric oxide produces peroxynitrite, a very strong oxidant and nitrating agent. Nitric oxide is a vasodilator resulting from the breakdown of arginine to citrulline, in a reaction catalysed by a family of NADPH-dependent enzymes called nitric oxide synthases.

**Since NO$\bullet$ formation requires oxygen, the rate at which it is produced varies with the intramitochondrial oxygen concentration.** (Alvarez et al, 2003)

The mitochondrial matrix contains a specific form of SOD, with manganese in the active site, which eliminates the $O_2^-\bullet$ formed in the matrix or on the inner side of the inner membrane. The expression of MnSOD is further induced by agents that cause oxidative stress, including radiation and hyperoxia, in a process mediated by the oxidative activation of the nuclear transcription factor NF$\kappa$B.

**The steady-state concentration of $O_2^-\bullet$ in the intermembrane space is controlled by three different mechanisms.**

**Firstly,** this compartment contains a different SOD isozyme which contains copper and zinc instead of manganese (CuZnSOD) and is also found in the cytoplasm of eukaryotic cells.

**Secondly,** the intermembrane space contains cytochrome $c$ which can be reduced by $O_2^-\bullet$ ($k = 10^7$ M$^{-1}$ s$^{-1}$, regenerating oxygen in the process. The reduced cytochrome $c$ can then transfer electrons to the terminal oxidase. Thus, some of the electrons that escaped the respiratory chain producing $O_2^-\bullet$ may re-reduce cytochrome $c$ and still contribute to energy production by providing the energy needed to pump H$^+$ through Complex IV.

**Finally,** the spontaneous dismutation of $O_2^-\bullet$ in the intermembrane space is facilitated by the lower pH in this compartment, resulting from the extrusion of H$^+$ coupled to respiration.

Hydrogen peroxide, the product of $O_2^-\bullet$ dismutation and the main precursor of OH$\bullet$ in the presence of reduced transition metals, is mostly decomposed by the enzyme glutathione peroxidase.

In the liver, mitochondria account for about one third of the total glutathione peroxidase activity.

**Catalase, a major $H_2O_2$ detoxifying enzyme found in peroxisomes, is also present in heart mitochondria**. However, this enzyme has not been found in mitochondria from other tissues, including skeletal muscle.

In addition to cytochrome $c$, other electron carriers appear to have a detoxifying role against EMODs. Ubiquinol ($QH_2$) has been shown to act as a reducing agent in the elimination of various peroxides in the presence of succinate but it can have prooxidant activity.

Thus, coenzyme Q is a source of $O_2^-\bullet$ when partially reduced (semiquinone form) and an antioxidant when fully reduced.

**The inner mitochondrial membrane also contains vitamin E**, a powerful antioxidant that interferes with the propagation of free radical-mediated chain reactions.

**Apoptosis (or programmed cell death)** is the mechanism used by mammals, plants and other organisms to eliminate redundant or damaged cells. Apoptosis may be triggered by extracellular signals (extrinsic pathway) or by intracellular processes (intrinsic pathway).

An increased mitochondrial formation of EMODs triggers the intrinsic pathway by increasing the permeability of the outer mitochondrial membrane through the opening of transition pores.

**The gradual loss of cytochrome $c$ from the intermembrane space during apoptosis favors the mitochondrial formation of $O_2^-\bullet$ in two ways**: (1) cytochrome $c$ is a scavenger of $O_2^-\bullet$ and (2) as cytochrome $c$ is released, the respiratory chain becomes more reduced because electron flow between Complex III and Complex IV slows down.

> **"The cell's intracellular cytoplasmic sea is**
> **an ocean of symphonic motion awash with**
> **incomprehensible complexity."**
> R. M. Howes, M.D., Ph.D.
> 1/24/04

## Mitochondrial EMODs, hyperoxia and hypoxia

**As predicted, the mitochondrial production of $O_2^-\bullet$ must increase with oxygen concentration.**

The proportion of oxygen converted into $O_2^-\bullet$ *in vitro* ($[O_2] = 220\ \mu M$) accounts for about 1-2 % of the overall oxygen consumption. **RMH Note: amounts vary according to investigators.**

*In vivo*, particularly in tissues not exposed to atmospheric oxygen, the proportion of oxygen converted $O_2^-\bullet$ is likely to be smaller since the intramitochondrial oxygen concentration is between 3 and 30 $\mu M$.

**As oxygen concentration increases, the rate of mitochondrial $O_2^-\bullet$ production increases linearly.** (Turrens et al, 1982)

**I believe this is very important in the case of hyperbaric oxygen therapy.**

**However, the release of $H_2O_2$ from mitochondria is biphasic, increasing at a faster rate above 60 % $O_2$.** (Turrens et al, 1985)

The slower release of $H_2O_2$ at lower $P_{O2}$ suggests that the mitochondrial antioxidant defenses can compensate for sudden increases in the concentration of this peroxide. **Apparently these defenses become overwhelmed at higher $P_{O2}$, which explains the mitochondrial alterations observed in the lungs of animals exposed to oxygen concentrations around 60 % or higher.** (Crapo et al, 1983)

Under normobaric hyperoxic conditions, the only organs affected by EMOD formation are the lungs, since they the only ones in direct contact with atmospheric oxygen. However, **under hyperbaric conditions**, more oxygen is dissolved in the plasma, and therefore other tissues become exposed to a hyperoxic environment. Under these conditions, **the brain is the first organ to show the effects of an increased ROS (EMOD) formation, resulting in convulsions.**

Interestingly, this phenomenon was proposed to be associated with oxygen free radicals 15 years before the discovery of $O_2^-\bullet$ as a normal intracellular metabolite. (Gerschman et al, 1954)

The formation of EMODs should decrease with hypoxia, since this activity is proportional to ROS. Yet, **various groups have reported**

**a paradoxical increase in oxidative stress under moderately hypoxic conditions** (1.5 % $O_2$, equivalent to an oxygen concentration of around 16 μM.

The proposed increase in EMOD formation during hypoxia is difficult to explain.

Given the high affinity of cytochrome oxidase for oxygen, at low $P_{O2}$ any remaining oxygen should be reduced to water by the terminal oxidase.

Several xenobiotics interact with the mitochondrial electron transport chain, increasing the rate of $O_2^-\bullet$ production through two different mechanisms. Some of these compounds stimulate oxidative stress because they block electron transport, increasing the reduction level of carriers located upstream of the inhibition site.

Other xenobiotics may accept an electron from a respiratory carrier and transfer it to molecular oxygen (redox cycling), stimulating $O_2^-\bullet$ formation without inhibiting the respiratory chain.

**The mitochondrial respiratory chain constitutes the main intracellular source of EMODs in most tissues.**

The steady-state concentration of these oxidants is maintained at non-toxic levels by a variety of antioxidant defenses and repair enzymes. The delicate balance between antioxidant defenses and EMOD production may be disrupted by either deficient antioxidant defenses, inhibition of electron flow or exposure to xenobiotics.

## My way of thinking

Let me introduce you to my overall thinking.

**Radicophobes can ignore the truth or
they can reject the truth or
deny the truth but
they can not change the magnificent truths
regarding the crucial role
of EMODs in the life process
of all aerobes
or the inherent splendor of oxygen.**
R. M. Howes M.D., Ph.D.
1/26/09

**Normal redox homeostasis may be pathologically disturbed by overzealous use of antioxidants.**

**My UTOPIA (Unified Theory Of Oxygen Participation In Aerobiosis) and ROSI syndrome theories (Reactive Oxygen Species Insufficiency) present a new perspective more correctly informed by the most contemporaneous experimental findings and most reliable clinical studies.**

The ideal drug to treat cancer would be not only potent and highly selective for tumors but also broken down quickly into harmless compounds and excreted from the body. **This is exactly what my singlet oxygen delivery system does!**

**The average person breathes in about 6 pounds of oxygen a day,** which is about the same amount by weight of food and water intake. **Six has always been my lucky number.**

**We breathe 21,600 times per day. I believe that our strongest drive is not to acquire food or sex; instead, it is to keep breathing...to keep taking in essential oxygen quantities on a continual basis throughout our lifetime!**

**To distribute oxygen throughout the body, the heart beats 100,000 times per day and pumps 5,000 gallons of blood. This alone emphasizes the crucial role played by oxygen in our everyday survival.**

**The free radical theory teaches the nonsense/nonscience approach that all of this effort is to bring a toxic agent (i.e., oxygen) into the body and distribute it to all aerobic cells on a continuous basis.**

**Thus, I believe that the free radical theory is not based on sound scientific reasoning and that it flies in the face of all teachings of Darwinian evolution.**

**During a single hour of HBOT (hyperbaric oxygen therapy), a person will take in about 2.4 pounds of oxygen. This increases the oxygen content of the tissues by a factor of 10-15.** Please remember this point for our later in depth discussions of HBOT.

The radio airways are filled with nonscience/nonsense regarding antioxidants, energy production and oxidation. I was recently listening to a station promoting antioxidant sales, with claims that antioxidants will cure damned near every disease out there. It claimed that CoQ 10 is like putting an internal ice pack on an inflamed joint. It claimed that one will get an incredible energy boost from antioxidants.

Please remember that it was the founder of the free radical theory, Denham Harman, who told Jack Chelam that taking too many anti-oxidants would cause fatigue, not an incredible energy boost. Even Harman was aware of the dangers of excessive antioxidant levels.

**Energy production goes toward enzyme production and half the protein produced in the body every day is enzymes and our endogenous antioxidant superoxide dismutase (SOD) is the fifth most abundant protein in the body.**

SOD generates hydrogen peroxide from the dismutation of superoxide anions.

**The brain uses 20% of our inspired oxygen and must produce and use 20% of the body's total ATP production in order to maintain normal function.**

**Researchers are using other technologies to determine how the loss of oxygen affects the functions of genes in the brain.**

**Of the approximately 30,000 genes investigated to date, at least 6,000 are either inactivated or highly activated when a stroke reduces the oxygen in the brain (hypoxia).**

Future work will explore the ramifications of those changed gene func-tions. **I believe that this illustrates the absolutely crucial role of adequate oxygen levels, EMOD levels and the redox status of the cell.**

### Howes ratiocinations

### The Howes ratiocination of EMOD insufficiency and disease allowance.

**EMODs do not cause wanton destruction to cells or within cells.**

**Epidemiology teaches that every statistical association has only 3 possible explanations: a) bias, b) chance, and c) cause. However, I impugn this statement and would add to this 1)**

partial fabrication of data, 2) unscrupulous manipulation of data and 3) completely made up data, i.e., bald-faced liars.

In actuality, free radicals perform many crucial roles in normal, healthy physiological processes like our immune system and promote beneficial oxidation.

It is important to realize that many vitamins and supplements classified as antioxidants (or so-called antioxidants) are actually *redox agents*, meaning that they act as antioxidants in some instances and pro-oxidants in others.

Both prooxidants and antioxidants are designed to exist in alternating redox states. This markedly increases the difficulty of intrepreting redox data and is seldom addressed or mentioned in the literature or considered in arriving at so-called scientific conclusions.

Unfortunately, many believe that correlation equals causation. But, they are wrong.

As of 2015, the continued non-acceptance of the null findings of over 500 clinical trials on vitamin and antioxidant supplements has **no scientific basis or biochemical plausibility**.

The underlying principles of the free radical theory have been proven to be unsound.

**Nick Nolte's ravaged face**

**Nick reportedly has a thousands-of-dollars-a-week vitamin habit.**

**He takes 60 supplements a day!**

**Angelina Jolie's suprapubic tattoo**

*"Quod me nutrit me destruit"*

translates as "That which nourishes me, destroys me".

It bears a resemblance to some lines by Shakespeare: Consum'd with that which it was nourished by' (Sonnet 73) and 'A burning torch that's turned upside down; / The word, *Qui me alit, me extinguit* [Who feeds me extinguishes me]' (Pericles, II.ii.33).

**And the biggest loser comment goes to Bruce Ames' who infamously said, "The thing we need most, oxygen, is what is killing us."**

**Forrest Gump could figure that such a statement is nonscience/ nonsense.**

In my opinion, this whole scenario is a quintessential example of 21$^{st}$ century snake oil salesmanship!!! Snake oil now flows faster than Texas crude.

**At worst, antioxidant supplements have dangerous consequences and at best, they are a waste of money. (RMH 1-5-09)**

**In the absence of a proven vitamin deficiency, these supplement products are basically useless and do not have the same biochemical effect as the nutrients being obtained from a healthy diet.**

**With such a large portion of the population using antioxidant vitamins, even a small effect from antioxidant restriction could have a big negative public health impact. This should be combined with increasing overall oxidative capacity. RMH 1-26-10**

Certainly, research findings have not been sufficiently compelling to convince most cellular biochemists that the free radical theory and overall disease causation are functionally linked. In fact, recent studies undermine this link.

**A comprehensive literature review shows that antioxidant therapies have enjoyed unjustified support in preclinical studies across disparate animal models, but have shown little or no benefit in human intervention studies or clinical trials.**

A total reassessment of the role of antioxidant vitamins in human health is in order.

**It has previously been believed that knockout of various antioxidant defense enzymes raises oxidative damage levels and promotes age-related cancer development in animals.** In explaining this, most attention has been paid to direct oxidative damage to DNA by certain RS, such as hydroxyl radical (OH*).

**However, increased levels of DNA base oxidation products such as 8OHdg (8-hydroxy-2'-deoxyguanosine) do not always lead**

**to malignancy**, although malignant tumors often show increased levels of DNA base oxidation. Hence additional actions of ROS must be important, possibly their effects on p53, cell proliferation, invasiveness and metastasis.

Chronic inflammation predisposes to malignancy, but the role of ROS in this is likely to be complex because **ROS, EMODs can sometimes act as anti-inflammatory agents** (Halliwell, 2007) (Oxidative stress and cancer: have we moved forward? B. Halliwell. Biochem J (2007) 401: 1-11). **I believe that this discounts and nullifies the suggestions that EMODs are both carcinogenic and inflammatory agents.**

## Cancer cells and (so-called) oxidative stress

### Abstract

Reactive oxygen species (ROS, EMODs) formation are a constant element of a cell's oxygen metabolism.

**They are its normal products and in physiological concentrations they play important roles in a variety of cell processes**.

Allegedly, disturbances in the balance between EMOD formation and the efficiency of antioxidant mechanisms lead to oxidative stress. Oxidative stress may cause damage to important macromolecules, such as DNA, proteins, and lipids.

Some believe that the evidence indicates the participation of EMODs in the cancerous transformation of cells. So-called oxidative stress was also found in cancer cells, but the mechanisms responsible for its induction have not been definitively explained. It is known that they include inflammation and cytokine action, oncogenic signals, intensive metabolism related to constant proliferation, mutations in mitochondrial DNA, and malfunction in the respiratory chain.

A high level of EMODs in cancer cells may lead to a variety of biological responses, such as cell adaptation, increased proliferation rate, formation of DNA mutations and genetic instability, and resistance to some drugs used in anticancer therapy. Therefore, **it can be useful in the search for new therapeutic strategies of cancer treatment**. (Scibior-Bentkowska, Czeczot, 2009)

**RMH Note: Such is the case with my tumoricidal singlet oxygen system. Actually, EMODs add to the effectiveness of chemotherapeutic drugs, and they are blocked by excessive levels of antioxidants.**

**Paracelsus stated,** "Practice should not be based on speculative theory; theory should be derived from practice. Experience is the judge; if a thing stands the test of experience, it should be accepted; if it does not stand this test, it should be rejected." **RMH Note: This could well refer to the situation with antioxidants. In theory, they should work but in practice, they do not. Ergo, they should be rejected.**

Antioxidants are (allegedly) especially important in the mitochondria of eukaryotic cells, since the use of oxygen as part of the process for generating energy produces reactive oxygen species.

The process of aerobic metabolism requires oxygen because oxygen serves as the final resting place for electrons generated by the oxidation steps of the citric acid cycle (i.e. **oxygen is the final "electron acceptor"** of the redox reactions). However, the superoxide anion is produced as a by-product of this reduction of oxygen in the electron transport chain.

Specifically, the reduction of coenzyme Q in complex III is currently believed to be the major source of superoxide anion, since a highly reactive free radical is formed as an intermediate ($Q^{\cdot}$). This unstable radical can lead to electron "leakage": instead of moving along the well-controlled reactions of the electron transport chain, the electrons jump directly to molecular oxygen, forming the superoxide anion (Finkel and Holbrook 2000). (http://articles.gourt.com/en/Antioxidant).

**I interpret this to mean that oxygen is not ripping electrons away from reducing agents, but it is "accepting" electrons. Ripping is very aggressive process, whereas, accepting is passive. Please remember that oxygen is the "ultimate electron acceptor."**

> **"It, and its kindred, stands as the singular barrier**
> **between health and sepsis,**
> **between normal and cancerous,**
> **between living and dead.**

> **This astonishing anomaly, of the periodic table,
> offers unsolicited chemical solace
> to the vulnerable collective of living creatures.
> Thank you, most beloved
> oxygen."**
> R. M. Howes, M.D., Ph.D.
> 11/25/04

## EMODs (Electronically Modified Oxygen Derivatives)

It is also time to discard ROS, RONS, OS, ROI, ROM, AOS, etc. and utilize a more meaningful and accurate term. I propose the term **"electronically modified oxygen derivative(s)" (EMODs).**

This term does not imply charge, radicality, or reactivity. **It merely indicates that an electron(s) of oxygen has (have) been altered or changed from it ground state orbit.** This avoids all of the inaccuracies of terms such as reactive oxygen species, reactive oxygen metabolites, or oxygen intermediates, all of which should be discarded from usage.

Thus, EMODs include superoxide anion, singlet oxygen, hydrogen peroxide, hypochlorous acid, peroxynitrite, hydroxyl radical, nitric oxide, alkyl radicals, alkoxyl radicals, etc. The term does not limit itself to oxygen covalent bonding or hydrogen abstraction and addition. Thus, oxygen-containing sulfates, nitrates, phosphates, etc. would also qualify as EMODs.

Further, it includes all of the nitrative and oxidative forms of oxygen. If one wishes to further delineate biochemical or biological EMODs, one could use the term, **BEMODs,** which would be the closest acronym to the old designation of RONS, but would not be burdened with its inaccuracies. Nonetheless, the BEMODs designation has specific, but limited meaning.

During periods of normalcy or good health, we exist in an **EMOD sufficiency state (EMOD-SS).**

The cumulative cellular damage that is blamed on **EMODs** is frequently seen only in *in vitro* experiments and consequently, biochemical conditions bear little resemblance to the conditions existing in **the living/ breathing cell.** Most people live a normal life, free of disease, to die of attrition through programmed senescence, just as all other living things do (viruses are not considered to be alive).

**I believe that the most predictable consequence of life is death. In other words, life is the number one cause of death, especially if viewed, as suggested by the free radical theory.**

## Ubiquitous Free Radicals

Reactive oxygen species are grouped together in a meaningless manner. Not all of the reactive oxygen species (ROS) are "reactive" and many are not free radicals. The **reactive oxygen species must be considered on an individual molecular basis** because of vastly differing one electron reduction potentials (redox potentials), rate constants, and chemical reactivities. I believe that **it is no longer acceptable to "lump" ROS together under one incorrect grouping, heading or classification.** (Refer to UTOPIA I$^{st}$ ed., Vol. I, pg. 70).

In the US, we spray 1.2 billion pounds of pesticides on our food crops, feed 9 million pounds of antibiotics to our farm animals, and dump 90 billion pounds of toxic wastes into 55,000 toxic waste sites annually.

There are 5 million registered chemicals in the world and humans contact 70,000 of which 20,000 are considered carcinogens.

Exogenous sources of free radicals are from environmental toxins in the water, air, smog, ozone, chemicals, drugs, pesticides, herbicides, cigarettes, radiation, and trace metals (e.g., lead, mercury, iron and copper). Yet, **our average lifespan continues to increase!**

Is this increase due to the increase in EMODs from environmental factors?

## The Free Radical Fairy Tale

**Perpetually repeated false impressions and exaggerated inaccuracies have led to the acceptance of flawed theories and disproved hypotheses. Yet, the inaccuracies and the theories, relative to oxygen free radicals, appear to live on and they are**

now, more than ever, erroneously referred to in the scientific literature as proven facts.

Sadly, the Free Radical theory of oxidative stress and aging seems to be indelibly tattooed into the frontal lobes of the minds of current medical scientists, who have accepted and embellished this fairy tale rumor with the zeal of a child embracing the perceived reality of Snow White, Mickey Mouse and Jolly Old St. Nick.

It appears to me that the oxy-morons are an insular group, who can not accept the inaccuracies of their predictions and who are stuck with the limitations of their imaginations. They need to rid themselves of the burdens of the erroneous Free Radi-Crap theory and open their minds toward the beneficent sufficiency of cellular electronically modified oxygen derivatives (EMODs). RMH 4-7-05

Many authors have stated that, "In the past several years, unprecedented progress has been made in the recognition and understanding of roles of reactive oxygen species in many diseases. These include atherosclerosis, vasospasms, cancers, trauma, stroke, asthma, hyperoxia, arthritis, heart attack, age pigments, dermatitis, cataractogenesis, retinal damage, hepatitis, liver injury, and periodontitis, which are age related." (Lee, Koo, Min, 2004)

Unfortunately, **they have implied a cause and effect relationship between reactive oxygen species (EMODs) and over 100 diseases (now some authors say over 200 diseases, actually it is as many diseases as they can think of), including aging.**

I do not agree with their assessment and a review of the literature will readily reveal that the evidence linking these conditions to reactive oxygen species is **clearly circumstantial**. Proof is lacking.

Data is confusing and contradictory, such that arriving at scientific proof is impossible, and following the faint truth-trail, in search for the scientific Holy Grail of cellular biochemical reality, is rife with difficulty.

**Separating "fact from factitious" has become increasingly challenging.**

**Extrapolations of data obtained from in vitro studies to the living/breathing cell have been occasionally disastrous and frequently erroneous. The complexities in the living/breathing cell are light years removed from the simplicity of test**

**tube studies, which are clearly laden with countless "dead" artifacts.**

Perhaps the most important aspect of these artifacts is due to the fact that **in vitro studies take place outside of the living totality of a respiring aerobic organism and are conducted in the glass-casket test tube, housed inside the sterile confines of the laboratory-morgue.**

**This is, indeed, a far cry from the beautifully integrated complex of a living cell and its incorporation into a living and fully functional organism.**

> **"The master's guard dogs were characterized**
> **as pernicious, rapacious and only capable of**
> **uncontrollable violence.**
> **Yet, they only acted instinctively, with the innate loyalty of**
> **an ever-dedicated protector.**
> **And, so it is, with the**
> **maligned reactive oxygen species;**
> **truly, man's best friend."**
> R. M. Howes, M.D., Ph.D.
> 11/25/04

Man is an electromagnetic being. Information gathered from all five of our senses is converted into electro-chemical signals for central processing. Our brains assimilate and electromagnetically analyze this data, following which, it electro-chemically formulates a response.

This response is then electro-chemically transmitted throughout our bodies for action or reaction.

Our existence is dependent upon the passage, the flow, or the movement of electrons, which we can measure by electrocardiograms and electro-encephalograms. Equally or even more importantly, the flow of electrons, via oxygen and the **electronically modified oxygen derivatives (EMODs),** is essential for energizing our state of being alive. Without the flow of electrons we cease to live.

Oxygen free radicals are designed to provide for the flow of electrons and I believe that antioxidants are designed as a possible assistant (not preventative) for this electron flow.

By design, the shift back and forth between two oxidation states, via single-electron-transfer reactions, is the property that makes iron and copper such essential components of the hemeproteins and enzyme complexes. Transition metals can exist in several spin-states and are able to relieve the π-electron spin restrictions of dioxygen. The coordination of biomolecules by transition metals almost always involves the d-orbitals of the metal.

As with oxygen, **certain atoms and molecules are designed to promote vital electron flow.**

Thus, the vast majority of so-called autoxidation reactions are most likely metal catalyzed. Iron and copper can serve as prooxidants and deficiency states of both are associated with an increased incidence of cancer, infections and arthritis.

Many researchers say that oxygen free radicals are causative of between 100-200 diseases and of aging, culminating in death. In my view, many diseases, such as cancer, atherosclerosis, diabetes, obesity, arthritis and cataracts, appear to be interdigitated and to occur in clusters or to coexist.

Clustering illustrates my principle that **"one good free radical deficiency or insufficiency (EMOD) disease deserves another."**

Researchers have used the in vitro analogy of milk or butter becoming rancid to illustrate the manner in which oxygen free radicals react with lipids inside a living/breathing cell. However, one only needs to remember that **the best way to prevent butter from becoming rancid is to keep it in the cow.**

Frequently, in vitro studies have minimal relevance to complex biochemical processes, which are constantly occurring in exponential numbers, within the synchronized and segmentalized living/breathing cell.

The followers of the **free radical theory (FRT)** of oxidative stress and aging say that, "oxygen is killing us." They have engendered a societal "cult following" of radicophobes, who are unknowingly and dangerously trying to block basic salutary prooxidative processes with hyped vitamin and dietary supplemental nostrums.

The pendulum of homeostasis has swung to a precarious position in its arc of rationality, as it encroaches and moves into the zone of irrationality.

The brain is an $O_2$ sponge. $H_2O_2$ is produced in dopamine nerve terminals by **monoamine oxidase (MAO). Catalase** quantities are low and superoxide dismutase levels are high in the brain. Both of these situations further increase $H_2O_2$ levels in the brain and at neural terminals. In the vulnerable brain, EMODs rule, normally, with the appearance of very few of the predicted harmful effects of the FRT.

Additionally, exercise, which generates 10-20 times normal levels of EMODs, is good for the brain. Exercise improves concentration and cognitive abilities and I believe that it is due to the increase in EMODs, which are critical to normal brain function.

If EMODs were harmful to the brain, it seems to me that Darwinian principles would have evolved with much higher levels of antioxidant enzymes in the brain and lower levels of prooxidant iron.

## Harman's free radical five points

**Dr. Harman believes that support for the free radical theory is stated in the following five points:**

1) "Studies of the origin and evolution of life"
   **By definition, this is a mega SWAG (scientific wild a$$ed guess) and is, at best, fanciful speculation.**
2) "Studies of the effect of ionizing radiation on living things"
   **Comparing the energetics for the metabolic formation of oxygen free radicals to those products produced by ionizing radiation is as unreasonable as comparing products produced by the flame of a cup cake candle to those generated by the fusion fire of the sun. The energies involved are remarkably and significantly different between the two processes.**
3) "Dietary manipulations of endogenous free radical reactions"
   **Vitamin and dietary supplements have repeatedly been shown to cause harmful consequences, including increases in cardiovascular disease, strokes, cancer and in overall mortality.**
4) "The plausible explanations it provides for aging phenomena"
   **Presently, there is no plausible explanation for the aging phenomena. There have been over 300 unproven and unsupported "possible" explanations or theories put forth.**
5) "The growing number of studies that implicates free radical reactions in the pathogenesis of specific diseases"

**Results from double blind, randomized studies involving hundreds of thousands of patients from the past two decades, have primarily shown that antioxidants do not effectively control or reverse diseases which have been attributed to oxygen free radicals (EMODs). Implicating oxygen free radicals in disease causation has proven to be inaccurate, misleading and unfounded.**

### My rebuttal

If one is allowed to be prejudicially selective from the world's scientific literature, one can offer biased support that electronically modified oxygen derivatives (EMODs) cause disease, that EMODs are not directly related to disease or that EMODs make no difference at all in disease occurrence or in the aging phenomenon.

I have tried to follow the precarious pathways leading to **scientific truth** and to avoid corridors of confusion.

**"Poor selection of terminology" could be the mantra of redox biochemistry**.

Frequently repeated and false impressions and embellished inaccuracies have led to the acceptance of flawed theories and disproved hypotheses. Yet, the inaccuracies and the unsupported theories, relative to EMODs, are now, more than ever, erroneously referred to as being firmly established facts.

Followers of the free radical theory and the mitochondrial theory of aging say that aging is a stochastic (random) disease of accumulation of damaged products of oxidation and I say that aging and disease are the result of deficiency states, especially of EMODs.

Others have said that disease is a problem of oxygenation but I say that it is, specifically and in particular, a problem of oxidation.

The magic of oxygen's unique reactivity lies in the individual reactivities of the various EMOD derivatives. **Aging and EMOD formation are occurring simultaneously but they do not causally relate. Aging is a universal phenomenon occurring in all known entities, not just living beings on planet Earth. To stop aging in man would represent a unique and singular cosmological exception.**

**As I have said, "If you think oxygen is the cause of aging, just try aging without it. Oxygen allows us to age."**

**First**, and contrary to the teachings of the free radical theory, one must realize that oxidants or EMODs are essential for good health.

**Second**, one must appreciate the fact that antioxidants can be harmful and **third**, that EMODs serve to aid redox cycling.

**Fourth**, the constant presence of high concentrations of steady state levels of EMODs is a strong argument for their obvious low toxicity.

**Fifth**, huge clinical studies have shown that dietary supplements of vitamins and antioxidants produced increases in heart disease, stroke and cancer and an early demise.

I believe that this is a strong argument for the importance of a sufficiency state of EMODs, i.e., conditions which substantially decrease EMOD levels "allow" for the manifestation of a wide array of diseases.

With aging, after the 2nd and 3rd decades of life, we gradually and progressively have decreases in oxygen consumption, decreased ability to transport oxygen to our cells and decreased abilities for our cells to generate EMODs and adenosine triphosphate (ATP). EMOD production is believed to be stoichiometrically related to $O_2$ consumption.

Thus, with increasing age, while there is progressive decreasing $O_2$ consumption, we see increasing incidences of cancer, cardiovascular disease, atherosclerosis, diabetes, arthritis, cataracts, tissue hypoxia, pain and susceptibility to all diseases.

In fact, **those who seem to have the best health are the individuals who exercise and who metabolize the highest levels of oxygen and generate the highest levels of EMODs.**

**This is exemplified in my book entitled, *Cancer and Longevity: Naked Mole Rats, Exercise, and EMODs (ROS)*, 2015.** (Howes RM, 2015, Naked mole rats)

**A lack of oxygenation leads to a lack of oxidation, which leads to or "allows" for disease manifestation. Ground state oxygen lacks the reactivity necessary to participate in the complex biochemical reactions required to maintain**

**homeostasis, to protect us against pathogens and to sustain our health.**

**EMODs are sufficiently reactive to protect and to heal us.**

Our bodies instinctively know of their dire need for adequate oxygen levels. Oxygen consumption per kilogram in a normal fetus is almost double the consumption of the adult.

I believe that this high fetal $O_2$ consumption rate argues against the alleged toxicity of $O_2$ and its derivatives. **The evolutionary process has chosen to double the $O_2$ consumption during this most crucial fetal growth period and sensitive time of human development.**

I say that these oxygen radicals are responsible for health and life of the living/breathing cell. **The primary process which stands between us and constant or perpetual infections or manifestations of neoplasia, is our ability to generate oxidative events in the form of EMODs, which forms a major part of our "intrinsic defense system."**

Cyclic neutropenia, chronic granulomatous disease and spontaneous regression of cancer illustrate my point.

Neutrophils produce pathogen protective EMODs. It appears that the key players, among others, in the immune system, in preventing infections and cancer, are antibodies, macrophages, lymphocytes, neutrophils, T-cells and Interleukin-2. **All of these** can and do generate or stimulate **EMOD** production.

Antibodies can generate hydrogen peroxide ($H_2O_2$) from singlet molecular oxygen ($^1O_2^*$). Antibodies produce up to 500 mole equivalents of $H_2O_2$ from $^1O_2^*$, without a reduction in rate. There is an enormous potential for $H_2O_2$ production by antibodies.

**I believe that this inter-relationship between $^1O_2^*$, $H_2O_2$ and $O_3$ will prove to have great significance in the generation of a DOA (deadly oxidative assault) and prooxidant protection towards cancer and disease.**

The Cercospora nicotianae SOR1 (singlet oxygen resistance) gene has been identified as a gene involved in the resistance of this fungus to singlet-oxygen-generating phototoxins. **I believe it indicates that mammals have a basic need for $^1O_2$, otherwise, we would have evolved a similar gene to block it....but, we have not!**

I believe that these EMODs are the fundamental basic elements for prooxidant protection from pathogens and neoplasia and that they are responsible for oxidative self-healing and for staving off death. They keep countless pathogens and neoplastic cells continually in check and they await bodily injury, such that they can assist in collagen synthesis and wound healing.

**Just as the body has the fibrinolytic system which continually keeps blood from clotting intravascularly, the body has oxidative systems which keep cancer from growing, plaques from forming, herpetic lesions from developing and cataracts from coalescing.**

My review of the literature revealed that spontaneous regression is also seen in arteriosclerosis, cataract formation, a wide range of cancers, HIV/AIDS, arthritis, etc. This gives strong support to the position that we must have in place an intrinsic system to hold in abeyance or reverse these conditions or they would remain or progressively get worse.

**Estimates are that human cells produce up to 10 million EMODs/mitochondria/day.**

Mitochondria are present in all eukaryotic cells in varying numbers, from hundreds to thousands and the body contains between 75-100 billion cells.

EMODs, especially superoxide anion, $H_2O_2$ and nitric oxide, serve as messengers to the cytosol, the nucleus and all areas within the cell and in its immediate environs.

Consider the issue of the alleged toxicity of EMODs. It is estimated that the mitochondria produce 15% of the EMOD generation by aerobic cells. The endoplasmic reticulum produces 45% and the peroxisomes produce 35%.

Further, it has been found that EMODs are produced by all nucleated cells, glial cells, and by platelets. The have been found to be produced within the cell by the lysosomes, phagolysomes, the nucleus, and the plasmolemma. Based on accepted calculations of EMOD production, **the body is literally internally bathed in steady state levels of oxygen free radicals (EMODs).**

This is particularly true for tissue or organs, which have high levels of oxygen consumption, such as the heart and the brain. Instead of being destroyed by these high levels of EMODs, these organs thrive and are dependent on the essential presence of these crucial EMODs.

Prof Randolph M. Howes MD, PhD

They say that **antioxidants** counter or block the harmful effects of EMODs, but I say that they are designed to assist EMODs in the passage of these electrons and that they actually act, at least in part, as co-oxidants or co-prooxidant protective agents. All antioxidants can become prooxidants.

**Antioxidants are major assistants and participants in redox cycling (e.g.,** vitamin C, $\alpha$-tocopherol, glutathione, sulfhydryl groups, etc.). I believe that this allows for the continual electron flow and provides for the presence of adequate levels of EMODs, for uninterrupted pathogen and neoplasia protection, and decreases the possibility of excesses of EMODs.

In a sense, **EMODs and antioxidants work together**; otherwise, one can not explain the prooxidant activity of antioxidants. Thus, I have referred to antioxidants as co-oxidants or pre-oxidants.

Further, I believe that EMODs participate in self-regulation and feedback control mechanisms. We must keep in mind that superoxide and hydrogen peroxide are the two main products of mitochondrial and microsomal metabolism and the other EMOD derivatives are primarily derived from them. I believe that EMODs and antioxidants work in a coordinated modulating system to establish homeostatic redox levels.

Experiments to test the effectiveness of antioxidants in the prevention of disease and for curtailing aging have largely failed to do so, when tested in double blind, randomized cohort studies.

Stated simply and logically, antioxidants do not prevent the alleged "EMOD-caused diseases or aging" because these conditions are not caused by oxidation. Thus, **the free radical theory of oxidative stress and aging has been invalidated.**

A new paradigm of predictability must be theorized, which will more correctly explain current scientific and clinical observations. In my many tomes on this subject, I have done just that.

Additionally, EMODs surround us externally in the atmosphere and on the skin, secondary to reactions of $O_2$ with UV light.

We inhale and exhale EMODs, we drink them, we eat them in raw and cooked foods, we generate them in the digestion of foods and we find them present in the excretory organs of the gastrointestinal tract and the urinary system.

96

Once $O_2$ enters the vascular system, 3% of hemoglobin produces superoxide and all layers of the vascular wall are constantly generating EMODs.

Further, within the vascular system, the red blood cells, the platelets and the white blood cells are all producing EMODs at varying levels throughout the diurnal cycle or in response to injury or disease. **Hyperoxic or hypoxic inhalation respectively regresses or aggravates the development of atherosclerotic lesions, not by an indirect action on blood lipid concentrations but by a direct action on the vascular wall.**

I believe that this indicates that EMODs, derived from hyperoxia, are present in and on the arterial wall and are responsible for the maintenance of a plaque-free intima and media. An EMOD insufficiency state allows for plaque formation and augmentation of the lesion.

As a result of our healing process, type VI plaque lesions can return to type V morphology. I believe that this indicates that plaques are frequently "repaired" by our self-cure system, which is responsible for normally keeping plaque formation under control.

The mere fact that lesions can spontaneously regress, or be healed, is classic evidence that we normally possess the ability to keep plaques in abeyance and/or to decrease or heal plaques already formed.

**Our body protects us with the primary way that it has available to it, which is through oxidation.**

Contrary to expectation, **all major antioxidant enzymes showed a significant upregulation before plaque formation**, reaching a peak roughly coinciding with the onset of intimal thickening. Increased antioxidant enzymes reduced EMOD levels such that atherosclerotic lesions were "allowed" to develop.

Thus, **the cause of the lesion formation was due to an EMOD insufficiency state in the vascular wall**. Further, it has been shown that there is a "surprising high content of low-molecular weight antioxidants, such as vitamin E, ascorbate, and urate" **in human atherosclerotic plaques**. Also, there is a weak glutathione-related enzymatic antioxidant shield in human atherosclerotic plaques.

In studying the problem of human bacterial infections following cardiac valve replacement, with prosthetic valves or xenografts, these sites have a peculiarity which makes them vulnerable to pathogenic bacterial growth. I believe that the lack of endothelial cells and their production of EMODs "allows" for this pathogenic growth.

This is expressed as **bacterial endocarditis and vegetations**.

I came to realize that all layers of the vascular wall continuously generate EMODs and I feel that this is the primary protective modality which normally prevents endocarditis and vegetations. In other words, the vascular system is frequently seeded with pathogenic organisms but EMOD production by the vascular endothelial cells and the vascular smooth muscle cells prevents them from being a suitable site for pathogen growth.

It is stated that bacteria are allowed into the vascular system from faulty dentition, cuts or abrasion in the skin or following bowel movements.

The presence of bacteria has proven to be very high in arteriosclerotic and atherosclerotic lesions. This is especially true for Chlamydia. I feel that this is because the presence of a plaque or calcification is a site which has diminished abilities to produce EMODs and thus, it is a logical fertile site for bacterial growth.

Additionally, I believe that deficiencies of EMODs at this site allow for increased aggregation of circulating atheromatous materials.

**The association between cigarette smoking, atherosclerosis and systemic diseases is well established.** Smoking produces EMOD deficiency levels in the arterial wall, which then "allows" for the development of atherosclerosis. A few puffs on a cigarette will reduce your oxygen absorbing capability by about 25%.

**Cigarette smoke exposure results in an acute decrease in delivery of oxygen to the artery wall during cigarette smoke exposure and a chronic, persistent decrease in delivery of oxygen to the artery wall with long - term cigarette smoke exposure.**

It seems most important that aortae from old animals still act like old vessels when transferred to young ones. **To me, this indicates that the deficiency states of EMOD production in the older animals persists even after it has been transplanted**. There has apparently been a modification of an intrinsic vascular wall defense system, i.e., EMOD production.

Human studies have shown that **cigarette smoking decreases tissue and systemic oxygen supply.** Thus, I would expect systemic problems. Cigarette smoking alters endothelial cell structure similar to that found in models of systemic hypoxia and increases endothelial cell permeability to many substances including cholesterol.

Cigarette smoking acutely decreases the delivery of oxygen to the artery wall during each exposure to cigarette smoke and this effect occurs along with a corresponding decrease in arterial blood oxygen content.

The decreased levels of ground state oxygen lead to deficiency states of EMODs, which in turn "allows" for the development of systemic diseases, neoplasia and atheromatosis.

Man does not synthesize the many antioxidants that are available to the plant world, such as the carotenoids, tocopherols, polyphenolics, vitamin C, lycopenes, and the flavonoids.

According to the free radical theory, the body should be making these antioxidants by the pound, such that we are protected from **these alleged most-damaging and critical toxins, i.e., oxygen and its derivative metabolites...but, we do not.**

Over 80-90% of $O_2$ that living organisms breathe is used in the mitochondria to generate our fuel in the form of ATP. The crucial importance of $O_2$ for human existence is readily apparent.

Oxidative and antioxidative agents (redox agents) work in amazing synchrony to perpetuate electron movement and to utilize the full complement and potential of all metabolically generated electrons. **At least 127 genes and signal transducing proteins have been reported to be sensitive to reductive and oxidative (redox) states in the cell.**

I do not believe that antioxidants are present in the cell or that they are created to prevent the formation of needed free radicals, because they are themselves turned into free radicals, after reacting with a free radical. Furthermore, nearly all antioxidants can be prooxidants. If the free radical theory is correct, then antioxidants become what they fear most, i.e., free radicals.

It has been shown that supplementation with antioxidant vitamins will not lower serum lipid and lipoproteins or blood pressure. Moreover, a recent study, conducted in more than 20,000 subjects, found that vitamin E, vitamin C, and beta-carotene supplementation resulted in small but significant increases in serum total cholesterol, low density lipoprotein-cholesterol, and triglyceride concentrations.

In another study, no significant differences were found in serum lipid, lipoprotein, and C-reactive protein concentrations, blood pressure, or intima-media thickness between vitamin supplemented and non-supplemented subjects. **Three large trials, ATBC, GISSI, and HOPE, involving thousands of subjects failed to show a reduction of cardiovascular events when vitamin E was used at doses ranging from 50 to 400 IU per day.**

Some studies show that individuals with iron overload do not suffer from premature atherosclerosis.

By taking into account the fact that many people live healthy and normal long lifespans, it is abundantly clear that so-called EMOD toxicity is extremely low or no one would be capable of attaining old age in relatively good health and with a properly functioning brain.

However, one must take into consideration "the Paracelsus principle," which states that anything in extremes can be harmful. It is also well known that **hypoxia is pathognomonic of disease, illness, inflammation or injury.**

Anaerobic metabolism is favorable to many pathogenic organisms and hypoxia is the predominant condition within cancerous cells. **Hypoxia allows cancer cells to be more aggressive, to metastasize and impairs the effect of radiation, which is based on the generation of tumoricidal EMODs.**

Conditions which substantially decrease the amount of oxygen available to the cell, at the EMOD production level in the electron transport chain and oxidative phosphorylation, will predictably cause or result in the manifestation of disease and/or cell death.

**Hyperthermia increases the effectiveness of cancer therapy dramatically.** As the body's natural response to heat, **hyperthermia increases blood flow and oxygenation and increases rates of chemical reactions**, overcoming tumor resistance to radiation and chemotherapy.

Hyperthermia also improves the performance of certain anti-cancer drugs, many of which generate EMODs.

Clinical scenarios, which have intentionally produced EMODs in tens or hundreds of thousands of patients, such as irrigation of wounds with hydrogen peroxide or phototherapy for hyperbilirubinemia, have proven that the intentional stimulated production and utilization of EMODs is safe and without long term adverse effects.

Hydrogen peroxide has been used for over a century and phototherapy has been successfully applied for over half of a century. Conversely, **conditions which have used classic antioxidants, such as $\alpha$-tocopherol or $\beta$-carotene, have been shown to cause increased rates of strokes, cardiovascular disease and overall mortality.**

Some studies have even indicated significantly increased rates of cancer with the use of $\beta$-carotene. Yet, investigators desperately try to make their data fit the invalidated and erroneous free radical theory.

I believe that it is possible that the current US epidemics of cancer, diabetes, obesity and fatigue are worsened by increased ingestion of vitamins and dietary supplements, which are routinely found as additives or fortifiers of many foods.

These agents likely interfere with our prooxidant protective system and with energy production. The negative effects of antioxidant vitamins and dietary supplements will likely be magnified in immunocompromised patients.

Therapeutic remission of rheumatoid arthritis (RA) has been obtained following intra-articular administration of superoxide dismutase (SOD). Please remember that SOD generates $H_2O_2$ with great efficiency. Also, rheumatoid joints have been successfully treated by direct injection of $H_2O_2$.

Ironically, **gouty joints** have all of the signs of "inflammation," all of which are caused by the so-called super antioxidant, **uric acid**. Another natural antioxidant, **bilirubin**, is responsible for kernicterus and permanent brain damage.

Considerable bodily harm can be caused by natural and synthetic antioxidants.

I was first struck by the importance of EMODs when my studies, with Dr. Richard Steele, in the early 1970's revealed that mammalians are capable of generating electronic excitation states with the microsomal mixed function oxidases and cytochrome P450.

Later, I became aware that singlet oxygen could selectively kill cancer cells via photodynamic therapy (PDT). PDT is used to treat diseases ranging from cancer to psoriasis and utilizes injectables or ointments, which are light-activated to produce singlet oxygen. Long-persisting photoproducts continue the initiation of apoptosis for about 100 minutes following irradiation.

**The resulting singlet oxygen causes little damage to a mammalian cell, because it is well prepared for oxidizing reactions.** It has been shown that phagocytic cells can kill cancer cells with the respiratory burst, when there is a sufficiency of EMODs.

**Ultimately, this led me to develop an orthomolecular singlet oxygen cancer therapy generating system**, which I have used to selectively kill human squamous cell carcinoma in athymic mice and human basal cell skin cancer.

Further, in the literature, I was struck by Dr. William Coley's work, at the beginning of the 20$^{th}$ century, with **spontaneous regression of cancer**.

He demonstrated that when the body developed an infection and followed it with a massive reaction to the pathogen, apparently, the markedly increased levels of EMODs produced by drastically stimulating the respiratory burst, resulted in tumoricidal activity at both the cancer's primary and its metastatic locations.

In the 1960's and the 1970's, a group at Baylor University Medical Center found that intra-arterial and intravenous administration of **hydrogen peroxide** would aid in killing cancer, pathogens and in the regression of arteriosclerotic plaque.

**I believe that hydrogen peroxide is the most prevalent, and perhaps the most significant EMOD in the body**, even exceeding the well recognized importance of nitric oxide.

Subsequent work done with PDT has revealed that the use of fiber optics and photosensitizers, which generate EMODs, will also dissolve arteriosclerotic plaque and kill cancer cells.

**Now, it is realized that EMODs represent our most important means of defense against bacteria, viruses, fungi, protozoans and neoplasia**. True, there is considerable debate as to the identity of the most potent bactericidal EMOD but clearly EMODs are of primary protective importance.

The currently accepted tortured logic of the free radical theory teaches that oxygen and its radicals are highly toxic, even lethal. I believe that the overall data shows that they are wrong. I believe that these EMODs are primarily "protective prooxidants."

Further, I believe that they are of low toxicity, considering the fact that all of our aerobic cells are continually bathed in steady state levels of EMODs, throughout our entire lifetimes.

The **chemotherapeutic drugs** doxorubicin, mitomycin C, etoposide and cisplatin are superoxide generating agents. The anti-estrogen tamoxifen, used in breast cancer therapy, induces oxidative stress within carcinoma cells. This adds support to the results seen with PDT and with the Howes Singlet Oxygen Cancer Therapy System.

Radiotherapy and photodynamic therapy generate oxygen radicals within the carcinoma cell. In my opinion, **this is adequate to show that EMODs are, indeed, tumoricidal.**

**Photosensitization reaction of drugs**, including many antibiotics, leads to the formation of reactive oxygen species ($^1O_2^*$) under ultraviolet radiation and oxidation plays a major rule in the actions of some antibiotics.

Many of the diseases treated with **interferon** have been postulated to have been caused by excessive levels of EMODs and yet, they have been treated, with varying degrees of success, with interferon, an immune cytokine known to increase EMOD levels.

**Skin cancer** is the most common type of cancer in the United States. **I believe that hydrogen peroxide is the most prevalent, and perhaps the most significant EMOD in the body,** even exceeding the well recognized importance of nitric oxide. I believe that it this is related to relative hypoxia and subsequent deficiency of EMODs, thus, "allowing" the manifestation of neoplasia.

Aging skin receives less oxygen than young skin. I believe that this argues that the skin in aged patients has decreased abilities to produce EMODs and is more susceptible to infection, injury, necrosis and cancer.

Skin tumors called keloids have decreased and narrowed vessels, which likely reduces oxygen perfusion and which allows the keloids to develop due to a deficiency of EMODs.

By definition, **granulomas are tumors.** Chronic granulomatous disease patients can not generate an oxidative EMOD respiratory burst. According to the Free Radi-Crap theory of aging, they should live longer....but, they die at younger ages from infections. They have EMOD deficiency levels, which I believe serve to "allow" for the manifestation of tumors and frequent infections.

If **chronic inflammation** is causative of cancer, as is argued by the followers of the Free Radi-Crap theory of oxidative stress and aging, then steroids, which inhibit inflammation, should reduce cancer rates or prevent cancer formation.

In actuality, just the opposite happens, in that **steroids cause patients to develop infections, cataracts and tumors** more frequently than normal and cessation of the steroid intake, can stop the infections and result in spontaneous remission of cancer.

Type 2 diabetes is increasing at epidemic rates and is beginning to appear in children and adolescents, just as is arteriosclerosis. I believe that the fats accumulated in young obese patients serve as a trap for EMODs and this "allows" for the development of diabetes and atherosclerosis.

There is a decrease in the immune system which is seen in obesity and may be related to the presence of double bonded fats, which act as a sink (trap) for EMODs. **It seems obvious that all of these factors are interrelated.** Obesity is like a chronic inflammation of the adipocytes and these areas have lower levels of oxygen and consequently, lower levels of EMODs.

Thus, low EMOD levels "allow" for the manifestation of many diseases. It is rare for any of this cluster of diseases to occur in a patient as a single disease entity and not be associated with other diseases of this EMOD deficiency group.

Routine **exercise** is widely recognized as one of the most important adjuncts for disease prevention and maintaining overall good health, **even though it generates extreme quantities of EMODs in humans. Risk reduction for chronic degenerative diseases** can even occur with low levels of **exercise** as was made clear in consensus statements published by the Centers for Disease Control and Prevention and the ACSM.

I believe that the most common denominator for the body's responses to exercise, are an increase in oxygen consumption and oxygen utilization, both of which result in increased levels of EMODs.

**Oxygen consumption increases up to 20 times greater with exercise** than the resting level, resulting in an elevated flow of oxygen through the mitochondrial electron-transport chain and a stoichiometric increase in EMOD production. According to the free radical theory, **the presence of the alleged damaging EMODs** would promote increases in diseases and aging....but, that does not happen!

Regular physical activity helps reduce the incidence of the "EMOD deficiency cluster of diseases" and the severity of related co-morbidities such as cancer, diabetes, hypertension, dyslipidemia and obesity.

Exercise promotes the release of neutrophils into the circulation and studies suggest that neutrophils mobilized after exercises have an enhanced capacity to generate some forms of **EMODs**.

Exercise is a physiologically relevant source of so-called oxidative stress. I believe that we should consider exercise to be a medicine and that each episode of exercise is equivalent to a substantial dose of EMODs.

Presently, **no consensus exists as to the cause of aging.**

Available **data about age-associated changes in free-radical processes are discrepant, conflicting and inconsistent. It has been assumed by the sycophants of the free radical theory that the production of oxygen free radicals increases with age but that is not necessarily the case.**

Data on age-associated changes in the activities of CuZn-superoxide dismutase (SOD) and peroxidation of lipids and proteins in different tissues are contradictory. SOD activity was significantly lower (by 46.8%, $p<0.001$) in the brain of aged rats compared with young rats. This follows my belief that SOD is a primary generator of EMODs, e.g., $H_2O_2$, and I would expect aging to result in a relative deficiency state of EMODs, which is reflected by decreased SOD in the brain. The total antioxidant activity of brain did not decrease with increased age in these studies.

**Noteworthy is the fact that in either the liver or blood serum, generation of EMODs significantly decreases with increasing age in humans.**

**Aging** is associated with a reduction of physical activity and fitness and cognitive decline goes hand in hand with advancing age. The brain, which is composed of post-mitotic cells, has high lipid content, low levels of antioxidants, high iron content and very high levels of EMOD production.

Yet, it can function normally for a lifetime. Human aging is also associated with decreased glucose metabolism, and glucose metabolism is reliant on a sufficient and continuous supply of oxygen.

Maximum breathing capacity decreases approximately 40% during this period and individuals with chronic lung diseases, such as emphysema, suffer a more significant decline. Lung capacity decreases 5% with every decade of life. Cardiovascular function declines approximately one half of one percent each year, starting around age 30.

There is a 40-50% decline in muscle mass and a similar decline in bone mass, along with a simultaneous increase in body fat in both men and women. The metabolic rate also declines with age and is primarily affected by muscle mass. After 25 years of age, we tend to gain one pound per year as we age. Hormone production declines with age.

Involution of the thymus begins early in life and by mid-life it is about 15% of its maximum size, with the cellular mass of the thymic cortex having fallen by 75 to 80 percent. As the body ages, the immune system decreases.

I believe that the body has to respond with or by attempting to increase EMOD levels, including $^1O_2$, $H_2O_2$ and $O_2^-$ in order to provide adequate prooxidant protection. Yet, with aging, there is a relative EMOD deficiency state. The prevalence of both cancer and anemia increases with age.

**The amount of oxygen moving in and out of the lungs and to the muscles may decrease 40% between 30 and 65 years of age.** The cardiac muscle progressively decreases in size and strength and it pumps less, and the amount of blood flow throughout the body is slowed to about 70% that of a 30 year-old.

The whole alveolar tree becomes less elastic as we age and there is a decrease in the alveoli surfaces after age 20 of 3 square feet/year. There is less lung blood flow, less elasticity and 40% less air moving in and out of the lungs. The **cell oxygen consumption decreases progressively with age.** However, this **diminution of the cellular oxygen consumption is neither regular nor uniform.**

Alveolar macrophages freshly harvested from non-sensitized aged rats produce less $O_2^-$ than those from young animals. The activity of CuZn-superoxide dismutase (SOD) was found decreased in the brain of aged rats (30 months old) by 46.8% as compared to young animals.

**Collectively, I believe that these are the reasons for the changes seen with aging and with the appearance of EMOD deficiency diseases, such as cancer, arteriosclerosis, diabetes, arthritis, susceptibility to infections and cataracts.**

**Caloric restriction** (CR) apparently not only increases longevity and life span but it also postpones age-related diseases, decreases the rate of aging, and delays development. Shifting a diet's relative amounts of nutrients, such as carbohydrates, protein, and fat, while only modestly cutting calories, extends the lifespan just as much as a drastic calorie cut does.

Peroxisomal oxidation of fatty acids has been recognized as an important source of $H_2O_2$ with prolonged starvation. This may be involved in increased longevity with caloric restriction. One common feature of animals, such as mice, rats, and monkeys, under CR is a lower body temperature.

The energy consumption theory is contradicted by studies which showed that mice kept at lower temperatures, eat 44% more than control mice and yet do not age faster. CR results in profound and sustained beneficial effects on the major atherosclerosis risk factors, serum total cholesterol, LDL-C, HDL-C, triglycerides and blood pressure. Reportedly, CR provides a powerful protective effect against obesity and insulin resistance, provides evidence for a decrease in inflammation and lowers the risk of developing atherosclerosis.

Extensive volunteer studies in humans are warranted for CR, due to the possibility of its being the first method to actually increase the lifespan and slow aging in man.

One recent study, in *Drosophila,* found that lowering EMOD leakage from the mitochondria did not result in extended longevity and it failed to find differences in EMOD production in CR flies despite their living longer.

Both *Drosophila* and *C. elegans* are mostly composed of post-mitotic cells, which may explain why results from these invertebrates are much more supportive of the free radical theory of aging than results from mice.

Oxidation is implicated in cataractogenesis. However, the protein-bound chromophores, which increase with aging in the human avascular lens, act as UVA sensitizers, producing almost exclusively singlet oxygen in vitro. Direct irradiation of whole, aged human lenses with high intensity UVA light, **failed to produce singlet oxygen damage**. Thus, low oxygen levels in the lens prevent singlet oxygen damage in vivo.

In conclusion, the predominance of the scientific evidence, which I have presented, does not lend support to the free radical theory of oxidative stress and aging. I have proposed a new paradigm to explain the metabolism of oxygen and its electronically modified derivatives.

Basically, my Unified theory emphasizes the fundamental role of EMODs in prooxidant protection from pathogens and neoplasia, the maintenance of homeostasis and in providing the key elements for a lifetime of normal self-healing.

## Cumulative Oxidative Therapy (COT)

I am developing an emerging concept which suggest that it will require **"cumulative oxidative therapy" (C.O.T. or COT)** to effectively treat conditions of far advanced diseases such as terminal or disseminated cancer, severe diabetes, advanced rheumatoid arthritis, Alzheimer's disease or atherosclerosis. Each oxidative modality will have to be instituted to adequately muster a successful oxidative assault upon these advanced diseases. Modalities consist of exercise, peroxide orally or by infusion, sodium hypochlorite orally or by infusion, PDT, artemisinin, hypericin, iron along with vitamin C, 100% oxygen inhalation, hyperbaric oxygen, ozone therapy, UV light blood treatment, possibly altered glucose to facilitate EMODs production, etc.

## Possible Ways to Increase Oxidative-Cure:

-take $H_2O_2$ orally
-$H_2O_2$ soak/baths
-take $H_2O_2$ IV
-take $O_3$ IV
-take Fe++ and Vit. C orally
-take Ca++ orally
-avoid diets high in antioxidants
-avoid antioxidant supplements
-take NaOCl orally
-take NaOCl IV

-take Vancomycin (a chloramine) and $H_2O_2$ to produce $^1O_2$
-take vit. K (a quinone) redox cycler to produce $^1O_2$
-take chloramine T (N-chloro-p-toluene-sulfonamide)
-take redox cycler – quinones – such as ubiquinone
-take redox cycler – quinones – such as tetracycline
-ingest ethanol daily in moderation
-consumption of caffeine

Theophylline and caffeine (methylxanthines) are now among the most commonly prescribed drugs in neonatal intensive care. (Lesko, Epstein, Mitchell. 1990)

Long-term **administration of caffeine in preterm infants is associated with an increase in oxygen consumption and with a reduction of weight gain.** This may have implications for clinical practice as nutritional regimens need to be adjusted during this therapy. (Bauer et al, 2001)

> "It, and its kindred, stands as the singular barrier
> between health and sepsis,
> between normal and cancerous,
> between living and dead.
> This astonishing anomaly, of the periodic table,
> offers unsolicited chemical solace
> to the vulnerable collective of living creatures.
> Thank you, most beloved
> oxygen."
> R. M. Howes, M.D., Ph.D.
> 11/25/04

## Misnomers Which Convey Mis-Information

The **literature on antioxidants is filled with inaccuracies, which become perpetuated as facts.** It is well known that **inaccuracies which are frequently repeated seem to be ultimately accepted as facts, if they are repeated enough.** If we are ever to reach a real point of enlightenment, concerning health and disease, this nonsense must stop.

**Just as with reactive oxygen species, antioxidants must be considered on a one to one identity basis.** The biochemical reactivities and chemical redox characteristics of antioxidants are as diversified as those of reactive oxygen species and should not be "lumped" under vast all-encompassing categories.

It is difficult to develop a term to encompass the proper meaning for such varied such varied chemical species, which have erroneously been referred to as reactive oxygen species, reactive oxygen metabolites or reactive oxygen intermediates.

Perhaps, they could more accurately be **called "electronically-modified ground state oxygen derivatives" (EMGSOD)** or, if it is assumed that it is referring to ground state oxygen, **"electronically-modified oxygen derivatives" (EMOD).**

**Thus,** EMOD is not disclosing reactivity, number of electrons altered, excited states vs. electron additions or removals, etc. It only tells you that oxygen's electrons have been modified. Then, each EMOD could be considered for its own specific chemical and biochemical properties and reactivities.

Similarly, **antioxidants need to be considered on an individual chemical basis because the term "antioxidant" is misleading and frequently chemically incorrect, especially when the same substance can act as a prooxidant.**

Furthermore, **the time to abandon the overly simplistic and confusing term of "oxidative stress" is long overdue.** I submit that there is no more a reality of cellular oxidative stress than there is for potassium stress, chloride stress, cyclic AMP stress, thyroxine stress, insulin stress, sterol stress, sulfide stress, glutathione stress, or any other so-called stress, which someone can dream up or draw into a cute little pathway or diagram.

Logically, it follows that, if we can not determine which cellular oxidizing or reducing molecules are the so-called reactive oxygen species, or if we can not determine which antioxidants are anti- or pro-oxidants, then **I do not believe that we can place any degree of reliability on so-called measures of total antioxidant capacity or of "oxidative stress."** However, I can say that oxidative systems tend to be for protection, healing and the perpetuation of a state of homeostasis.

Ergo, **I feel that oxidative processes are a good thing and not the settings for cellular disasters that have so frequently and erroneously been attributed to them.**

I believe that we must be constantly aware that **we are electromagnetic beings and that the passage and flow of electrons is essential for our very existence.** Without the flow of electrons, our system of energy production (ATP) would cease and we would die.

Most movement of electrons involves the participation of "free radicals" which possess the electromotive forces necessary to drive a system of energy production and to initiate proton (motive) gradient forces. Thus, many free radicals are not our mortal enemies but are, to the contrary, our greatest allies.

**A system "free of free radicals," which does not promote electron movement and/or chemical reactions, is basically a dead biological system.**

Fortunately, **electron potential differences exist between molecules, between intracellular organelles, between the inside and the outside of the cell, between individual cells, between tissues, between organs, between me and you and between you and me and our environment.** It is a system of flux, a system of movement, a system of change and a system of life. **A system without electron movement, is a dead system.**

**Keep in mind that toxicologists use the following definitions relative to oxygen:**

**Oxidizer.** A substance that gives up oxygen readily. Presence of an oxidizer increases the fire hazard.

**Oxygen deficiency.** That concentration of oxygen by volume below which atmosphere supplying respiratory protection must be provided. It exists in atmospheres where the percentage of oxygen by volume is less than 19.5 percent oxygen.

**Oxygen-enriched atmosphere.** An atmosphere containing more than 23.5 percent oxygen by volume.

### Biochemical Busy Bodies

Gravid (pregnant) females frequently refer to the beautiful feeling of "life within them" but **we all have life within us.** Most all of the trillions of cells, that make each and everyone of us, are alive and constantly carrying on cross-talk and they are in a constant state of electron flux and change.

**Each and every cell is a "buzzing biochemical beehive" of chemical activity, with bees that can carry out millions of homeostatic molecular functions per second.**

We are all **truly "busy bodies"** in a biochemical sense. It is a beautiful process and not something to be feared, trivialized or extinguished. Furthermore, many of the very molecules within our cells are "alive" in a real sense of the word. The Merriam-Webster dictionary **defines "alive" as being in force or operation, sensitive or animated.**

Thus, many of our biochemically complex molecules are, indeed, alive and I believe that this quality extends down to considerably simpler molecules, atoms and subatomic particles, such as our electrons and our protons.

**These biochemical molecules are the very ones, which collectively act to make our decisions, arrive at conclusions or chose which path to take.** They determine our moods, our attitudes and create our drives.

In fact, they determine just about everything about us because, **"They are "us."**

**You or I, as a distinct organism,
may represent a cumulative puppet,
displaying the antics, desires and drives of our
lesser molecular and atomic constituents;
for better or worse, for richer or poorer and
in sickness or in biochemical homeostasis.
Yes, it's a heavenly molecular marriage.**
R. M. Howes, M.D., Ph.D.
5/12/05

**Paracelsus**

**Paracelsus postulated in the 16th century the following:**

- Experimentation is essential in examination of responses to chemicals

- One should make a distinction between therapeutic and toxic properties of chemicals
- These properties are sometimes, but not always, indistinguishable by dose (Casarett, Bruce, 1980). We should heed his words today.

In a time, during which we are nearly plowed under by a scientific informational tsunami, we must strive to stay afloat during this data deluge and use thoughtful insight to try to get our minds around the entirety of the problems we are studying.

We must gladly approach fearless discussions of our beliefs and theories with excitement.

We must be willing to expend studious time in self-imposed exile, for the sake of discovery and the betterment of mankind.

## Paradox of Ventilatory Control

This **paradox of ventilatory control** is significant in that it provides clues into the fundamentally important role of reduction-oxidation (redox) reactions, oxidative enzymes, and highly reactive end products, which include EMODs, in central control of breathing. (Droge, 2001)

**A similar role for redox signaling and EMODs has been identified in $O_2$ sensing by peripheral chemoreceptors.** (Parbhakar, 2000)

**Redox signaling and EMODs are a general mechanism employed by many cell types to optimize matching between $O_2$ demand and $O_2$ supply in various organs.** (Acker, 1994)

The fact that hyperoxic hyperventilation occurs at all suggests that **brain stem neurons regulating breathing are sensitive to oxidative environments.** (Mulkey et al, 2003)

Many neurons in respiratory control nuclei of the brain stem contain oxidative enzymes and $O_2$-derived second messengers that are thought to participate in normal cell-signaling pathways. Mulkey reported that **hyperoxia, EMODs, and cellular oxidation directly stimulated firing rate of putative central $CO_2$**

**chemoreceptors in the solitary complex (SC) in rat brain stem slices**. In this context, recall that hyperoxia is a commonly used experimental protocol in studies of oxidative stress at normobaric pressure and hyperbaric pressure.

When subjects are **breathing HBO$_2$, the cumulative effects of EMODs are well recognized because of their role in CNS O$_2$ toxicity; yet, adverse reactions to HBO$_2$ are rare.** (Demchenko et al, 2003) (Demchenko et al, 2001) (Tibbles, Edelsberg, 1996) (Torbati et al, 1992) (Torbati et al, 1989)

Accumulating evidence supports the notion that **the CNS responds to a continuum of O$_2$ tension at both normobaric and hyperbaric pressures.** The direct effects of O$_2$ on the brain stem need to be considered when hyperoxia is used.

Dripps and Comroe first introduced the use of normobaric hyperoxia (100% O$_2$, 8-min exposure) as a tool for physiological denervation of the carotid body chemoreceptors. They emphasized, however, the following caveat:"It must be remembered that a stimulant effect of oxygen which tends to increase respiration may be acting simultaneously to limit the extent of this immediate depression of minute ventilation." (Dripps, Comroe, 1947)

**"The verity of the nature of oxygen radicals can only be realized by acknowledgement of the condition resultant to their absence: death and rigor mortis. The way of the radical is the way of life."**
R. M. Howes, M.D., Ph.D.
6/11/04

### Hyperoxia Increases EMODs

The present working model is that **hyperoxia increases EMODs,** which inhibit a potassium channel(s), although the specific ionic targets have not been identified.

**Levels of O$_2$ in *in vitro* preparations of the CNS that are often referred to as hypoxia are in fact physiological (PtiO$_2$ <35 Torr), and accounting for this fact may alter our interpretation of the responses of the brain to true hypoxia.**

Classical oxygen and its free radical offspring
are the cross-pollinating butterflies of biological molecules,
which transfer exponential numbers of sweet electrons.
They are the skillful molecular humming birds,
acrobatically darting to-and-fro to obtain their fill of
electron-nectar.
They are the colorful, cross-pollinating honey bees of aerobic
life,
busily buzzing to overcome adversity and to endure.
They are the hurried cellular pony-express,
lathered and riding hard
to furnish intricate lines of intra-organismal communication
necessary to sustain living animation.
R. M. Howes, M.D., Ph.D.
5/26/05

## Oxygen Toxicity and Antioxidants

Out of necessity, **the body creates free radicals and oxygen re-active species relentlessly and continuously.** Antioxidants are compounds which provide our body with a means of reacting with molecules to continue the passage of electrons throughout the cell. By definition an antioxidant is a compound that is able to react with free radicals, forming harmless unreactive molecules and protecting other biological molecules from damage.

**However, I believe that these compounds, which are referred to as antioxidants, may be better describe as compounds which assist EMODs and should be called "co-oxidants."**

Antioxidants are either reactive chemicals such as vitamin E or special-ized enzymes such as catalase. The body produces enzymatic antioxi-dants but it cannot make antioxidant chemicals such as vitamin E, C and flavonoids. These antioxidant chemicals protect the sites in the body which the enzymatic systems cannot reach.

**We obtain these antioxidant chemicals from our diet but they are rapidly turned over in the body and need to be constantly replenished.**

Vitamin E is an antioxidant which dissolves in our body's fats and oils. **Any radicals formed in the fats will react with vitamin E to form a vitamin E radical. This vitamin E radical lacks the energy to** cause any further damage but will react with vitamin C in the blood to regenerate the vitamin E. The breakdown product of vitamin C is then removed by the kidneys. In this way radicals formed in fats are removed from the body by transfer to vitamin E then to vitamin C and out through the kidneys as urine. Vitamin C also reacts with a number of water soluble radicals formed in the blood.

Thus far, results with antioxidants have been very disappointing and have failed in the major studies to prevent or curtail cancer and heart disease.

Scientists cannot measure these radicals directly but must look for the damage they cause as an indication they are present. Unfortunately, free radical reactions are at best described as being messy.

The hydroxyl radical can form over a hundred different products when it reacts with a protein. The situation is even more complex with fats. Many of the products of free radical damage to fats are unstable and break down into even more complex compounds.

The measurement of one of these compounds in the blood does not always mean that body is being damaged permanently as the body may be dealing with the damage successfully by removing it. To make the task more complex, diseases such as heart disease develop very slowly, over many years, at rates impractical to model in the test tube.

"You are being radically misled
by antioxidant vitamin fraudsters.
Someone is trying to radically mislead you
concerning antioxidant vitamins and
antioxidant supplements,
such that you will make
a radical mistake."
R.M. Howes M.D., Ph.D.
3/22/06

Disease and Decreased Oxygen Availability

Curiously, the major diseases occur at a time during aging when $O_2$ levels have dropped. I believe that this is much more than coincidence and that it is a causal relationship.

**Cancer, atherosclerosis, arthritis, stroke, Alzheimer's, cataracts and diabetes all occur with increasing frequency as $O_2$ availability becomes deficient.** I believe that this $O_2$ deficiency leads to an **EMOD** deficiency state, which "allows" for the manifestation of these diseases.

**Thus, a lack of oxygenation leads to a lack of oxidation, which leads to disease manifestation.**

Further, it is believed that SOD decreases in the 3rd and 4th decades of life and this decrease is associated with the major diseases. However, I **believe that it is the lack of $H_2O_2$ generated by the SOD, which is responsible for the "allowance" of these major diseases.**

Dr. Charles Farr, a pioneer in peroxide therapy, used to say that, "hydrogen peroxide therapy is an effort to deliver oxygen for the purpose of oxygenation, not oxidation." **I believe that the whole purpose of oxidative therapy should be for the delivery of EMODs and for increasing the prooxidant status of the body.**

Cells are equipped to varying degrees with internal mechanisms to deal with the oxidative effects produced by internal "leaks" of oxygen and it radicals. Remember, that **I do not consider the generation of EMODs as a mistaken leak or accidental spillage but as a "purposeful productive pathway" for the production of EMODs.**

The antioxidant enzymes, such as catalase, superoxide dismutase and glutathione peroxidase represent means to neutralize excess amounts of **EMODs** and there are other reparative enzyme systems to correct the oxidative effects of **EMODs.**

Curiously and ironically, **man does not synthesize the many antioxidants that are available to the plant world, such as the carotenoids, tocopherols, polyphenolics, vitamin C, lycopenes, and the flavonoids.**

If they are so important, I ask, "Why not?" Is this another super screwup of mother-nature? If you are an oxy-moron, you must surely think that it is.

Some 2.5 billion years following the introduction of oxygen into the environment by the utilization of sunlight by blue-green algae, the body should be making these antioxidants by the pound, such that it could protect itself for **this alleged most-damaging and critical toxin,**

**oxygen.** The appearance of oxygen allowed evolving organisms the use of a highly efficient system in deliverance of more energy for less food.

**Over 80-90% of $O_2$ that living organisms breathe is used in the mitochondria to generate ATP**, the universal cellular energy currency.

**The "essential poison" paradox is not limited to oxygen but also includes glucose and iron.**

Glucose is a vital metabolic fuel for the brain, nervous system and red blood cells, but prolonged hyperglycemia causes widespread tissue damage, as in diabetes and can result in the excessive production of EMODs. Excess levels of free iron can reportedly result in excessive generation of the hydroxyl radical in the presence of $H_2O_2$.

**I do not believe that any one of these (glucose, iron or oxygen) is an essential poison. This is more nonscience/nonsense. They are vital for survival. Basically, anything in extremes of excess can serve as a poison.**

Edwards and Hart (1974) examined the effects of **hyperbaric oxygen administration on healthy elderly outpatients and found substantial improvements** in performance on tests of short term memory and visual organization, but their conclusions are tentative due to the lack of a comparative control group.

Most organs in the body are able to utilize many substrates present in the blood. They are able to absorb and metabolize a wide range of amino, keto and fatty acids for example, in addition to glucose, and the supplies of all these substances are fully adequate to maintain normal function. Such is not the case for **the brain which relies solely on the oxidative metabolism of glucose for its energy requirements** (Siesjo 1978).

**RMH Note: Other authors state that the brain prefers fats as an energy source.). At rest the brain consumes 17 calories per 100 grams of brain tissue per minute.**

(Siebert et al. 1986). Kadekaro et al. (1985) demonstrated that electrical stimulation of the sciatic nerve produced increases of up to 150% in metabolic rate where the afferent terminals made synapses with dendrites. This indicates that local activation leads to large scale changes in local metabolism, and by virtue in glucose and oxygen utilization.

**The normal arterial concentration of glucose is 5.5mM/L, and the normal level of oxygen is equivalent to 0.12mM/L.**

As **6 molecules of oxygen are required to oxidize 1 molecule of glucose,** then from the standpoint of supplying these metabolic needs, **the concentration of glucose is 275 times greater than that of oxygen** in the extracellular fluid at the surface of the cell.

Thus, **oxygen turnover is the highest amongst the essential nutrients** (Forster and Eastabrook (1993). Such times of high cellular demand for energy as mentioned above, (and more importantly in terms of this thesis, during cognitive processing) may outstrip the supply of oxygen and the cells may have to fall back (to some degree) on anaerobic metabolism.

This provides less energy and leads to the accumulation of toxic end products, but allows a level of baseline cellular metabolism until physiological responses can restore supply to the required levels (Rose 1966).

Once **glucose** has entered cells it undergoes the process of glycolysis in the cytosol, thereafter **pyruvate**, the main product of glycolysis, enters the tricarboxylic cycle in mitochondria. It is through these complex series of reactions that **ATP the 'universal energy currency of nature'** is produced.

To maintain the oxidative metabolism of glucose then, **the brain needs a constant supply of oxygen.** Certain metabolic intermediates e.g. lactate and pyruvate can substitute for glucose as alternative substrates for metabolism (Sokoloff 1989); however there is no such alternative for oxygen, and as **the brain does not store oxygen,** even a transient disruption of supply can have deleterious consequences.

**Glucose utilization by the brain proceeds at a rate of 31m mol/100gm/min, and oxygen consumption at 160m mol/100gm/min** (Sokoloff 1960).

With a global brain blood flow of 57ml/100gm/min, **the brain extracts approximately 50% of available oxygen and 10% of glucose from arterial blood under resting conditions.** It should be noted that **a limited proportion of the oxygen supply is consumed for other neural processes** than the production of energy, including interactions with oxidases and hydroxylases, which are key regulatory enzymes in the metabolic pathways of a number of neuroactive pathways, and the recently discovered nitric oxide (NO) synthase pathway also consumes oxygen.

Currently it is not known exactly how much oxygen is consumed during neural activation.

In summary, it is generally accepted that **altitudes above 10,000 ft.**, lead to profound effects on human cognitive performance, and that these effects result from hypoxia induced by the low levels of available oxygen. Limited evidence also suggests that such decrements in performance may be reversed through oxygen administration.

It is well known that **cognitive decline goes hand in hand with advancing age** (albeit not inevitably). Kuhl et al. (1984) and Reige et al. (1985) reported that **human aging is also associated with decreased glucose metabolism,** and it is possible that the two are inextricably linked.

As has been stated above, **glucose metabolism is reliant on a sufficient and continuous supply of oxygen,** and any compromise in this delivery system may be responsible, at least in part, for any resultant cognitive decline.

**EMODs are continuously being generated in neurons during normal metabolism and neuronal activity.**

**Oxidative damage of DNA** usually involves damage to single **bases.** It is estimated that **at least 35 different base modifications are formed in reactions with reactive oxygen species.** (McBride et al, 1991)

### The "Free Radi-Crap" Theory of Aging and Oxidative Stress

In spite of the promotion and predominance of **"tabloid science,"** I will do my best to set the record straight.

**The prevailing prejudice against reactive oxygen species (EMODs) is manifestly illustrated in the November 2003 issue of Readers Digest. In quoting Dr. Bruce Ames, a highly respected biochemist at University of California at Berkley, he states, "free radical oxidation doesn't just rise with aging--it causes it.**

**The more that mitochondria 'leak' free radicals (i.e., oxygen radicals) the more those radicals end up damaging the mitochondria, which in turn leak even more free radicals."** In bold print, the article states, "The ultimate irony: The thing we need most to live--oxygen--is what's killing us."

Statements such as this, which appear in both the lay press and in scientific publications, point out the currently accepted dogma which states that oxygen and its radicals are highly toxic, even lethal.

I believe that the overall data shows that they are wrong.

I believe that these EMODs are primarily "protective prooxidants." Further, I believe that they are of low toxicity, considering the fact that all of our aerobic cells are continually bathed throughout our entire lifetimes in steady state levels of EMODs.

Obviously, without oxygen, man would not develop diseases or age but unfortunately, he would be dead.

It appears to me that **the body has adapted (over million of years) to its advantage, the "leak" of electrons in the electron transport chain, by converting them to the superoxide anion and thus, to hydrogen peroxide; although I also believe that this is a purposeful design of nature and not a mistake or a leak** (the RSVP pathway referred to in Vol I, UTOPIA). (Howes, 2004, UTOPIA)

This is analogous to the use of a turbo charger, to take advantage of the exhaust gases of internal combustion engines, to improve the function of the engine, in which a leaking, waste product is used to a great advantage. Ergo, the perceived waste product is not a waste product at all but is instead a product to increase the overall efficiency of the engine or organism.

### Exercise

Exercise in humans helps to counteract the impairment of endothelium-mediated vasodilatory capacity normally seen with aging. Interestingly, **exercise in the lower extremities may affect endothelial vasomotion in remote organs such as the arm**, suggesting that exercise has **systemic** and possibly sustained beneficial effects. (Green et al, 2002)

I have been saying all along that **exercise introduces a large dose of EMODs and this is responsible for the salutary effects and systemic effects of exercise.** This therapeutic role of regular **physical activity helps reduce the incidence and the severity of related co-morbidities such as diabetes, hypertension, dyslipidemia and obesity.** (Barton, Furrer, 2003)

Usually, **aging is associated with a reduction of physical activity and fitness.** (Mazzeo, Tanaka, 2001)

When it comes to countering aging, **nutritional additives such as vitamins, appear to be largely ineffective in interfering with age-dependent functional changes associated with aging.**

## Hyperbaric Oxygen (HBO)

**Hyperbaric oxygen (HBO)** treatment of cholesterol-fed rabbits **dramatically reduces the development of arterial lesions despite having little or no effect on plasma or individual lipoprotein cholesterol concentrations.**

Compared with no treatment in cholesterol-fed animals, **HBO** treatment also substantially **reduces the accumulation of lipid oxidation products (conjugated dienes, trienes and thiobarbituric acid-reactive substances) in plasma,** in the low density lipoprotein and high density lipoprotein fractions of plasma, in the liver, and in the aortic tissues.

In addition, **HBO treatment prevents the decrease in plasma paraoxonase activity** observed in rabbits fed cholesterol-rich diets.

Similarly, in regression studies, **HBO treatment** has no effect on the rate of plasma (or lipoprotein) cholesterol decline but **significantly accelerates aortic lesion regression** compared with no treatment.

Direct measures of aortic cholesterol content support these morphological observations. Repeated, but relatively short, exposure to **HBO induces an antioxidant defense mechanism**(s) that is responsible for retarding the development or accelerating the regression of atherosclerotic lesions. (Kudchodkaar et al, 2000)

In this case, **I believe that the authors made some extremely valuable observations but they came to the wrong conclusion.**

**The plaque regression was not due to increased antioxidants but was due to increased EMODs, which are well known products of HBO$_2$. Further, administration of HBO$_2$ should, according to the Free Radi-Crap theory, cause increased lipid oxidation and plaque formation. Whereas, just the opposite is the result in experimental animals, whereby *HBO$_2$* causes increased regression of plaque and decreases accumulation of lipid oxidation products.**

**This is one of my most important observations.**

### HBO$_2$ and Hydrogen Sulfide Toxicity

In the past HBO has been used to treat toxicity of ingested hydrogen sulfide but now some researchers are **advocating hydrogen sulfides (H$_2$S) as a means of inducing a state of hibernation or suspended animation.**

US scientists at the Fred Hutchinson Cancer Research Center have for the first time eased mice in and out of hibernation, a possible procedure for treating critically ill and injured humans. **A study exposed the mice to high levels of hydrogen sulfide to put them into hibernation, suspending most metabolic activity,** Science magazine said. Later the mice were revived showing no significant ill effects, said the scientists. "We are, in essence, temporarily converting mice from warm-blooded to cold-blooded creatures, which is exactly the same thing that happens naturally when mammals hibernate," said lead investigator Mark Roth. "We think this may be a latent ability that all mammals have -- potentially even humans -- and we're just harnessing it and turning it on and off, inducing a state of hibernation on demand," said Roth.

In a hibernation-like state, cellular activity almost stops completely, **reducing the organism's need for oxygen.**

Applied to humans, this could gain valuable time for critically ill patients in operating rooms, injured soldiers on battlefields, and those awaiting organ transplants. It could help people suffering from severe fever, and also possibly help in treating cancer, by protecting normal cells during radiation and chemotherapy, according to Roth.

For the mice, the artificial hibernation was induced using hydrogen sulfide, a chemical normally produced in humans and animals that scientists believe helps regulate body temperature and metabolic activity. The mice' respiration and temperatures plunged drastically as they appeared to lose consciousness, the study noted. They were then **revived with little apparent effect.**

"Today, physicians have no way of dealing with uncontrolled fever other than literally putting people on ice. Well, we believe we know how to flip the breaker on the patient's furnace. If they have a fever, we believe we know how to stop it on a dime," Roth said.

**Hyperbaric oxygen** treatment has also been tested and presents positive outcomes, as it reduces ischemia and reperfusion injuries and improves microcirculation. (Haapaniemi et al, 1996) (Sirsjo et al, 1993)

## Oxygen Metabolism

Despite the demonstrated presumed role of antioxidants in cellular and animal studies, **the ineffectiveness of antioxidants in reducing cardiovascular death and morbidity in clinical trials has led many investigators to question the importance of oxidative stress in human atherosclerosis.**

**Antioxidants are ineffective in reducing cardiovascular death despite evidence for oxidative stress (OS) in cardiovascular diseases (CVD) from animal and human investigations.** (Madamanchi et al, 2005)

It is with this introduction that I would like to begin an in-depth discussion of **cardiac function, atherosclerosis, arteriosclerosis, hyperoxia, hypoxia and hyperbaric oxygen.**

## Mammalian Heart Facts

Some of the following materials was adapted, excerpted or modified from the following article: (Giordano, 2005)

The **mammalian heart is an obligate aerobic organ.** At a resting pulse rate, **the heart consumes approximately 8-15 ml $O_2$/ min/100 g tissue.** This is **significantly more than that consumed by the brain (approximately 3 ml $O_2$/min/100 g tissue)** and **can increase to more than 70 ml $O_2$/min/100 g myocardial tissue during vigorous exercise.** (West, 1991) (Braunwald, 2001)

**Mammalian heart muscle cannot produce enough energy under anaerobic conditions to maintain essential cellular processes;** thus, **a constant supply of oxygen is indispensable to sustain cardiac function and viability.** The story of oxygen in the heart is complex and goes well beyond its role in energy metabolism.

**Oxygen is a major determinant of myocardial gene expression,** and **as myocardial $O_2$ levels decrease,** either during isolated hypoxia or ischemia-associated hypoxia, **gene expression patterns in the heart are significantly altered.** (Huang et al, 2004)

Is there a relationship between ventricular geometry, oxygen, **EMODs** and cardiac function?

Ventricular geometry is a major determinant of cardiac function and is also a critical determinant of myocardial oxygen consumption. Myocardial oxygen consumption is proportional to ventricular wall tension, and by Laplaces' law, ventricular wall tension is proportional to P **X** r / 2π (where P is pressure, r is the radius of curvature of the ventricle, and π is ventricular wall thickness). Thus, at any given pressure and myocardial thickness, **a larger ventricle will consume more oxygen per gram tissue than a smaller one.**

Therefore, irrespective of the etiology, **a failing dilated heart requires more oxygen per gram tissue than a non-failing smaller heart. I believe that this also means that it will be more susceptible to the decreasing levels of $O_2$, which are available to it, which are seen with aging and consequently, decreasing levels of EMODs are going to be produced, which will "allow" the progressive development of coronary atherosclerosis.**

**Oxygen is indispensable for cardiac energy metabolism** and plays a central role in other biochemical processes that can be determinants of cardiac function, including the generation of **EMODs** and the determination of cardiac gene expression patterns.

Although their role in the pathogenesis of clinical heart failure remains **unclear, EMODs have been implicated by most authors to have a significant effect on cardiac function, including:**

-hypertrophy
-ion flux and calcium handling
-EC coupling
-extracellular matrix configuration
-vasomotor function
-metabolism
-gene expression
-and downstream signaling of several growth factors and cytokines.

**Clinical trials based on antioxidant therapy have been, however, generally disappointing.** (Giordano, 2005)

**Once again, I believe that the predictions of the Free Radi-Crap theory are wrong. If the Free Radi-Crap theory had been correct, we could have controlled the alleged harmful effects of EMODs and heart disease, including atherosclerosis, and they would be a thing of the past, instead of the current pandemic and the number one killer in the United States.**

**Oxygen participates in the generation of NO, which plays a critical role in determining vascular tone, cardiac contractility,** and a variety of additional parameters. Oxygen is also central in the generation of reactive oxygen species (EMODs), which can participate as **benevolent molecules** in cell signaling processes or can allegedly induce irreversible cellular damage and death. Oxygen is thus both vital and deleterious. (Davies, 1995)

**The heart can utilize a variety of metabolic fuels, including fatty acids, glucose, lactate, ketones and amino acids.** In the fed state, **fatty acids are the preferred fuel**, accounting for up to 90% of the total acetyl-CoA provided to cardiac mitochondria. (Jafri et al, 2001)

**Fatty acids are metabolized by β-oxidation, producing acetyl-CoA, NADH and $FADH_2$. The acetyl-CoA enters the Krebs cycle, producing more NADH and $FADH_2$.**

**Glucose** is metabolized initially via the glycolytic pathway, producing a relatively small amount of ATP and also pyruvate, which enters the Krebs cycle, producing NADH and $FADH_2$. **In the absence of oxygen, the total amount of energy produced by these processes is insufficient to meet cardiac needs.** The cardiac energy requirement is met, however, by entry of the resultant NADH and $FADH_2$ into **the electron transport chain, which generates ATP by oxidative phosphorylation in the mitochondria.**

Oxygen serves as the terminal electron acceptor in the electron transport chain, and **in the absence of sufficient oxygen, electron transport ceases and cardiac energy demands are not met. If oxygen is not supplied, death ensues.**

**EMODs can be formed in the heart** by a variety of mechanisms, including generation during oxidative phosphorylation in the mitochondria as **a byproduct of normal cellular aerobic metabolism.** Thus, the major process from which the heart derives sufficient energy can also result in the production of **EMODs.**

Molecular oxygen, $O_2$ is characterized as diradical, a property that allows liquid oxygen to be attracted to the poles of a magnet. This property also dictates that full reduction of oxygen to water as a terminal event in the electron transport chain requires four electrons. The sequential donation of electrons to oxygen during this process can generate **EMODs** as intermediates, and **"electron leakage"** can also contribute to the formation of **EMODs.**

**Singlet oxygen ($^1O_2$),** a very short-lived and reactive form of molecular oxygen in which the outer electrons are raised to a higher energy state, can be formed by a variety of mechanism, including the Haber-Weiss reaction ($H_2O_2 + O_2^- \rightarrow \cdot OH + OH^- + {}^1O_2$) (Toufekstian et al, 2001)

Please remember that other investigators have determined that, **under physiological conditions, the Haber-Weiss reaction does not occur. Its reaction kinetics are too slow to be of practical importance.**

**EMODs can be formed in the heart**, and other tissues, by several mechanisms:

-they can be produced by xanthine oxidase (XO), NAD(P)H oxidases
-cytochrome P450
-by autooxidation of catecholamines

Prof Randolph M. Howes MD,PhD

-by the action of cytokines and growth factors
-and by uncoupling of NO synthase (NOS).

NO contains an unpaired electron, and under certain conditions can react with $O_2^-$ to form peroxynitrite ($ONOO^-$), a powerful oxidant.

**EMODs have important roles in biological processes, including the oxidative burst reaction essential to phagocytes.** (Hensley et al, 2000)

**They are involved in a variety of cellular signaling pathways, acting in some instances as second messengers downstream of specific ligands, including TGF-$\beta$1, PDGF, ATII, PGF-2, endothelin, and others.**

**EMODs are also involved in modulating the activity of specific transcription factors, including NF-$\kappa$B and activator protein-1 (AP-1).**

NF-$\kappa$B, for example, becomes more transcriptionally active in response to the contribution of ROS to the degradation of I$\kappa$B, the inhibitory partner of NF-$\kappa$B that sequesters it in the cytosol. Thus, **EMODs can play an important role in modulating inflammation.**

General aging and age-related alteration in the cardiovascular system have been attributed to the long term cumulative effects of **EMODs,** although **the relative contribution of EMODs to the aging process remains the subject of debate.** (Sinclair, 2002)

Experimental evidence **suggests** that **EMODs** can mediate apoptosis by a variety of mechanisms, including direct mediation of genotoxicity. (von Harsdorf et al, 1999)

Interestingly, **whether or not apoptosis is induced in cardiomyocytes by oxidative stress appears to be dependent upon the level of EMODs produced.** (Kwon et al, 2003)

**EMODs can target L-type calcium channels on the sarcolemma and suppress the $Ca^{2+}$ current.** (Guerra et al, 1996)

**EMOD generation can also alter the function of cardiac sodium channels, potassium channels and ion exchangers, such as Na/Ca exchanger.** (Goldhaber, 1996)

**Physical activity (exercise) is tantamount to
electron activity, whereby triplet oxygen
is empowered, such that it can
achieve its missions
of pathogen and cancer protection
and energy production.**
R. M. Howes, M.D., Ph.D.
1/25/15

**"Exercise deficiency diseases"
are the same thing as
"EMOD insufficiency diseases"**
R. M. Howes, M.D., Ph.D.
1/7/15

# SECTION FOUR

## HBO AND HYPEROXIA

### Hyperoxia and Hyperbaric Oxygen (HBO)

Some of the following material was excerpted, abstracted or modified from: (Neubauer, Walker, 1998)

Hyperbaric Oxygen Therapy (**HBOT**) involves the use of pure oxygen at higher-than-atmospheric pressure to help overcome disease associated with a lack of oxygen in the tissues or organs. Unfortunately, this treatment is no longer considered beneficial by doctors in the United States for use in routine heart surgery, as an adjunct to cancer chemotherapy, or in the reversal of senility.

American doctors accept HBOT for use in **wound healing, bone infection, carbon monoxide intoxication, and air emboli, or air bubbles in the bloodstream due to decompression sickness, open-heart surgery,** and other sources. HBOT can also be used for conditions such **as coma resulting from head injuries, bruising of the spinal cord, stroke, and neurological disorders such as multiple sclerosis.** These additional applications have yet to be recognized by the medical establishment in the U.S.

Oxygen under pressure not only dissolves in the plasma but in all the body's fluids, such as the lymph and the fluid surrounding the brain and spine, as well as in bone marrow.

Nature has dictated that healing cannot take place in aerobic organisms without appropriate oxygen levels in the body's tissues. In many cases, such as those involving circulatory problems and strokes, **adequate oxygen can't reach the damaged area, and the body's natural healing process fails to function properly.**

All of the body's major components – water, protein, carbohydrate, and fat – contain oxygen **and its amount exceeds all other elements of the body combined**. Second, oxygen helps bring about certain chemical reactions within the body that result in energy production, ATP production. Energy is needed for functions such as circulation, respiration, and digestion and to power enzymatic reactions. Energy is also used to maintain a constant body temperature in man.

This extra oxygen helps the healing process. It enhances the white blood cells' ability to fight infection. It can promote the development of new capillaries, the tiny blood vessels that connect arteries to veins by a process called **angiogenesis.** It helps the body build new connective tissue through **collagen synthesis**.

Doctors now realize **there are other many uses for HBOT, including treatment of non-healing wounds, carbon monoxide poisoning, various infections, damage caused by radiation treatments, and all types of diving accidents**. (Sukoff, Gottlieb, 1998) (Neubauer, Kagan, Gottliev, 1989) (Gottlieb, 1989) (Gottliev, Neubauer, 1988)

**For more than three hundred years, people have been breathing pressurized air for its therapeutic effect.**

**A British physician named Henshaw is believed to have been the first, in 1664, to use compressed air in a specially equipped room called a domicilium.**

Henshaw believed that breathing vigorously inside the domicilium improved both digestion and respiration.

**One atmosphere absolute is the average atmospheric pressure exerted at sea level, or 14.7 psi.**

## Cerebrovascular Accidents (strokes)

**Stroke is the third most frequent cause of death in the United States** and the major cause of disability among Americans. **One third of those who suffer a stroke do not survive the initial attack,** and another third enter nursing homes.

Only one third improve, and many of these patients are left with disabilities that hinder their capacity to resume their pre-stroke lives. Stroke care in the United States costs more than $30 billion a year and is fraught with pain and suffering.

Packed within the soft mass of the brain are more than 10 billion interconnected nerve cells, called neurons. Though the brain is protected against danger from without by the skull, danger can lurk from within in the form of a **blockage** or rupture in one or more of the brain's thousands of blood vessels.

**A cutoff of blood circulation can occur for one of three reasons: ischemia, emboli and cerebral hemorrhage, including aneurysms.** It is estimated that approximate 35 of every 100 persons who experience a transient ischemic attack (TIA) will suffer a lethal or incapacitating stroke within five years.

After the ischemic cascade associated with a stroke, the brain goes through a reorganization phase, which lasts for about a week. After the reorganization, the brain enters a fairly stable phase, which may last anywhere from a week to three months. Preliminary results suggest that **HBOT is not as useful during the reorganization phase as it is before or after this phase.**

**Most neurologists believe that little or no further recovery will occur after three months.**

**HBOT decreases swelling and reawakens the stunned neurons within the penumbra by providing them with oxygen.** (Simon, 1976) (Astrup et al, 1981)

**Drugs can reduce edema but they cannot supply the brain with needed oxygen.**

Studies demonstrate HBOT's effectiveness in treating stroke. **Eight of nine animal studies showed positive results when HBOT was used.** (Smith et al, 1961) (Whalen, Heyman, Saltzman, 1966) (Moore et al, 1966) (Corkill et al, 1985) (Shiokawa et al, 1986) (Burt, Kapp, Smith, 1987) (Weinstein et al, 1986) (Reiten et al, 1990)

In another study, 122 patients with strokes caused by blood clots were treated with HBOT. Of the 122, 79 were treated from five months to ten years after their initial attacks – beyond the time that spontaneous recovery is believed to take place. Many of the patients had received various conventional physical therapies. They underwent HBOT at 1.5 to 2.0 atmospheres absolute, with duration and frequency of treatment adjusted as each patient improved. **Of the 79 patients, 65% reported improvement in their quality of life.** The HBOT patients spent much less time in the hospital – an average of 177 days compared with 287 days for conventionally treated patients. It is noteworthy that **all of the HBOT patients were able to go home,** while a number of the other patients had to enter rehabilitation centers. That represents a significant conservation of resources, in both emotional and financial terms, for the HBOT patients (Neubauer, End, 1980)

**Unfortunately, this approach is under utilized in the U.S.**

Head injuries deprive certain areas of the brain of oxygen by swelling or hemorrhage. HBOT can, at times, break this cycle by constricting the brain's blood vessels, yet **delivering more oxygen.** This seems like a contradiction, but **HBOT can increase oxygen levels because the increased pressure forces oxygen into the blood plasma,** the liquid part of the blood that normally carries only 3% oxygen, and into the cerebrospinal fluid that surrounds the brain. The plasma and cerebrospinal fluid can then reach areas that the red blood cells, which normally carry oxygen, cannot penetrate. With HBOT, oxygen in the capillaries is pushed further into the adjacent tissues than when oxygen is administered at standard pressure. **HBOT can also stabilize and repair what is called the blood-brain barrier,** a protective layer of cells that keeps many toxins or noxious materials from reaching the brain. This barrier is often greatly disturbed when a head injury occurs. Often, this increased oxygenation helps to restore the patient to a conscious state. (DeVolder et al, 1990)

Prompt use of HBOT is important because the more time a patient spends in a coma, the poorer his or her chances are of making a good recovery. **Post-coma psychosis is known to occur at a higher rate for coma patients who are not treated with HBOT.**

The spinal cord is made up of similar types of nerve tissue as that found in the brain. Therefore, when it is bruised, it tends to undergo the same type of damage to which the brain is subject. That is, **swelling causes a cutoff of the blood supply, which in turn causes the cells to die from lack of oxygen** and from being poisoned by their own waste.

**Studies have shown HBOT's effectiveness in cases where spinal damage is associated with injuries.** (Jain et al, 1990) (Morgami et al, 1969) (Holbach, Wassmann, Kolberg, 1974) (Artu et al, 1976) (Sukoff, Ragatz, 1982) (Rockswold, Ford, 1985)

## Migraine Headaches

**During the first phase of a migraine, blood flow may be reduced by an average of 36%.** Reduced blood flow results in **lack of oxygen** in the tissues, along with changes in the brain's chemistry. This, in turn, causes the release of substances that greatly dilate the blood vessels. Local tissue injury and **swelling occur** as a result. It is at this time that migraine pain strikes the patient. **Many migraine patients who receive HBOT find that the interval between attacks is significantly increased.**

## Macular Degeneration

**There is some evidence that HBOT can reverse age-related macular degeneration (AMD),** the leading cause of severe visual loss in people over the age of fifty.

In a study by Dr. L. Bojic and colleagues, 4 patients who had nearly total loss of eyesight from macular degeneration received HBOT. **Three of the patients experienced a doubling of visual acuity, while the fourth experienced almost a fourfold increase in acuity.** The doctors who treated the patients thought that the hyperbaric oxygen helped increase the amount of oxygen in the retinal tissue, which allowed the retina to renew itself without causing a buildup of waste material. They thought this waste material interfered with cell function and led to macular degeneration. (Bojic et al, Split Naval Medical Institute pp 1-4)

## Multiple Sclerosis

There are approximately half a million **multiple sclerosis (MS)** patients in the United States, with about 10,000 Americans newly diagnosed each year. In MS, the nerve fibers in the brain and spinal cord gradually lose their protective covering, which is made of a **fatty substance called myelin**. Nerve impulses are basically electrical impulses, so myelin covers and insulates a nerve in the same way insulation covers an electrical wire. A nerve that is covered **with myelin conducts impulses more rapidly** than a nerve that isn't covered.

As a result of MS, hardened, scarred patches called **plaques** may develop throughout the brain and spinal cord, although affected areas do not always form plaques. Yet, even before these scars develop, **MS can cause swelling and a lack of oxygen** in the tissues which, in turn, can produce many different symptoms. MS may cause a number of secondary problems, such as inflammation of the membranes covering the brain and spinal cord, problems with nerves beyond the brain and spinal cord, changes in the retina, loss of nerve cells, blood spots in the skin, and blood vessel changes. **No one is sure what causes MS.**

A variety of treatments have been developed in an effort to reverse, or at least relieve, the symptoms of MS. These come out of two theories about what causes MS – viral infection and autoimmune dysfunction. Numerous investigations have done studies in which **neither theory was found to be valid.** (Chattaway, 1989) (Gottlieb, Neubauer, 1988) (McDonald, 1985)

**HBOT was the safest and most effective treatment available for MS.**

**The Gottlieb-Neubauer theory, proposing that MS is caused by lack of oxygen, has been supported by research showing that HBOT, which overcomes a lack of oxygen, is an effective treatment method.**

**Seventy percent of the treated MS patients either did not deteriorate, had their conditions stabilize, or showed small improvements.** (Davidson, 1989)

### Injuries

Each year, Americans make about 25 million visits to emergency rooms because of injuries caused by everything from car accidents to falls to acts of violence. Many of the most severe injuries cause equally severe blood-circulation problems, which in turn bring on **oxygen starvation** in the body's tissues. Such under-oxygenation can disrupt the body's normal functioning almost as much as the actual injuries themselves.

Sometimes, there is a lack of oxygen in the tissues due to a disruption in the blood supply. This disruption arises after the blood that generally flows from a wound starts to clot. Such clotting interferes with the circulation in the wound areas by blocking the blood vessels. Such blockages **reduce the area's oxygen supply** and prevent removal of wastes produced by the cells. The affected tissues begin to swell. Even when the circulation is restored, the swelling may persist or get worse. That further **cuts off the supply of blood and oxygen** to the area, and traps even more waste within the tissues. The oxygen depletion and waste buildup combine to kill cells, and the presence of dead cells, in turn, leads to even more oxygen depletion and waste buildup.

A lack of oxygen in the tissues can reduce the injured person's defense against infection by decreasing the activity of infection-fighting white blood cells and lead to immunosuppression. **A wound's chances of becoming infected are directly related to how little oxygen there is in the affected tissues.** (Hunt, 1979)

**Under-oxygenation can also reduce the body's ability to heal the wound, especially since healing tissue needs even more oxygen than does healthy tissue.** (Niinikoski, Hunt, Zederfeldt, 1972)

A **lack of oxygen** can deactivate the cells that produce granulation tissue, the tissue that covers a wound before the new skin grows. It can **also interfere with the production of collagen,** the basic building material of which new skin is made, and any collagen that is produced is likely to be of poor quality. (Hohn, 1977) (Hunt, Pai, 1972) (Hunt, Niinikoske, Zederfeldt, et al, 1977) (Silver, 1984)

**The creation of capillaries, the tiny blood vessels that connect arteries to veins, requires both collagen and oxygen.** (Knighton, Silver, Hunt, 1981) (Ketchum, Thomas, Hall, 1969)

**If either is lacking, new capillaries cannot be created, and wound healing cannot occur.** Thus, **a lack of oxygen in the wounded tissues interferes with the entire wound healing process.** (Wells et al, 1977)

As the swelling increases, the fluid pressure can become so severe that it brings about a partial or complete collapse of the capillary circulation within the affected tissues.

**HBOT is the best way of increasing the oxygen content of under-oxygenated tissues.** (Sheffield, 1985) (Strauss et al, 1983) (Strauss et al, 1986) (Skyhar et al, 1986) (Nylander, et al, 1986)

**HBOT can put more oxygen in the body's fluids, and thus is able to deliver more oxygen to under-oxygenated tissues.** (Peirce, 1969) (Tan et al, 1984)

The use of **HBOT is a very valuable way of treating difficult wounds.** (Hunt, van Winkle, 1976) (Sheffield, 1985) (Sheffield, 1984) (Kindwall, Goldmann, 1984)

**Under-oxygenation makes a wound more susceptible to infection, which slows the rate of healing.** (Niinikoski, 1969) (Hunt, Cononlly et al, 1979) (Hunt, Pai, 1972)

**Swelling reduces the number of white blood cells and other infection fighters that can reach the affected tissues, and those cells that do find their way to the area cannot act very effectively without oxygen.**

Some of the most dangerous microbes in wounds are anaerobic, which means that they thrive in the absence of oxygen. **HBOT can help counteract infection indirectly by providing the white blood cells with the oxygen** they need. It can also act directly by **killing anaerobic organisms**, stopping their multiplication, and neutralizing the toxins that some of them produce. (Jones, 1984) (Hohn, 1980)

**HBOT also helps antibiotics such as sulfa drugs work more effectively.** (Van Meter et al, 1986) (Keck, Gottlief, Conley, 1980) (Adams, Sutton, Mader, 1987) (Adams, Mader, 1987) (Norden, Kleti, 1980)

**Oxygen is essential in the creation of granulation tissue, the pink, fleshy tissue that first grows over a healing wound.** (Hunt, Zederfeldt, Goldstick, 1969)

**Granulation tissue can be seen within seven to ten days of starting a patient on HBOT.**

By thirty days, this tissue becomes densely supplied with blood vessels. (Winter, Perrins, 1969)

**Oxygen also promotes the growth of collagen,** the material of which skin and connective tissue are formed. Collagen, in turn, forms the bed on which new capillaries are created. Therefore, the more collagen is produced, the more quickly the new skin's blood supply is created.

**It encourages bone repair**. Bone repair depends on the action of osteoclasts, cells that dispose of dead bone, and osteoblasts, cells that create new bone. In turn, **these cells depend on a rich supply of oxygen.**

**HBOT's effectiveness in minimizing tissue death, reducing swelling, and promoting healing has been proven in the laboratory.** (Strauss et al, 1986) (Nylander et al, 1985) (Kivisaari, Niinikoski, 1975)

**Seven teams of researchers published reports in English language medical journals about the successful use of HBOT for crush injuries and compartment syndrome.** All the patients – including 93 trauma cases – showed extensive benefits. And a series of reports from the Eastern European medical literature, 634 cases in all, also **attested to the benefits of HBOT.**

**The earlier and more frequently HBOT is used, the more likely it is that severely injured body parts will be saved.** (Strauss, Hart, 1984) (Shupak et al, 1987)  (Strauss, Hart, 1989)

One of the most respected trauma surgery units in the world is the Department of Microsurgery at the University of Liege Hospital in Belgium. The **Liege doctors were convinced that HBOT helped them heal difficult wounds** and save reattached limbs that would otherwise have not been healed or saved.

## Infection's Therapeutic Adjunct

Throughout the course of human history, infection has been one of the leading causes of death. Infectious diseases such as bubonic plague have decimated civilizations.

Humankind began to win the war on infection with the **development of sulfa drugs in the 1930s and penicillin in the 1940s.** HBOT has proven itself to be a useful treatment for some of these infections. **Oxygen acts as a potent antibiotic.** Oxygen dissolved in the blood improves the ability of special scavenger white blood cells, called phagocytes, to rid the body of bacteria and other foreign proteins. Since

HBOT forces oxygen into the body's tissues, it has a distinct antimicrobial effect that is equal to or better than that of numerous antibiotics.

**HBOT helps fight all microorganisms, but especially those that thrive in the absence of oxygen. There is evidence that HBOT, because of its immune system-enhancing effects, can help the body fight these microbes.** (Gotlieb et al, 1964) (Gottlieb, Pakman, 1968) (Gottlieb et al, 1974) (Keck, Gottlieb, Conley, 1980) (Adams, Sutton, Mader, 1987) (Adams, K.R., Sutton, T.E. and Mader, J.T. In vitro potentiation of tobramycin under hyperoxic conditions. Undersea Biomed Res 1987; 14(suppl): 37) (Adams, Mader, 1987) (Norden, Kleti, 1980) (Jones, 1984) (Hohn, 1980)

**Gas gangrene** is a painful condition in which the body's soft tissues are destroyed by toxins produced by bacteria. It is usually caused by microbe called **Clostridium perfringens, which is implicated in 80 to 90% of all cases of gas gangrene.** About 1,100 Americans die of gas gangrene each year.

Injury results in hypoxia, or lack of oxygen in the tissues. The bacteria thrive under these conditions, and produce toxins that cause swelling. The swelling further diminishes the supply of both blood and oxygen to the area. That keeps the immune system from functioning properly, which in turn allows the disease to spread and produce even more toxins.

**The high levels of oxygen, with HBOT, lead to the death or inactivation of the microbes.** However, dead tissue creates toxins that can keep HBOT from doing its job, which is why surgery is often necessary for HBOT to work most effectively. Once the dead tissue is removed, the oxygen can act freely against the bacteria. (Fischer et al, 1988) (Van Unnik, 1965) (Schoemaker, 1964) (Kivisaari, Niinikoski, 1973) (Sheffield, 1988) (Demello, 1970)

**More than 4,000 cases of gas gangrene treated with HBOT have been reported in medical journals. Here are conclusions taken from just a few of these studies:**

- In one study, there was a survival rate of 88.3% among 248 patients who received HBOT. (Bakker, 1988)
- A study by Dr. M.E. Ellis and Dr. B.K. Mandal analyzed the cases of 58 patients who had failed to respond to antibiotics and surgery, and who were considered to have poor prognoses. After these patients received HBOT, there was a survival rate of 84%. Survivors showed a marked improvement in their conditions. (Ellis, Mandal, 1971)

- In another study of 139 patients treated with HBOT, there was a survival rate of 70%. Eighty percent of the survivors were able to avoid amputations (some patients had more than one limb involved). (Hart, Lamb, Strauss, 1983)

## Lyme Disease

**Lyme disease** is a tick-borne illness with a wide array of symptoms. It is **named for the town of Old Lyme, Connecticut, where it was first describe in 1975.**

Lyme disease is caused by a corkscrew-shaped bacterium called a **spirochete**, usually **Borrelia burgdorferi**. The spirochete is carried by the deer tick, a tiny creature that in the adult stage is about the size of a sesame seed.

The first sign of Lyme disease is a usually **painless skin rash called erythema migrans** at or near the site of the bite. This rash, which generally has **a bull's-eye appearance**, develops within a week after the bite occurs.

If the disease is not detected early, the body's own cells tend to protect the Lyme spirochete against antibiotics. Thus, even when very strong drugs are used, the spirochete may not be completed destroyed.

**Studies suggest that HBOT works against Lyme disease by attacking the spirochete itself.** (Austin, 1993) (Burgdorfer, 1996) (Schwan, 1996)

Preliminary evidence of HBOT's effectiveness against Lyme disease in humans was provided by a pilot study conducted by Dr. William Fife and Dr. Donald Freeman at Texas A&M University. (Fife, Freeman, 1997)

The use of HBOT in the treatment of Lyme disease is a relatively recent development. Therefore, no standard treatment plan yet exists. Nevertheless, the study by Dr. Fife and Dr. Freeman, preliminary as it is, indicates great promise for the use of HBOT in this area.

HBOT can be employed to treat a variety of other infections. Three of those infections are **streptococcal infections, leprosy and actinomycosis**.

In deeper tissues, a streptococcal infection can cause necrotizing fascitis, a severe infection of the body's connective tissue, or myositis, a muscle infection.

**Leprosy, also known as Hansen's disease,** is a chronic bacterial disease that, contrary to common belief, is not very contagious. It affects mainly the peripheral nerves and the skin. **Leprosy was the first infectious disease to be treated with HBOT: in 1938,** doctors in Brazil gave it to 9 patients, with good results. (Ozorio, Costa, 1938)

Two later studies showed positive results. (Duenas, 1969) (Wilkinson, et al, 1970)

**Actinomycosis, or lumpy jaw**, is an infection caused by a bacterium called **Actinomyces israelii.** It mostly occurs among those who work with animals, as both cattle and hogs can transmit the disease to human beings.

**HBOT has proved to be a superb therapy for this fungal infection.** (Manheim et al, 1969)

### Burns

Each year, over 40,000 Americans are burned badly enough to require skin grafts for survival. There are also 80,000 burn victims each year who don't need skin transplants but who do need medical assistance. **HBOT can help burn patients heal faster with fewer complications.** (Wada et al, 1965) (Grossman, 1978)

**HBOT usefulness in aiding burn recovery has been shown in animal studies.** (Wells, Hilton, 1977) (Ketchum, Thomas, Hall, 1969) (Ketchum et al, 1967) (Arzinger-Jonasch et al, 1978) (Kaiser et al, 1985)

A 1974 study by Dr. G.B. Hart and colleagues looked at 191 human burn patients. **The researchers concluded that while HBOT is not a cure-all for burn patients, it can play a significant role in a total burn-treatment program.** (Hart et al, 1974)

Burn expert and plastic surgeon, Dr. Richard Grossman, developed an HBOT treatment program at Sherman Oaks Community Hospital in Sherman Oaks, California, in which HBOT is given within four hours of the patient's admission to the burn unit. Dr. Grossman also uses HBOT both before and after operating on burn patients. (Grossman, 1978)

## Bone Disorders

Every day, people from all walks of life suffer bone injuries. A bone has three layers of tissue: a spongy inner layer, a rigid middle layer and a tough outer layer. Bones are rigid because of the minerals, mainly calcium, that are found in the middle and outer layers.

The **osteoclasts depend on oxygen for proper functioning**. However, injury often results in hypoxia, or a lack of oxygen in the body's tissues. **Osteomyelitis has been linked to a lack of blood vessels at the site of a bone infection.** (Harrelson, Hills, 1970) (Niinikoske, Hunt, 1972)

**HBOT helps to heal bone disorders by stimulating both the osteoclast and the osteoblasts.** (Hunt, Zederfeldt, Goldstick, 1969) (Strauss, 1987)

Doctors first discovered HBOT's effectiveness in the treatment of osteomyelitis back in 1968, in studies done with laboratory rats. **The animals were cured of bone infections – with symptoms that included sinus infections, abscesses and bony deterioration – through the use of HBOT alone.** No antibiotics were used, and surgery was not performed. (Hamblin, 1968)

Dr. Jefferson C. Davis, a leading figure in the early days of hyperbaric medicine, studied two groups of patients – 98 in 1977 and 38 in 1986 – at Southwest Texas Methodist Hospital. These patients had refractory chronic osteomyelitis of the spine, extremities, pelvis, skull and chest wall.

**In over half of all these patients, the infections cleared up completely as a result of receiving HBOT**. They remained cured long after a five-year follow-up study was completed. (Davis, Hunt, 1977) (Davis et al, 1986)

In another study, 40 patients suffering from chronic osteomyelitis were treated with HBOT as an adjunct to surgery and antibiotics. **The cure rate at the two-year follow-up examination was 85%.** (Morrey et al, 1979) (Mainous, Boyne, Hart, 1973) (Evans et al, 1976)

## Aseptic Bone Necrosis (ABN)

Under certain circumstances, bones can become inflamed without being infected. Such an inflammation is called aseptic bone necrosis (ABN). This painful condition occurs most often among professional divers. Osgood-Schlatter has no known cause, and neither does spontaneous ABN. **ABN is essentially a blood-supply problem.** (Neubauer, Kagan, Gottlieb, 1989)

It stands to reason that putting more oxygen in the affected tissues will help halt further deterioration and promote healing. **There is evidence that HBOT does indeed help** patients with ABN.

## Fracture Nonunion

**HBOT works to heal fracture nonunion by stimulating the production of collagen**, a tough, fibrous material that fills in the space between the two broken ends of bone. Collagen production, in turn, stimulates the production of capillaries, the tiny blood vessels that connect arteries to veins. The more blood vessels there are in the area, the more oxygen and nutrients can be brought to the site of the break. This additional oxygen and nutrient supply reinvigorates the cells that break down old bone and form new bone, and stimulates the formation of calcium deposits within the newly formed bone. (Mainous, 1982) (Mainous, Boyne, Hart, 1973) (Strauss, Malluche, Faugere, 1982) (Mainous, 1982)

**HBOT leads to greater cartilage production** (cartilage is the material that separates bones from each other, such as in the knee) and increased bone formation. (Davis, Hunt, 1977) (Kulagin et al, 1981) (Tikhilow, Akimov, Lotovin, 1980) (Sepnov, Uglova, 1979)

**Adding HBOT to conventional orthopedic methods shortened the process of bone regeneration and wound healing by ten to twelve days.** (Zavesa, 1977)

## Complications of Radiation Treatment and Skin Surgery

Each year, Americans undergo over 20 million radiation treatments, at an average of twenty-four treatments a patient. **Radiation treatment damages cells** by interfering with their ability to reproduce. If the cells cannot reproduce, they eventually die. That is why radiation treatment is used to treat cancer in the first place – cancer cells reproduce much more rapidly than normal cells do, and are thus more susceptible to radiation than normal cells are.

**Radiation damage, called radionecrosis**, may be the result. Radionecrosis can be easily induced by injury or surgery (even tooth extraction) after the patient has undergone radiation treatment.

Until recently, there has been no satisfactory treatment of radiation damage. HBOT fills this long-standing need. **Radiation damage causes hypoxia, or a lack of oxygen in the body's tissues. Hyperbaric oxygen helps fight this damage by increasing the amount of oxygen within the tissues.** (Mainous, 1977) (Greenwood, Gilchrist, 1973)

**Radiation myelitis and radiation encephalopathy are two potential nervous-system complications of radiation treatment.** Myelitis is an inflammatory disease that affects the entire spinal cord. This inflammation results in a loss of the cord's ability to transmit nerve impulses, much as if the cord had been severed. (Boden, 1948)

However, **HBOT, if used too soon after radiation treatments are given, can aggravate the effects of radiation.** (Luk, Baker, Fellows, 1978) (Hopewell, 1979)

Varying degrees of improvement was observed in all of the patients. (Torubarov et al, 1983)

**At least eight months should pass following the last radiation treatment.** (Hart, Strauss, 1986)

48 patients underwent surgery after receiving radiation treatment to the head and neck. Their surgical wounds opened up because of radiation-induced damage to the tissues. These patients were given **HBOT and all except one of the patients improved.** (Hart, Strauss, 1986)

15 patients had radiation damage to the bladder. Remissions took place in an average of twenty-four months, and **only one patient failed to respond.** (Weiss, Neville, 1989)

HBOT was used to treat 20 patients who had radiation damage of the soft tissues. In **16 of these patients, the injuries healed.** (Glassburn, Brady, Plenk, 1977)

Radiation can also damage bone. Since bone is 1.6 times denser than soft tissue, it absorbs a larger portion of a radiation dose than does soft tissue.

HBOT has proven its worth in **the treatment of radiation-induced jawbone damage**. Hart and Strauss reported on 206 patients who received HBOT as an adjunct treatment. Of these patients, **72% responded with excellent results**, 10% with good results and 15% with fair results. The remaining 3% did not respond. (Hart, Strauss, 1986) (Marx, Johnson, Kline, 1985)

Another fairly common site of **radiation-induced bone damage is the spinal column,** which is made up of 33 vertebrae. These vertebrae are divided into four groupings – neck, chest, lower back and tailbone – and the location of the damage depends on where the cancer under treatment is located. Such damage causes back pain. There may also be impairment to the spinal cord itself. In a 1986 study, 4 patients with radiation-induced vertebrae damage were given HBOT, and some damaged tissue was removed. All four patients recovered. (Hart, Strauss, 1986) (Marx, Johnson, 1988)

**HBOT can help assure that skin grafts** take hold and scars don't reveal themselves. Healing takes place three times faster than before HBOT became available to plastic surgeons. HBOT tends to improve the chances that a graft will take, both by supplying oxygen directly to the graft and by encouraging quick capillary growth.

In the case of a **pedicle graft, it is important that HBOT be employed before what little circulation that is present develops blood clots.** (Champion, Mcsherry, Goulian, 1967) (Boerema, 1961) (Perrins, 1966) (Perrins, 1967) (Perrins, 1970) (Shulman, Krohn, 1867) (Wilmeth, Gazau, 1982)

**HBOT can also help speed the healing of skin ulcers,** especially chronic ulcers caused by a lack of oxygen. It has been known since 1969 that even moderately elevated levels of oxygen may be effective in such situations. (Bass, 1970) (Fischer, 1969) (Olejniczak, 1969) (Rosenthal, 1970)

**HBOT not only helps the body develop new circulation in the wound area, as it does in skin grafts, but also inhibits or kills surface bacteria on the ulcers.**

## Carbon Monoxide Poisoning

Carbon monoxide – a colorless, odorless gas – is the most common cause of death by poisoning. **Thousands of American die of carbon monoxide poisoning every year**, and more than 10,000 people miss at least one day of work because of exposure to carbon monoxide. The gas is produced by motor vehicles, defective gas appliances, and factories. It is also produced during fires and mining accidents, and by propane-powered equipment. Also, **methylene chloride**, the active ingredient in paint thinner, is converted to carbon monoxide by enzymes in the liver.

Animal studies clearly demonstrated that **hyperbaric oxygen could drive carbon monoxide out of its bonds with hemoglobin.** (Valois, Schade, 1967) (Araki, Nashimoto, Takano, 1988)

**Children, the elderly and pregnant women are more susceptible to the effects of carbon monoxide**. All of these people can be helped by HBOT. A pregnant woman is especially prone to the effects of carbon monoxide because the fetus, which absorbs carbon monoxide through the placenta, eliminates the gas slowly.

**Hydrogen sulfide** is a highly toxic gas that is readily recognized by its characteristic "rotten eggs" odor. In high concentrations, it can cause death. At lower concentrations, it can irritate the eyes, throat and lungs. Hydrogen sulfide can also cause headache, weakness, convulsions, a feeble pulse and a fall in both body temperature and blood pressure. Chronic low-level exposure can bring on headache, nausea, confusion, insomnia, dry mouth, tearing, abdominal cramps and throat and chest irritation.

Hydrogen sulfide has a number of industrial applications, including use as a bleaching agent. Most poisoning cases result from industrial exposure. Like carbon monoxide, **hydrogen sulfide ties up the hemoglobin** in the body's oxygen carrying red blood cells, which **reduces the amount of oxygen that reaches the tissues**. This loss of oxygen produces swelling of the brain, which can cause brain damage.

Many chemicals can produce methemoglobinemia, a condition in which red blood cells cannot carry their normal amount of oxygen because hemoglobin, the oxygen-bearing chemical they contain, is damaged or occupied by an interfering molecule other than oxygen. **This condition degrades the ability of the body's tissues to get all the oxygen they need.** Chemicals that can produce methemoglobinemia include nitrites and nitrates, used as preservatives in food and medicines, potassium chloride, used in fertilizer, potassium permanganate, used in dyes and deodorizers, drugs such as phenacetin, nitroglycerine and local anesthetics; and aniline dyes.

Methemoglobinemia usually produces no symptoms, but is associated with collapse, coma and death when it affects more than 65% of the blood's hemoglobin. While such deaths are rare, nonfatal levels of methemoglobinemia can cause people to function at less than full capacity.

The heart and the major blood vessels, such as the aorta, make up only half of the circulatory system. The other half is made up of thousands of blood vessels throughout the body. When disease occurs in these blood vessels, it is called **peripheral vascular disease (PVD)**. PVD may be a sign of a serious underlying condition, such as diabetes or heart disease. PVD can also have serious consequences, such as limb loss. (Dawber, 1980)

In the United States, according to the Department of Labor, **PVD is responsible for more than 6 million person-days a year of lost work time.** (Dinkel, Bochner, Pampuro, 1986)

HBOT helps patients with PVD in several ways. The use of **hyperbaric oxygen leads to the development of new capillaries, tiny blood vessels linking arteries and veins**. This dissolved oxygen is more readily used by the body than the oxygen that is normal carried by the red blood cells. (Fredenucci, 1983) (Fredenucci, 1982)

As a result of the **additional oxygen, the tissues functional more normally**. The effects of HBOT can readily be seen in the way the patient's skin and nail beds steadily turn pink or red in color. (Kindwall, 1979)

HBOT also improves the blood's chemical properties and appears to **reduce the blood's tendency to clump.**

In the 1980s and into the 1990s, additional doctors found HBOT to be useful in treating PVD. In France, Dr. P. Fredenucci worked with 2,021 patients between 1966 and 1983, and found that **proper blood flow to under-oxygenated parts of the body was revived in 40% of the patients treated with HBOT**.

**Other studies found that HBOT healed skin ulcers.** (Gerad et al, 1967)

## HIV infection

The rate of progression from the **initial HIV infection to fully developed acquired immune deficiency syndrome (AIDS)** depends upon the individual; it can take from eighteen months to more than 10 years. **Women tend to develop AIDS more quickly than men.** A patient has AIDS when the level of T-cells, a type of immune-system cell, drops **to less than 200 in every milliliter of blood**.

HIV and its cofactors (the viruses that often accompany HIV) also impair the cells that line the blood vessels. This damage can result in blockages of both small and large vessels. These obstructions can reduce the flow of blood to the limbs, brain and heart. Indeed, transient ischemic attacks (TIAs), strokes, and heart attacks are common among patients with AIDS. Daily TIAs increase as the disease progresses, resulting in mental impairment, loss of muscle control, decreased memory and reduced independence.

**The blood vessel blockages produced by herpes and other viruses have been relieved by HBOT for decades.** (Jain, 1995)

**Kaposi's sarcoma has been linked to one of the many human herpes viruses** by Patrick Moore and Yuan Chang. It is an opportunistic viral infection that attacks both externally and internally. It is usually treated with chemotherapy and, often, radiation.

**HBOT is recommended as an adjunct treatment to reduce the side effects of these therapies in the management of certain cancers.** (Jain, 1995, 446)

And, as Michelle Reillo has documented in AIDS Under Pressure (Hogrefe & Huber, 1997), HBOT is extremely beneficial in the treatment of Kaposi's sarcoma in patients with HIV/AIDS. (Reillo, 1997, 51)

Michelle Reillo has found that patients with AIDS who regularly use preventative HBOT and drug therapy develop PCP less often. (Reillo, 1997)

**Research into HIV history also reveals the astonishing complexity of the virus and its ability to mutate and recombine with other strains -- continually producing "new and improved" versions that outpace mankind's efforts at treatment, he said.** "What we know about how the virus evolves is not very good news for therapies and vaccines ... it is going to be very difficult," Sharp said.

## HIV: ROS, enveloped viruses and HBO

**Abstract** (Note: ROI is interchangeable with ROS or EMODs by some authors)

This paper demonstrates that there are many examples in the literature of contradictory data concerning reactive oxygen intermediates (ROIs), responsible for producing cellular oxidative stress (OS), and their enhancement or diminution of viral replication. Nevertheless, ROIs repeatedly have been shown to be virucidal against enveloped-viruses, like the human immunodeficiency virus (HIV).

**Hyperbaric oxygen therapy (HBOT) increases the production of ROIs throughout the body, leaving no safe harbor for the virus to hide outside the genome.** This technique already has been tried on acquired immune deficiency syndrome (AIDS) patients, with exciting results.

Historically, the biggest setback to demonstrating HBO's antiviral effects has been the investigator's folly of studying non-enveloped viruses or failing to initiate ROI production.

**ROIs (EMODs) specifically attack areas of unsaturation occurring in the polyunsaturated fatty acids of cell membranes and viral envelopes.** Moreover, it consistently has been shown that a peroxidized viral envelope breaches, and a breached viral envelope causes viral disintegration. (Baugh, 2000)

**I believe this illustrates the anti-HIV/AIDs (and all other lipid coated viruses) potential for EMODs and hyperbaric oxygen.**

## HIV antiviral effects of HBOT

### Abstract

Researchers have speculated that hyperbaric oxygen (HBO) therapy has an antiviral effect in HIV infection. To determine HBO's antiviral effect, the authors performed ex vivo and in vivo quantitative assays on HIV-infected plasma and peripheral blood mononuclear cells (PBMCs) at baseline and after treatment. The authors also HBO-treated uninfected PBMCs and then exposed them to HIV at ambient pressure.

**HIV viral load was decreased in the infected cells, and few viruses entered uninfected peripheral blood mononuclear cells (PBMCs) exposed to HBO. The results of this study support the theory that HBO has an antiviral effect.** (Reillo, Altieri, 1996)

---

Some of the following was adapted from: (Zhang, Gould, 2014)

### HBO reduces MMP in ischemic wounds

**Hyperbaric Oxygen Reduces Matrix Metalloproteinases in Ischemic Wounds through a Redox-Dependent Mechanism.**

**Abbreviations:** ERK, extracellular signal–regulated kinase; GPx, glutathione peroxidase; HBO, hyperbaric oxygen; HBOT, hyperbaric oxygen treatment; H/N, HBO and NAC; $H_2O_2$, hydrogen peroxide; iNOS, inducible nitric oxide synthase; JNK, c-Jun N-terminal kinase; MAPK, mitogen-activated protein kinase; MMP, matrix metalloproteinase; NAC, N-acetylcysteine; 3-NT, 3-nitrotyrosine; ROS, reactive oxygen species; RNS, reactive nitrogen species; SA, superoxide anion; TIMP, tissue inhibitor of metalloproteinase

Little is known about the impact of hyperbaric oxygen treatment (HBOT) on matrix metalloproteinase (MMP) production in pre-existing high-oxidant wounds. This study aimed to investigate whether HBOT modulates reactive oxygen species (ROS) and MMP regulation in ischemic wound tissue. Using a validated ischemic wound model, Sprague–Dawley rats were divided into four groups for daily treatment: HBOT,

N-acetylcysteine (NAC), HBO and NAC, and control (normoxia at sea level).

High levels of inducible nitric oxide synthase (iNOS), gp91-phox, and 3-nitrotyrosine were detected in ischemic wounds, indicating high-oxidant stress.

**HBOT not only increased antioxidant enzyme expression, such as Cu/Zn-superoxide dismutase, catalase, and glutathione peroxidase, but also significantly decreased pro-oxidant enzyme levels, such as iNOS and gp91-phox, thereby decreasing net oxygen radical production by means of negative feedback.**

This effect was blocked by NAC treatment in ischemic wounds.

**HBO-treated ischemic wounds also manifested reduced phosphorylation of extracellular signal–regulated kinases 1/2, c-Jun N-terminal kinase, and c-Jun, indicating downregulation of mitogen-activated protein kinases (MAPKs).**

Furthermore, **HBOT decreased the expression of several MMPs while simultaneously increasing tissue inhibitor of MMP (tissue inhibitor of metalloproteinase 2).**

These results indicate that **HBOT acts via the ROS/MAPK/MMP signaling axis to reduce tissue degeneration and improve ischemic wound healing.** (Zhang, Gould, 2014)

**Hyperbaric oxygen treatment (HBOT) is an effective adjunct for wound healing that has both systemic and local effects.** (Kessler et al, 2003)

**At the tissue level, HBOT modulates cytokine release, accelerates microbial oxidative killing, reduces apoptosis, and modulates leukocyte activation and adhesion.** (Jon, 2000) (Thackham et al., 2007) (Sen, 2009)

Systemically, **hyperbaric oxygen (HBO) increases bone marrow–derived endothelial progenitor cell mobilization.**

Although direct evidence of homing to the wound is lacking, there may be a correlation between increased circulating EPC and enhanced wound healing in diabetic patients.

**It is understood that ROS signaling is fundamental to HBOT** but the exact manner in which HBOT modulates ROS signaling pathways in the wound and protects ischemic tissue from oxidative stress remains unclear. (Thom, 2009)

Although upregulation of antioxidant enzyme activity by HBO preconditioning has an important role in the generation of tolerance against brain and heart ischemia-reperfusion injury, a clear understanding of HBOT's cellular and molecular mechanisms in cutaneous wound healing is lacking. (Zhang et al., 2005)

**HBOT-induced MMP9 is known to be an important mediator for endothelial progenitor cell migration at the systemic level.** (Liu and Velazquez, 2008)

**HBOT is indicated for treating compromised flaps and grafts and to enhance healing in selected problem wounds, i.e., delayed effects of radiation and refractory diabetic wounds.**

In ischemic wounds, neutrophils and macrophages are the major source of EMODs, with gp91-phox (Nox 2) in phagocytes being the primary source of SA and iNOS producing high levels of NO. (Wlaschek and Scharffetter-Kochanek, 2005)

We propose that HBO treatment of ischemic wounds transiently increases EMOD levels, activating the negative feedback loop that downregulates the inducing enzymes (less production of EMODs) and upregulates the antioxidant enzymes (increased removal of EMODs) thereby limiting subsequent higher levels of EMOD production.

**HBOT corrected the dysfunction of ROS-related signals in ischemic wounds, changing the molecular pattern to closely resemble the acute non-ischemic wounds.**

In conclusion, high oxidative stress exists in ischemic cutaneous wound tissue. Although the complex and often contradictory nature of ROS/RNS signaling is difficult to explain and is highly dependent on local concentration and timing, we have demonstrated that **HBOT provides a stimulus that promotes endogenous antioxidants to establish a therapeutic balance of oxidants and antioxidants, decreasing net oxygen radical production by means of negative feedback.**

The effect of HBOT on the ROS/MAPK/MMP axis alters the MMP/TIMP balance to increase extracellular matrix deposition. (Zhang, Gould, 2014)

Prof Randolph M. Howes MD,PhD

## HBOT increases EMODs in blood of humans

**Hyperbaric oxygen therapy increases free radical levels in the blood of humans.**

### Abstract

It has been postulated that exposure to high concentrations of oxygen results in increased oxygen radical production which may account for the toxic effects of excessive exposure to oxygen.

**Examination of blood from persons undergoing hyperbaric oxygen (HBO) exposure, by low temperature electron spin resonance (ESR) spectroscopy, demonstrated a marked increase in the magnitude of a signal with properties consistent with a free radical** (g = 2.006).

The signal diminished to baseline levels within 10 minutes of cessation of HBO exposure.

**Further in vitro studies of blood revealed an ESR signal generated in red blood cells by oxygen, and dependent on oxyhaemoglobin, which had characteristics indistinguishable from those of the ESR signal of ascorbate radical and the signal in blood from persons undergoing HBO exposure.**

It is postulated that HBO exposure increases ascorbate radical levels in blood, which is likely to reflect increased ascorbate turnover in human red blood cells. (Narkowicz, Vial, McCartney, 1993)

## Oxygen in wound healing--more than a nutrient

### Abstract

This article provides an overview of the role of oxygen in wound healing. The understanding of this role has undergone a major evolution from its long-recognized importance as an essential factor for oxidative metabolism, to its recognition as an **important cell signal interacting with growth factors and other signals to regulate signal transduction pathways**. Our laboratory has been engaged in the study of animal models of skin ischemia to explore in vivo the

154

impact of hypoxia as well as the use of oxygen as a therapeutic agent either alone or in combination with other agents such as growth factors. **We have demonstrated a synergistic effect of systemic hyperbaric oxygen and growth factors that has been substantiated by Hunt's group.** Within the past 10 years research in the field of wound healing has given new insight into the mechanism of action of hypoxia and hyperoxia as modifiers of the normal time-course of wound healing. The article concludes with a discussion of why hypoxia and hyperoxia play an important role in wound healing. Hypoxia-inducible factor 1 is crucial in that interplay. (Tandara, Mistoe, 2003)

## HBOT for surgical and traumatic wounds

**Hyperbaric oxygen therapy is used for treating acute surgical and traumatic wounds.**

### Abstract

### BACKGROUND:

Hyperbaric oxygen therapy (HBOT) is used as a treatment for acute wounds (such as those arising from surgery and trauma) however, the effects of HBOT on wound healing are unclear.

### OBJECTIVES:

To determine the effects of HBOT on the healing of acute surgical and traumatic wounds.

### SEARCH STRATEGY:

We searched the Cochrane Wounds Group Specialised Register (25 August 2010), the Cochrane Central Register of Controlled Trials (CENTRAL) (The Cochrane Library 2010, Issue 3), Ovid MEDLINE (1950 to August Week 2 2010 ), Ovid MEDLINE (In-Process & Other Non-Indexed Citations August 24, 2010), Ovid EMBASE (1980 to 2010, Week 33) and EBSCO CINAHL (1982 to 20 August 2010).

### SELECTION CRITERIA:

Randomized controlled trials (RCTs) comparing HBOT with other interventions or comparisons between alternative HBOT regimens.

Prof Randolph M. Howes MD, PhD

## DATA COLLECTION AND ANALYSIS:

Two review authors conducted selection of trials, risk of bias assessment, data extraction and data synthesis independently. Any disagreements were referred to a third review author.

## MAIN RESULTS:

Three trials involving 219 participants were included. The studies were clinically heterogeneous, therefore a meta-analysis was inappropriate. One trial (48 participants with burn wounds undergoing split skin grafts) compared HBOT with usual care and reported a significantly higher complete graft survival associated with HBOT (95% healthy graft area risk ratio (RR) 3.50; 95% confidence interval (CI) 1.35 to 9.11). A second trial (36 participants with crush injuries) reported significantly more wounds healed with HBOT than with sham HBOT (RR 1.70; 95% CI 1.11 to 2.61) and fewer additional surgical procedures required with HBOT: RR 0.25; 95% CI 0.06 to 1.02 and significantly less tissue necrosis: RR 0.13; 95% CI 0.02 to 0.90). A third trial (135 people undergoing flap grafting) reported no significant differences in complete graft survival with HBOT compared with dexamethasone (RR 1.14; 95% CI 0.95 to 1.38) or heparin (RR 1.21; 95% CI 0.99 to 1.49). Many of the predefined secondary outcomes of the review, including mortality, pain scores, quality of life, patient satisfaction, activities daily living, increase in transcutaneous oxygen pressure (TcpO(2)), amputation, length of hospital stay and costs, were not reported. All three trials were at unclear or high risk of bias.

## AUTHORS' CONCLUSIONS:

There is a lack of high quality, valid research evidence regarding the effects of HBOT on wound healing. Whilst two small trials suggested that HBOT may improve the outcomes of skin grafting and trauma these trials were at risk of bias. Further evaluation by means of high quality RCTs is needed. (Eskes et al, 2010)

This is one of a few negative comments on HBOT and wound healing and skin grafting that I have seen.

### HBOT review in acute wounds

**Hyperbaric oxygen therapy: solution for difficult to heal acute wounds? Systematic review**

## Abstract

### BACKGROUND:

Hyperbaric oxygen therapy (HBOT) is used to treat various wound types. However, the possible beneficial and harmful effects of HBOT for acute wounds are unclear.

### METHODS:

We undertook a systematic review to evaluate the effectiveness of HBOT compared to other interventions on wound healing and adverse effects in patients with acute wounds. To detect all available randomized controlled trials (RCTs) we searched five relevant databases up to March 2010. Trial selection, quality assessment, data extraction, and data synthesis were conducted by two of the authors independently.

### RESULTS:

We included five trials, totaling **360 patients.** These trials, with some methodologic flaws, included different kinds of wounds and focused on different outcome parameters, which prohibited meta-analysis.

A French trial (n = 36 patients) reported that **significantly more crush wounds healed with HBOT than with sham HBOT**.

Moreover, **there were significantly fewer additional surgical procedures required with HBOT, and there was significantly less tissue necrosis.**

In one of two American trials (n = 141) **burn wounds healed significantly quicker with HBOT (P < 0.005) than with routine burn care**.

A British trial (n = 48) compared HBOT with usual care. **HBOT resulted in a significantly higher percentage of healthy graft area in split skin grafts**.

In a Chinese trial (n = 145) HBOT did not significantly improve flap survival in patients with limb skin defects.

### CONCLUSIONS:

**HBOT, if readily available, appears effective for the management of acute, difficult to heal wounds.** (Eskes et al, 2011)

## HBOT for traumatic brain injury

**Hyperbaric oxygen therapy aids the adjunctive treatment of traumatic brain injury.**

## Abstract

## BACKGROUND:

Traumatic brain injury is a common health problem with significant effect on quality of life. Each year in the USA approximately 0.56% of the population suffer a head injury, with a case fatality rate of about 40% for severe injuries. These account for a high proportion of deaths in young adults. In the USA, 2% of the population live with long-term disabilities following head injuries. The major causes are motor vehicle crashes, falls, and violence (including attempted suicide).

Hyperbaric oxygen therapy (HBOT) is the therapeutic administration of 100% oxygen at environmental pressures greater than 1 atmosphere absolute (ATA). This involves placing the patient in an airtight vessel, increasing the pressure within that vessel, and administering 100% oxygen for respiration. In this way, it is possible to deliver a greatly increased partial pressure of oxygen to the tissues.

**HBOT can improve oxygen supply to the injured brain, reduce the swelling associated with low oxygen levels and reduce the volume of brain that will ultimately perish**.

It is, therefore, possible that adding HBOT to the standard intensive care regimen may reduce patient death and disability. However, a concern for patients and families is that using HBOT may result in preventing a patient from dying only to leave them in a vegetative state, entirely dependent on medical care. **There are also some potential adverse effects of the therapy, including damage to the ears, sinuses and lungs from the effects of the pressure and oxygen poisoning**, so the benefits and risks of the therapy need to be carefully evaluated.

## OBJECTIVES:

To assess the effects of adjunctive HBOT for traumatic brain injury.

## SEARCH METHODS:

We searched CENTRAL, MEDLINE, EMBASE, CINAHL and DORCTHIM electronic databases. We also searched the reference lists of eligible articles, handsearched relevant journals and contacted researchers. All searches were updated to March 2012.

## SELECTION CRITERIA:

Randomized studies comparing the effect of therapeutic regimens which included HBOT with those that did not, for people with traumatic brain injury.

## DATA COLLECTION AND ANALYSIS:

Three authors independently evaluated trial quality and extracted data.

## MAIN RESULTS:

Seven studies are included in this review, involving 571 people (285 receiving HBOT and 286 in the control group). The results of two studies indicate use of HBOT results in a statistically significant decrease in the proportion of people with an unfavorable outcome one month after treatment using the **Glasgow Outcome Scale (GOS)** (relative risk (RR) for unfavorable outcome with HBOT 0.74, 95% CI 0.61 to 0.88, $P = 0.001$). This five-point scale rates the outcome from one (dead) to five (good recovery); an 'unfavorable' outcome was considered as a score of one, two or three. Pooled data from final follow-up showed a significant reduction in the risk of dying when HBOT was used (RR 0.69, 95% CI 0.54 to 0.88, $P = 0.003$) and suggests we would have to treat seven patients to avoid one extra death (number needed to treat (NNT) 7, 95% CI 4 to 22). Two trials suggested favorably lower intracranial pressure in people receiving HBOT and in whom myringotomies had been performed. The results from one study suggested a mean difference (MD) with myringotomy of -8.2 mmHg. The Glasgow Coma Scale (GCS) has a total of 15 points, and two small trials reported a significant improvement in GCS for patients treated with HBOT (MD 2.68 points, 95%CI 1.84 to 3.52, $P < 0.0001$), although these two trials showed considerable heterogeneity ($I(2) = 83\%$). Two studies reported an incidence of 13% for significant pulmonary impairment in the HBOT group versus 0% in the non-HBOT group ($P = 0.007$). In general, the studies were small and carried a significant risk of bias. None described adequate randomization procedures or allocation concealment, and none of the patients or treating staff were blinded to treatment.

Prof Randolph M. Howes MD,PhD

## AUTHORS' CONCLUSIONS:

**In people with traumatic brain injury, while the addition of HBOT may reduce the risk of death and improve the final Glasgow Coma Scale (GCS), there is little evidence that the survivors have a good outcome.**

The improvement of 2.68 points in GCS is difficult to interpret. This scale runs from three (deeply comatose and unresponsive) to 15 (fully conscious), and the clinical importance of an improvement of approximately three points will vary dramatically with the starting value (for example an improvement from 12 to 15 would represent an important clinical benefit, but an improvement from three to six would leave the patient with severe and highly dependent impairment). **The routine application of HBOT to these patients cannot be justified from this review.** Given the modest number of patients, methodological shortcomings of included trials and poor reporting, the results should be interpreted cautiously. An appropriately powered trial of high methodological rigor is required to define which patients, if any, can be expected to benefit most from HBOT. (Bennett, Trytko, Jonker, 2012)

## Can HBOT prevent deep infections in scoliosis surgery?

## Can hyperbaric oxygen be used to prevent deep infections in neuro-muscular scoliosis surgery?

### Abstract

### BACKGROUND:

The prevalence of postoperative wound infection in patients with neuromuscular scoliosis surgery is significantly higher than that in patients with other spinal surgery. Hyperbaric oxygen has been used as a supplement to treat post surgical infections. Our aim was to determine beneficiary effects of hyperbaric oxygen treatment in terms of prevention of postoperative deep infection in this specific group of patients in a retrospective study.

### METHODS:

Forty two neuromuscular scoliosis cases, operated between 2006-2011 were retrospectively reviewed. Patients who had presence of scoliosis and/or kyphosis in addition to cerebral palsy or myelomeningocele,

160

postoperative follow-up >1 year and posterior only surgery were the subjects of this study. Eighteen patients formed the Hyperbaric oxygen prophylaxis (P-HBO) group and 24, the control group. The P-HBO group received 30 sessions of HBO and standard antibiotic prophylaxis postoperative, and the control group (received standard antibiotic prophylaxis).

## RESULTS:

In the P-HBO group of 18 patients, the etiology was cerebral palsy in 13 and myelomeningocele in 5 cases with a mean age of 16.7 (11-27 yrs). The average follow-up was 20.4 months (12-36mo). The etiology of patients in the control group was cerebral palsy in 17, and myelomeningocele in 7 cases. The average age was 15.3 years (8-32 yrs). The average follow-up was 38.7 months (18-66mo). The overall incidence of infection in the whole study group was 11.9% (5/42). The infection rate in the P-HBO and the control group were 5.5% (1/18), and 16.6% (4/24) respectively.

**The use of HBO was found to significantly decrease the incidence of postoperative infections in neuromuscular scoliosis patients.**

## CONCLUSION:

In this study we found that **hyperbaric oxygen has a possibility to reduce the rate of post-surgical deep infections in complex spine deformity in high risk neuromuscular patients.** (Inanmaz et al, 2014)

## HBO, vasculogenic stem cells, and wound healing

### Abstract

### SIGNIFICANCE:

Oxidative stress is recognized as playing a role in stem cell mobilization from peripheral sites and also cell function.

### RECENT ADVANCES:

This review focuses on the impact of hyperoxia on vasculogenic stem cells and elements of wound healing.

## CRITICAL ISSUES:

Components of the wound-healing process in which oxidative stress has a positive impact on the various cells involved in wound healing are highlighted. A slightly different view of wound-healing physiology is adopted by departing from the often used notion of sequential stages: hemostatic, inflammatory, proliferative, and remodeling and instead organizes the cascade of wound healing as overlapping events or waves pertaining to reactive oxygen species, lactate, and nitric oxide. This was done because **hyperoxia has effects of a number of cell signaling events that converge to influence cell recruitment/chemotaxis and gene regulation/protein synthesis responses which mediate wound healing.**

## FUTURE DIRECTIONS:

Our alternative perspective of the stages of wound healing eases recognition of the multiple sites where oxidative stress has an impact on wound healing. This aids the focus on mechanistic events and the interplay among various cell types and biochemical processes. It also highlights the areas where additional research is needed. (Fosen, Thom, 2014)

### Ozone a new medical drug

12-1-12   by Velio Bocci

Oxygen-ozone therapy is a complementary approach less known than homeopathy and acupuncture because it has come of age only three decades ago. Bocci's book clarifies that, in the often nebulous field of natural medicine, the biological bases of ozone therapy are totally in line with classic biochemical, physiological and pharmacological knowledge.

**Ozone is an oxidizing molecule, a sort of superactive oxygen, which, by reacting with blood components, generates a number of chemical messengers responsible for activating crucial biological functions such as oxygen delivery, immune activation, release of hormones and induction of antioxidant enzymes,** which is an exceptional property for correcting the chronic oxidative stress present in atherosclerosis, diabetes, infections and cancer.

Moreover, **ozone therapy, by inducing nitric oxide synthase, may mobilize endogenous stem cells,** which will promote regeneration of ischemic tissues.

The description of these phenomena offers the first comprehensive picture for understanding how ozone works and why, when properly used as a real drug within the therapeutic range, not only **does not procure adverse effects** but yields a feeling of wellness. Half of the book describes the value of ozone therapy in several diseases, particularly cutaneous infections and vascular diseases where ozone really behaves as a "wonder" drug.

## Penn study finds HBOT mobilize stem cells

12-28-05

According to a study to be published in *The American Journal of Physiology-Heart and Circulation Physiology*, **a typical course of hyperbaric oxygen treatments increases by eight-fold the number of stem cells circulating in a patient's body**. Stem cells, also called **progenitor cells** are crucial to injury repair. The study is scheduled for publication in the April 2006 edition of the *American Journal*.

Stem cells exist in the bone marrow of human beings and animals and are capable of changing their nature to become part of many different organs and tissues.

In response to injury, these cells move from the bone marrow to the injured sites, where they differentiate into cells that assist in the healing process.

The movement, or mobilization, of stem cells can be triggered by a variety of stimuli – including pharmaceutical agents and hyperbaric oxygen treatments.

Where as drugs are associated with a host of side effects, **hyperbaric oxygen treatments carry a significantly lower risk of such effects.**

"This is the safest way clinically to increase stem cell circulation, far safer than any of the pharmaceutical options," said **Stephen Thom, MD, PhD**, Professor of Emergency Medicine at the **University of Pennsylvania School of Medicine** and lead author of the study. "This study provides information on the fundamental mechanisms for hyperbaric oxygen and offers a new theoretical therapeutic option for mobilizing stem cells."

"We reproduced the observations from humans in animals in order to identify the mechanism for the hyperbaric oxygen effect," added Thom.

**"We found that hyperbaric oxygen mobilizes stem/progenitor cells because it increases synthesis of a molecule called nitric oxide in the bone marrow.** This synthesis is thought to trigger enzymes that mediate stem/progenitor cell release."

Hopefully, future study of hyperbaric oxygen's role in mobilizing stem cells will provide a wide array of treatments for combating injury and disease.

**I believe that stem cell stimulation is a point of commonality with ozone therapy, hyperbaric oxygen therapy and PDT. Thom had been reporting this since 2005.**

# SECTION FIVE

## HBO MECHANISMS

The following paper was adapted from: (Thom, 2011)

### Hyperbaric oxygen – its mechanisms and efficacy

This paper outlines therapeutic mechanisms of hyperbaric oxygen therapy ($HBO_2$) and reviews data on its efficacy for clinical problems seen by plastic and reconstructive surgeons.

**Principal mechanisms of $HBO_2$ are based on intracellular generation of reactive species of oxygen (ROS, EMODs) and nitrogen (RNS).**

Reactive species are recognized to play a central role in cell signal transduction cascades.

Systematic reviews and randomized clinical trials support clinical use of $HBO_2$ for refractory diabetic wound healing and radiation injuries; treatment of compromised flaps and grafts and ischemia-reperfusion disorders is supported by animal studies and a small number of clinical trials.

### Conclusions

Clinical and mechanistic data support use of hyperbaric oxygen for a variety of disorders.

## Introduction

Hyperbaric oxygen ($HBO_2$) therapy is a treatment modality in which a person breathes 100% $O_2$ while exposed to increased atmospheric pressure. $HBO_2$ treatment is carried out in either a mono- (single person) or multi-place (typically 2 to 14 patients) chamber.

Pressures applied while in the chamber are usually 2 to 3 atmospheres absolute (ATA), the sum of the atmospheric pressure (1 ATA) plus additional hydrostatic pressure equivalent to one or two atmospheres (1 atmosphere = a pressure of 14.7 pounds per square inch or 101 kPa). Treatments are usually about 1.5 to 2 hours long, depending on the indication and may be performed one to three times daily. Monoplace chambers are usually compressed with pure $O_2$.

Multiplace chambers are pressurized with air and patients breathe pure $O_2$ through a tight-fitting face mask, a hood, or an endotracheal tube. **During treatment, the arterial $O_2$ tension often exceeds 2000 mmHg and levels of 200 to 400 mmHg occur in tissues**. (ATA, 1977)

The initial effect of pressurizing the human body is intuitively obvious - elevating hydrostatic pressure increases partial pressure of gases and causes a reduction in the volume of gas-filled spaces according to Boyle's law.

Gas volume reduction has direct relevance to treating pathological conditions in which gas bubbles are present in the body, such as arterial gas embolism and decompression sickness. The majority of patients who undergo $HBO_2$ therapy are not treated for bubble-induced injuries hence therapeutic mechanisms are related to an elevated $O_2$ partial pressure.

**It is well accepted that breathing greater than 1 ATA $O_2$ will increase production of reactive oxygen species (ROS, EMODs).** (ATA, 1977) (Thom, 1989)

This is critically important as it is the molecular basis for a number of therapeutic mechanisms. **ROS (EMODs) and also reactive nitrogen species (RNS) serve as signaling molecules in transduction cascades, or pathways, for a variety of growth factors, cytokines and hormones.** (Kemp, Go, Jones, 2008) (Circu, Aw, 2008) (Valko et al, 2007)

ROS is a collective and moderately imprecise term for $O_2$-derived free radicals as well as $O_2$-derived non-radical species such as hydrogen peroxide and hypochlorous acid.

**ROS (EMODs) are generated as part of normal metabolism** by mitochondria, endoplasmic reticulum, peroxisomes, various oxidase enzymes and phospholipid metabolism.

**ROS (EMODs) act in conjunction with several redox systems involving glutathione, thioredoxin and pyridine nucleotides, and play central roles in coordinating cell signaling and also anti-oxidant, protective pathways**. (Kemp, Go, Jones, 2008) (Circu, Aw, 2008) (Valko et al, 2007) (Zhang, Piston, Goodman, 2002)

This point is central to the ensuing discussion – **oxidative stress is not synonymous with oxygen toxicity**.

RNS include nitric oxide ( ·NO) and agents generated by reactions between ·NO, or its oxidation products, and EMODs (ROS).

Peroxide-dependent enzymes such as myeloperoxidase can catalyze reactions between nitrite, a major oxidation product of ·NO, and hydrogen peroxide or hypochlorous acid to generate oxidants such as nitryl chloride and nitrogen dioxide that are capable of nitration and S-nitrosylation reactions.

There are three nitric oxide synthase enzymes. The effect of hyperoxia on catalytic activity is reflected by values for the apparent Michaelis-Menten constant for $O_2$ and it differs among the three NOS isoforms. In part this is because enzyme activity is constrained by ferric-ferrous conversion at the active site. **As a general statement, however, hyperoxia augments RNS production**.

Consultation and advice on $HBO_2$ may be sought through the Undersea and Hyperbaric Medical Society and more locally with board-certified physicians. (Mathieu, 2006) (Neuman, Thom, 2008) (Gesell, 2008)

Undersea and Hyperbaric Medicine sub-specialty certification is obtainable through the American Board of Medical Specialists.

## Wound healing

---

**HBO$_2$ is used to treat refractory diabetic lower extremity wounds and delayed radiation injuries**. Clearly, the pathophysiology of these disorders differs but they share several elements include depletion of epithelial and stromal cells, chronic inflammation, fibrosis, an imbalance or abnormalities in extracellular matrix components and remodeling processes, and impaired keratinocyte functions.

Diabetic wound healing is also impaired by decreased growth factor production, while in post-radiation tissues there appears to be an imbalance between factors mediating fibrosis versus normal tissue healing.

### Clinical efficacy of HBO$_2$

Wound healing HBO$_2$ protocols involve daily treatments of 1.5 to 2 hours for 20 to 40 days. The effectiveness of HBO$_2$ as an adjuvant therapy for diabetic lower extremity ulcerations can be examined from the perspective of hastened healing and also reduced risk of major amputations.

This is the era of meta-analysis and despite drawbacks with these evaluations they are used regularly as a final judgment on efficacy of an intervention. According to the most recent evaluation, employing HBO$_2$ as a component to refractory diabetic wound management decreases risk of a major amputation with an odds ratio of 0.236 [95% confidence interval (CI) 0.133 – 0.418].

**Adjunctive use of HBO$_2$ as a component to diabetic wound care improves healing** with an odds ratio of 11.64. This analysis was based on clinical trials conducted through 2007.

The results continue to demonstrate that **HBO$_2$ markedly improves outcome**.

Another meta-analysis concluded that **only four patients needed to be treated with HBO$_2$ to prevent one amputation**. (Kranke et al, 2004)

Since this publication, two additional groups have reported benefits to use of $HBO_2$; one was a **double-blinded randomized trial**. (Duzgun et al, 2008) (Londahl et al, 2010)

The results continue to demonstrate that $HBO_2$ improves outcome. The double blinded trial was a single-center study that enrolled individuals with diabetes foot ulcers. Individuals were randomized to receive either $HBO_2$ (100% oxygen, 2.5 ATA for 85 minutes five days per week for 8-weeks) or control (room air, 2.5 ATA for 85 minutes five days per week for 8-weeks) and good wound care. **The outcome was a healed wound by 12 months after the commencement of therapy.** A total of 99 individuals were evaluated, 38 received HBO and 37 received control therapy. By one year of follow up 52% of those receiving $HBO_2$ healed and 29% of those receiving control (p=0.03).

**The benefit of $HBO_2$ for radiation injury also has been shown in randomized trials and its utilization supported by independent evidence-based reviews.** (Bennett et al, 2008) (Clarke et al, 2008) (Marx, Johnson, Kline, 1985)

It is important to state that for both diabetic wounds and radiation injuries, $HBO_2$ is used in conjunction with standard wound care management techniques.

## Mechanisms of action

**Animal trials have documented wound healing benefits of $HBO_2$.** (Marx et al, 1990) (Gallagher et al, 2007) (Zhang et al, 2008) (Goldstein et al, 2006)

The basis for its efficacy continues to be investigated and appears to be a combination of systemic events as well as local alterations within the wound margin.

Neovascularization occurs by two processes. Regional angiogenic stimuli influence the efficiency of new blood vessel growth by local endothelial cells (termed angiogenesis) and they stimulate the recruitment and differentiation of circulating **stem/progenitor cells (SPCs)** to form vessels de novo in a process termed **vasculogenesis**. (Carmekiet, 2000) (Hattori et al, 2001) (Tepper et al, 2005)

$HBO_2$ has effects on both these processes.

Bone marrow eNOS activity is required for SPCs mobilization and this is compromised by diabetes.

Radiation, chemotherapy and several other factors also diminish SPCs mobilization, although mechanisms for these effects are unclear. By stimulating ·NO synthesis in bone marrow, $HBO_2$ mobilizes SPCs in normal humans, patients previously exposed to radiation and in diabetics.

Importantly, in contrast to SPCs mobilization stimulated by infusion of growth factors; **$HBO_2$ does not concomitantly elevate the circulating leukocyte count which may be thrombogenic.** (Powell et al, 2005)

**In animal models, stem/progenitor cells (SPCs) mobilized by $HBO_2$ home to wounds and accelerate healing.** (Gu et al, 2008)

Separate from its effect on SPCs mobilization, **$HBO_2$-mediated oxidative stress at sites of neovascularization will stimulate stem/progenitor cells (SPCs) growth factor production.** (Hunt et al, 2007) (Milovanova et al, 2008)

This is due at least in part to augmented synthesis and stabilization of hypoxia inducible factors (HIF). (72–74) These transcription factors are heterodimers of HIF-$\alpha$ and a constitutively expressed HIF-$\beta$. It is well recognized that expression and activation of HIF-$\alpha$ subunits are tightly regulated and their degradation by the ubiquitin-proteasome pathway typically occurs when cells are replete with $O_2$.

However, whether hypoxic or normoxic conditions prevail, **free radicals are required for HIF expression.** (Semenza, 2001) (Dulak, Jozkowicz, 2003) (Schroedl et al, 2002)

$HBO_2$ elevates HIF-1 and -2 levels in vasculogenic SPCs because of increases in ROS.

**One consequence of ROS (EMOD)-mediated stress is augmented production of the antioxidant thioredoxin and one of its regulatory enzymes, thioredoxin reductase.** (Milovanova et al, 2008)

Thioredoxin can act as a transcription factor and in SPCs appears to be the proximal species responsible for promoting the expression and activity of HIFs. HIF-1 and -2 then stimulate transcription of many genes involved with neovascularization. A physiological oxidative stress that triggers the same pathway is lactate metabolism.

**Pluripotent mesenchymal stem cells were shown *in vitro* to be stimulated by HBO$_2$ to synthesize placental growth factor. This too is an EMOD-dependent phenomenon and will significantly increase cell migratory and tube formation functions.** (Shyu et al, 2008)

Microvascular endothelial cells exposed to HBO$_2$ in *ex vivo* studies up-regulate a variety of protein damage-control pathways that lead to enhanced oxidative stress resistance, cell proliferation and tube formation.

HBO$_2$ does not alter circulating levels of insulin, insulin-like growth factors, or pro-inflammatory cytokines [e.g. tumor necrosis factor (TNF)-$\alpha$, interleukin (IL)-6 and IL-8] in normal healthy humans.

Vascular endothelial growth factor (VEGF) and angiopoietin, as well as stromal derived factor (SDF-1) influence SPCs homing to wounds and SPCs differentiation to endothelial cells. **Synthesis of VEGF has been shown to be increased in wounds by HBO$_2$, and it is the most specific growth factor for neovascularization.** (Sheikh et al, 2000)

**HBO$_2$ also stimulates synthesis of basic fibroblast growth factor (bFGF) and transforming growth factor $\beta$1 by human dermal fibroblasts, angiopoietin-2 by human umbilical vein endothelial cells, bFGF and hepatocyte growth factor in ischemic limbs, and it up-regulates platelet derived growth factor (PDGF) receptor in wounds.** (Kang et al, 2004) (Lin et al, 2002) (Asano et al, 2007) (Bonomo et al, 1998)

**Extracellular matrix formation is closely linked to neovascularization and it is another O$_2$-dependent process.** (Hopf et al, 2005)

Enhanced collagen synthesis and cross-linking by HBO$_2$ have been described, but whether changes are linked to the O$_2$-dependence of fibroblast hydroxylases, alteration in balance of wound growth factors, metalloproteinases and/or inhibitors of metalloproteases, is as yet **unclear**.

Before leaving the subject of wound healing, mention should be made of conflicting data and where further work is needed. The influence HBO$_2$ has on HIF isoform expression appears to vary with different tissues and possibly with chronology [e.g. looking early or late after wounding or an ischemic insult].

One recent model showing accelerated wound healing by $HBO_2$ reported lower HIF-1 levels at wound margins, along with reduced inflammation and fewer apoptotic cells. In contrast, higher levels of HIF-1 have been linked to elevated VEGF in wounds in response to hyperoxia. (Hunt et al, 2007)

With regard to diabetes, there is a complex interplay present between ROS and RNS.

Impairments in eNOS function are related to hyperglycemia, insulin resistance, impaired enzyme synthesis, disordered caveolin associations and enhanced protein kinase C activity.

**Production of $O_2\cdot$ is augmented in diabetes and this will reduce bioavailability of $\cdot$NO because the two radicals react rapidly to generate alternative RNS.** (Koppenol et al, 1992) (Beckman, Kippenol, 1996)

Disordered balance between $O_2\cdot$ and $\cdot$NO is reflected by elevated levels of nitrotyrosine in plasma of type II diabetics. Data from diabetic animals and humans indicate that $HBO_2$ can overcome some aspects of eNOS inhibition but it is doubtful that all issues have been resolved. (Gallagher et al, 2007) (Thom, Milovanova, 2008)

To summarize, **$HBO_2$ can stimulate healing in refractory wounds and irradiated tissues.**

Therapy for refractory diabetic wounds is likely to reduce the risk of lower extremity amputation by 2 to 3 times, with an absolute rate of major amputation reductions of about 20% (e.g., 11% versus 32%) and a number needed to treat of about 4. With respect to cost-effectiveness, a study from Canada indicated that over a 12-year period, the use of $HBO_2$ should save about $9,000 in overall costs to the care of a patient with diabetes.

The common mechanistic theme for both indications is **oxidative stress responses improve neovascularization events.**

**Cells within the wound exhibit increased collagen synthesis, growth factors production, improved cell migration and tube-formation functions.**

**A separate free radical-based mechanism for augmentation of neovascularization by $HBO_2$ is through SPCs. Hyperoxia stimulates bone marrow SPCs mobilization and also improves their functions** once they home to peripheral sites.

## Compromised Flaps and Grafts

HBO$_2$ is used on occasion to treat compromised flaps and grafts, a practice supported by Guidelines from the Undersea and Hyperbaric Medical Society.

**A comprehensive review of HBO$_2$ use for flaps and grafts was recently published.** (Friedman et al, 2006)

There is no need to recapitulate the information except to say that there is one prospective, blinded clinical trial. **Administration of HBO$_2$ prior to and for three days following skin grafting led to a significant 29% improvement in graft survival.** (Perrins, Cantab, 1967)

A problem with this trial, however, is that the success in the control arm of the study was markedly less that one would expect in current practice. As was emphasized in the review, support for use of HBO$_2$ in flap/graft compromise comes from a very large number of animal studies. Comparative clinical trials support its use but more work is needed. (Roje et al, 2008)

## Reperfusion injuries and HBO$_2$

**Clinical studies have documented significant survival enhancement with HBO$_2$ for extremity re-implantation and free tissue transfer, and following crush injury.** (Bouachour et al, 1996) (Waterhouse et al, 1993)

As is the case with flaps and grafts, however, the amount of controlled clinical data is small and insufficient to perform an evidence-based assessment of HBO$_2$ efficacy. None-the-less, the breadth of clinical experience across a variety of disorders should spur closer assessment of its use.

**Clinical trials have shown that HBO$_2$ can reduce coronary artery re-stenosis after balloon angioplasty/stenting,** (Sharifi et al, 2004) (Sharifi et al, 2002) **decrease muscle loss after thrombolytic treatment for myocardial infarction,** (Dekleva et al, 2004) (Shandling et al, 1997) (Stavitsky et al, 1998) **improve hepatic survival after transplantation and lead to more rapid return of**

**donor liver function** (Mazariegos et al, 1999) (Suehiro et al, 2008) and **reduced the incidence of encephalopathy seen after cardiopulmonary bypass and following carbon monoxide poisoning.** (Alex et al, 2005) (Weaver et al, 2002)

In contrast to protocols for wound healing, **HBO$_2$ treatments for reperfusion injuries are done for just a few days rather than weeks; they are performed at higher O$_2$ partial pressures (~2.5 to 3.0 ATA) and may occur multiple times in the same day.**

An early event associated with post-ischemic tissue reperfusion is adherence of circulating neutrophils to vascular endothelium by $\beta_2$ integrins.

**When animals or humans are exposed to HBO$_2$ at 2.8 to 3.0 ATA for at least 45 minutes, the ability of circulating neutrophils to adhere to target tissues is temporarily inhibited.** (Kalns et al, 2002) (Labouche et al, 1999) (Thom, 1993) (Zamboni et al, 1993)

In animal models, HBO$_2$-mediated inhibition of neutrophil $\beta_2$ integrin adhesion has been shown to ameliorate reperfusion injuries of brain, heart, lung, liver, skeletal muscle and intestine, as well as smoke-induced lung injury and encephalopathy due to carbon monoxide poisoning.

It also appears that **benefits of HBO$_2$ in decompression sickness are related to the temporary inhibition of neutrophil $\beta_2$ integrins,** in addition to the Boyle's Law-mediated reduction in bubble volume as discussed in the introduction. (Martin, Thom, 2002)

**Exposure to HBO$_2$ inhibits neutrophil $\beta_2$ integrin function because hyperoxia increases synthesis of reactive species derived from iNOS and myeloperoxidase,** leading to excessive S-nitrosylation of cytoskeletal $\beta$ actin. (Thom, Bhopale, 2008)

This modification increases the concentration of short, non-cross-linked filamentous (F)-actin which alters F-actin distribution within the cell.

**HBO$_2$ does not reduce neutrophil viability and functions such as degranulation, phagocytosis and oxidative burst in response to chemoattractants remain intact.** (Juttner et al, 2003) (Thom, Mendiguren, Hardy et al, 1997)

Inhibiting $\beta_2$ integrins with monoclonal antibodies will also ameliorate ischemia-reperfusion injuries but **in contrast to HBO$_2$, antibody therapy causes profound immunocompromise.**

$HBO_2$ does not inhibit neutrophil antibacterial functions because the G-protein coupled 'inside-out' pathway for activation (such as that triggered by endotoxin) remains intact, and actin S-nitrosylation is reversed as a component of this activation process.

Probably the most compelling evidence that $HBO_2$ does not cause immunocompromise comes from **studies in sepsis models, where $HBO_2$ has a beneficial effect.** (Buras et al, 2006) (Ross, McAllister, 1965) (Thom, Lauermann, Hart, 1986)

**A separate anti-inflammatory pathway for $HBO_2$ involves impaired pro-inflammatory cytokine production by monocyte-macrophages.** This action has been shown in animal models and human beings. (Benson et al, 2003) (Lahat et al, 1995) (Weisz et al, 1997)

The effect on monocyte/macrophages may be the basis for reduced levels of circulating pro-inflammatory cytokines under stress conditions. **The molecular mechanism is unknown,** but could be related to $HBO_2$-mediated enhancement of heme oxygenase-1 and heat shock proteins (HSP). Hence, **once again, an oxidative stress response seems to occur.**

Finally, **$HBO_2$ has been shown in numerous models to augment ischemic tolerance of brain, spinal cord, liver, heart and skeletal muscle by mechanisms involving induction of antioxidant enzymes and anti-inflammatory proteins.** (Gregorevic, Lynch, Williams, 2001) (Hirata et al, 2007) (Kim et al, 2001) (Nie et al, 2006) (Yu et al, 2005)

A common theme among some studies is alterations in HIF-1 production but, as was the case in wound healing models, timing of $HBO_2$ application appears to influence cellular responses.

In several models, **exposure to $HBO_2$ ameliorates post-ischemic injuries by decreasing HIF-1 expression.** (Calvert et al, 2006) (Li et al, 2005)

When $HBO_2$ is used in a prophylactic manner to induce ischemic tolerance, however, its mechanism appears related to up-regulation of HIF-1 and at least one of its target genes, **erythropoietin.** (Gu et al, 2008)

In review, **oxidative stress responses triggered by $HBO_2$ improve outcome from a wide variety of post-ischemic/inflammatory insults.**

**HBO₂ also improves ischemic tolerance when used in a pro-phylactic manner.**

**Augmented synthesis of reactive species (EMODs) temporar-ily inhibits adherence/sequestration of neutrophils by inhibit-ing β₂ integrin function and in many tissues HBO₂ will induce antioxidant enzymes and anti-inflammatory proteins.**

## Treatment risks

This review has emphasized the positive aspects of HBO₂-induced reactive species, but **there is clearly a potential for negative effects.**

**The risks for O₂ toxicity depend on the concentration and in-tracellular localization of reactive species.**

Because exposure to hyperoxia in clinical HBO₂ protocols is rather brief, **studies show that antioxidant defenses are adequate so that biochemical stresses related to increases in reactive spe-cies (EMODs) are reversible.** (Narkowicz, Vial, McCartney, 1993) (Dennog et al, 1999) (Dennog et al, 1996) (Rothfuss, Radermacher, Speit, 2001)

Treatments often include so-called **air breaks,** where a patient breathes just air for 5 minutes once or twice through the course of a treatment.

This intervention has been demonstrated to enhance pulmonary O₂ tolerance. **CNS O₂ toxicity is manifested as a grand mal seizure. This occurs at an incidence of approximately 1 to 4 in 10,000 patient treatments.** (Hart, Strauss, 1987) (Davis, Dunn, Heimbach, 1988) (Plafki et al, 2000)

**Pathological changes in association with isolated O₂-mediated seizures have not been found in studies with guinea pigs, rab-bits and humans.** (Clark, 2008)

**Progressive myopia has been reported in patients who under-go prolonged daily therapy, but this typically reverses within 6 weeks after termination of treatments.** (Lyne, 1978)

**Development of nuclear cataracts has been reported with ex-cessive treatments that exceed a total of 150 to 200 hours, and**

**the change does not spontaneously reverse.** (Palmquist, Philipson, Barr, 1984)

## Summary

This brief review has highlighted some of the beneficial actions of $HBO_2$ and the data that **indicate oxidative stress brought about by hyperoxia can have therapeutic effects**. While there has been substantial advancement of the field in recent years, more work is required to establish the place of $HBO_2$ in 21st century medicine.

**An extended discussion on other indications for $HBO_2$ can be found in recent texts.** (Mathieu, 2006) (Neuman, Thom, 2008) (Gesell, 2008)

---

## HBOT for wound healing and limb salvage: a systematic review

### Abstract

This article is a systematic review evaluating published clinical evidence of the efficacy of hyperbaric oxygen therapy (HBOT) for wound healing and limb salvage. The data source is the Ovid/Medline database for key word "Hyperbaric Oxygenation" with search limits (human studies, 1978-2008). Results were combined by Boolean AND with 1 of the 3 following searches: (a) wound healing (10 permutations); (b) compromised flap or graft (3); and (c) osteomyelitis (1). The author evaluated 620 citations, of which 64 reported original observational studies and randomized controlled trials (RCTs) on HBOT and healing outcomes. All citations with 5 subjects were selected for full text review (44 articles) and evaluated according to GRADE criteria for high, medium, low, or very low level of evidence. A Cochrane review identified 1 additional study with a low level of evidence. This systematic review discusses and tabulates every article of high or moderate level of evidence. **For patients with diabetic foot ulcers (DFU) complicated by surgical infection, HBOT reduces chance of amputation (7 studies) and improves chance of healing (6 studies).**

Positive efficacy corresponds to HBOT-induced hyperoxygenation of at-risk tissue (7 studies) as measured by transcutaneous oximetry. **HBOT is associated with remission of about 85% of cases of refractory lower extremity osteomyelitis**, but an RCT is lacking to clarify extent of effect.

There is a high level of evidence that HBOT reduces risk of amputation in the DFU population by promoting partial and full healing of problem wounds. **There is a moderate level of evidence that HBOT promotes healing of arterial ulcers, calciphylactic and refractory vasculitic ulcers, as well as refractory osteomyelitis.**

**There is a low to moderate level of evidence that HBOT promotes successful "take" of compromised flaps and grafts.** (Goldman, 2009)

## HBOT promotes healing in diabetic foot ulcers

### IGF-1 Increases with HBOT and Promotes Wound Healing in Diabetic Foot Ulcers.

### Abstract

**Objectives.** To investigate insulin-like growth factor 1 (IGF-1) levels in response to hyperbaric oxygen therapy (HBOT) for diabetic foot ulcers and to determine whether IGF-1 is a predictive indicator of wound healing in patients with diabetic foot ulcers. **Design and Methods.** We treated 48 consecutive patients with diabetic foot ulcers with HBOT. Alterations of IGF-1 levels in patients whose wound healed with HBOT were compared with those in patients who did not benefit from HBOT.

**Results.** There was no significant difference in initial IGF-1 levels between the two groups (P = 0.399). The mean IGF-1 level increased with HBOT (P < 0.05). In the healed group, the mean IGF-1 increase and the final values were significantly higher (P < 0.05). In the nonhealed group, the mean IGF-1 increase was minus and the final values were not significantly different (P < 0.05). The increase in IGF-1 level with HBOT was significantly higher in the healed group (P < 0.001).

**Conclusions. IGF-1 increased significantly in the healed group. We believe that HBOT is effective in the treatment of diabetic foot ulcers, with an elevation of IGF-1.** This alteration seems to be a predictive factor for wound healing in diabetic foot ulcers treated with HBOT. (Aydin et al, 2013)

## Cognitive improvement with 100% oxygen

### Impact of breathing 100% oxygen on radiation-induced cognitive impairment.

### Abstract

Future space missions are expected to include increased extravehicular activities (EVAs) during which astronauts are exposed to high-energy space radiation while breathing 100% oxygen. Given that brain irradiation can lead to cognitive impairment, and that oxygen is a potent radiosensitizer, there is a concern that astronauts may be at greater risk of developing cognitive impairment when exposed to space radiation while breathing 100% O(2) during an EVA.

To address this concern, unanesthetized, unrestrained, young adult male Fischer 344 × Brown Norway rats were allowed to breathe 100% O(2) for 30 min prior to, during and 2 h after whole-body irradiation with 0, 1, 3, 5 or 7 Gy doses of 18 MV X rays delivered from a medical linear accelerator at a dose rate of ~425 mGy/min. Irradiated and unirradiated rats breathing air (~21% O(2)) served as controls.

Cognitive function was assessed 9 months postirradiation using the perirhinal cortex-dependent novel object recognition task. Cognitive function was not impaired until the rats breathing either air or 100% O(2) received a whole-body dose of 7 Gy. However, **at all doses, cognitive function of the irradiated rats breathing 100% O(2) was improved over that of the irradiated rats breathing air**. These data suggest that astronauts are not at greater risk of developing cognitive impairment when exposed to space radiation while breathing 100% O(2) during an EVA. (Wheeler et al, 2014)

Prof Randolph M. Howes MD,PhD

## Oxygen in acute and chronic wound healing

## Abstract

**Oxygen is a prerequisite for successful wound healing due to the increased demand for reparative processes such as cell proliferation, bacterial defense, angiogenesis and collagen synthesis.**

Even though the role of oxygen in wound healing is not yet completely understood, **many experimental and clinical observations have shown wound healing to be impaired under hypoxia.** This article provides an overview on the role of oxygen in wound healing and chronic wound pathogenesis, a brief insight into systemic and topical oxygen treatment, and a discussion of the role of wound tissue oximetry. (Scheml et al, 2010)

## Oxygen mechanisms in wound healing

## Oxygen in wound healing: nutrient, antibiotic, signaling molecule, and therapeutic agent.

## Abstract

Disturbances to healing observed under hypoxic conditions have given insights into the roles of oxygen. Wound hypoxia is more prevalent than generally appreciated, and occurs even in patients who are free of arterial occlusive disease. **There is a strong scientific basis for oxygen treatment as prophylaxis against infection, to facilitate wound closure, and to prevent amputation in wounded patients.** This article reviews extensive data from preclinical and human trials of supplemental inhaled oxygen, hyperbaric oxygen, and topical oxygen treatment. Oxygen supports biochemical metabolism and cellular function, and has roles in combating infection and facilitating the wound healing cascade. (Eisenbud, 2012)

## Hyperbaric oxygen for chronic wounds

### Abstract

Hyperbaric oxygen therapy (HBOT), the administration of pressurized 100% oxygen, is used as an adjunct to aid healing in selected chronic wounds. Though the therapy has had a controversial history, **research is now elucidating the mechanisms by which HBOT helps to heal wounds.**

**HBOT increases growth factors and local wound signaling, while also promoting a central stem cell release of endothelial progenitor cells from the bone marrow via nitric oxide pathways.**

**The clinical data continue to accumulate in support of HBOT to help hasten wound healing, and reduce the amputation rate in diabetic ulcers.**

In appropriate patients, **HBOT is an effective, noninvasive, adjunct modality that can be used to hasten chronic wound healing.** (Goldstein, 2013)

### Evaluation of HBOT for chronic wounds

### Abstract

### BACKGROUND:

Treating chronic wounds is challenging. Despite standard wound care, some chronic wounds fail to heal. Therefore, hyperbaric oxygen therapy (HBOT) was developed as an adjunct to standard wound care.

### OBJECTIVE:

To evaluate the efficacy of HBOT for treating chronic wounds due to a variety of causes at our institution.

## METHODS:

We reviewed the medical records of patients with chronic wounds treated with HBOT in addition to standard wound care at the Department of Dermatology, Nippon Medical School Hospital, from 2009 through 2012. Twenty-nine patients were reviewed (14 men and 15 women; mean age, 64.1±14.4 years). The cause of chronic wounds was diabetes mellitus (DM) in 13 patients, venous stasis in 10, polyarteritis nodosa cutanea in 2, and livedoid vasculopathy, pyoderma gangrenosum, chronic renal failure, and systemic sclerosis in 1 patient each. **The patients underwent HBOT for 60 minutes with 100% oxygen delivered via a mask in a hyperbaric chamber pressurized to 2.8 atmospheres of absolute pressure.** The response of the chronic wounds to HBOT was evaluated according to the following criteria:"excellent": more than 90% wound healing;"good": a greater than 30% reduction in wound size, and wound healing was confirmed on follow-up visits within 6 weeks;"fair": wound healing was achieved with a combination of further invasive interventions; and "poor": the wound showed a less than 30% reduction or worsened during HBOT, or wound healing had not been completed by follow-up visits within 6 weeks.

## RESULTS:

**The response to HBOT was "excellent" in 6 patients, "good" in 8, "fair" in 11, and "poor" in 4. All 4 patients with a "poor" response had DM and had undergone hemodialysis.**

## CONCLUSIONS:

**HBOT is an effective treatment for patients with chronic wounds, due to a variety of causes,** when used in combination with conventional standard therapy or further interventions. However, **HBOT is less effective in patients with DM than in patients with venous stasis because hemodialysis, which is more common in patients with DM, has negative effects on wound healing.** (Ueno et al, 2014)

# SECTION SIX

## HBOT

### Hyperbaric Oxygen therapy (HBOT)

Some of the following materials were excerpted, adapted or modified from the following article: (Delaney, Montgomery, 2001)

Hyperbaric oxygen ($HBO_2$) is used in a sports medicine setting to reduce hypoxia and edema and appears to be particularly effective for treating crush injuries and acute traumatic peripheral ischemias. When used clinically, $HBO_2$ should be considered as an adjunctive therapy as soon as possible after injury diagnosis. **Treatment pressures for acute traumatic peripheral ischemia range from 2.0 to 2.5 atmospheres absolute (ATA), with a minimum of 90 minutes for each treatment.**

In America, $HBO_2$ chambers were first used as a treatment for deep-sea divers who experienced decompression sickness. The Undersea and Hyperbaric Medical Society (UHMS) has evaluated the use and effectiveness of $HBO_2$ for different medical conditions. Currently, the UHMS approves $HBO_2$ for 13 medical conditions as follows:

Air or gas embolism

Carbon monoxide poisoning

Clostridial myositis and myonecrosis (gas gangrene)

Crush injury, compartment syndrome, and acute traumatic ischemia

Decompression sickness

Prof Randolph M. Howes MD,PhD

Enhancement of healing in selected problem wounds

Exceptional blood loss (anemia)

Intracranial abscess

Necrotizing soft-tissue infections

Osteomyelitis (refractory)

Radiation injury (delayed)

Skin grafts and flaps (compromised)

Thermal burns

Due to the technical and physiological problems inherent with OHP, studies were undertaken in Baylor University Medical Center laboratory to determine the feasibility of administering intravascular oxygen in a regional or systemic system. This approach employees dilute concentrations of hydrogen peroxide given by a variety of routes to provide oxygen. Hydrogen peroxide under the influence of catalase and peroxidases is degraded to oxygen and water. Human blood and tissues contain excess quantities of both enzyme systems. **Hydrogen peroxide provides from 3 to 8 atmosphere equivalents of oxygen which is administered in solution**, thus avoiding the necessity of lung transport. (Urschel et al, 1965)

Photodynamic therapy (PDT) is currently approved in the palliation of locally advanced cancers and a few early-stage diseases. **It should now be included for first-line treatment in early malignant and premalignant disease, adjuvant therapy for surgery, and interstitial treatment of deep-seated tumors.** Early observations indicate that **hypoxic or anoxic conditions almost completely reduce the antitumor effectiveness of PDT in vitro.** (Henderson and Fingar, 1987)

In other studies it was demonstrated that **hyperbaric oxygen can enhance the effects of PDT.**

**Normally, 97% of the oxygen delivered to body tissues is bound to hemoglobin, while only 3% is dissolved in the plasma. At sea level, barometric pressure is I ATA, or 760 mm Hg, and the partial pressure of oxygen in arterial blood ($P_aO_2$) is approximately 100 mm Hg. At rest, the tissues of the body consume about 5 mL of $O_2$ per 100 mL of blood.**

184

During $HBO_2$ treatments, **barometric pressures are usually limited to 3 ATA** or lower. **The oxygen content of inspired air in the chamber is typically 95% to 100%.** The combination of increased pressure (3 ATA) and increased oxygen concentration (100%) dissolves enough oxygen in the plasma alone to sustain life in a resting state.

**Under hyperbaric conditions, oxygen content in the plasma is increased from 0.3 to 6.6 mL per 100 mL of blood with no change in oxygen transport via hemoglobin.**

**$HBO_2$ at 3.0 ATA increases oxygen delivery to the tissues from 20.0 to 26.7 mL of $O_2$ per 100 mL of blood.**

Increased oxygen delivery to the tissues is believed **to facilitate healing** through a number of mechanisms.

**Hyperbaric oxygen, tissue levels may approach 1200 mmHg, in which increased production of superoxide, peroxide and other oxygen radicals occurs,** however, some organisms adapt by producing increased levels of superoxide dismutase. There is no direct antibacterial effect of enhanced oxygen on aerobic organisms. Indirect antibactericidal effects are related to improved PMN function in killing bacteria. (Delaney, Montgomery, 2001)

**Results with hyperbaric oxygen is similar to that obtained by the Baylor investigators using intra-arterial $H_2O_2$.**

**When subjects are breathing $HBO_2$, the cumulative effects of EMODs are well recognized because of their role in CNS $O_2$ toxicity; yet, adverse reactions to $HBO_2$ are rare.** (Demchenko et al, 2003) (Demchenko et al, 2001) (Tibbles and Edelsberg, 1996) (Torbati et al, 1992) (Torbati et al, 1989)

Accumulating evidence supports the notion that **the CNS responds to a continuum of $O_2$ tension at both normobaric and hyperbaric pressures.** The direct effects of $O_2$ on the brain stem need to be considered when hyperoxia is used. Dripps and Comroe (Dripps and Comroe. 1947) first introduced the use of normobaric hyperoxia (100% $O_2$, 8-min exposure) as a tool for physiological denervation of the carotid body chemoreceptors. They emphasized, however, the following caveat:"It must be remembered that a stimulant effect of oxygen which tends to increase respiration may be acting simultaneously to limit the extent of this immediate depression of minute ventilation."

**Hyperbaric oxygen (HBO) treatment of cholesterol-fed rabbits dramatically reduces the development of arterial lesions**

**despite having little or no effect on plasma or individual lipoprotein cholesterol concentrations.** (Delaney, Montgomery, 2001)

Similarly, in regression studies, **HBO treatment has no effect on the rate of plasma (or lipoprotein) cholesterol decline but significantly accelerates aortic lesion regression** compared with no treatment. (Kudchodkar et al, 2000)

In this case, **I believe that the authors made some extremely valuable observations but they came to the wrong conclusion. The plaque regression was not due to increased antioxidants but was due to increased EMODs, which are well known products of HBO$_2$. Further, administration of HBO$_2$ should, according to the Free Radi-Crap theory, cause increased lipid oxidation and plaque formation. But, it does not!**

**Whereas, just the opposite is the result in experimental animals, whereby HBO$_2$ causes increased regression of plaque and decreases accumulation of lipid oxidation products. This is one of my most important observations.**

**There is some evidence that HBOT can reverse age-related macular degeneration (AMD),** the leading cause of severe visual loss in people over the age of fifty. (Bojic et al, 2015)

Dr. L. Bojic treated 4 patients with advanced macular degeneration and severe vision loss in a clinical trial with HBOT. Three of the four patients experienced a doubling of visual acuity after HBOT. The fourth patient experienced a four-fold improvement.

It seems that a trial of thirty 90-minute treatments at 14 ATA in a monoplace HBO chamber, combined with other therapies such as laser and nutritional supplements, offers hope for additional benefit. Cells of the retina are specialized neurons that are actually extensions of the brain and retinal cells would be expected to respond to HBOT similar to brain-injury patients.

**Seventy percent of the treated multiple sclerosis (MS) patients either did not deteriorate, had their conditions stabilize, or showed small improvements.** (Davidson, 1989)

**A wound's chances of becoming infected are directly related to how little oxygen there is in the affected tissues.** (Hunt, 1979)

**Under-oxygenation can also reduce the body's ability to heal the wound, especially since healing tissue needs even more oxygen than does healthy tissue.** (Niinikoski et al, 1972)

**HBOT is the best way of increasing the oxygen content of under-oxygenated tissues.** (Sheffield, 1985) (Strauss et al, 1983) (Strauss et al, 1986) (Skyhar et al, 1986) (Nylander et al, 1985)

The use of **HBOT is a very valuable way of treating difficult wounds** (Hunt and van Winkle, 1976) (Sheffield, 1985.

**The earlier and more frequently HBOT is used, the more likely it is that severely injured body parts will be saved.** (Strauss and Hart, 1984) (Strauss and Hart, 1989)

One of the most respected trauma surgery units in the world is the Department of Microsurgery at the University of Liege Hospital in Belgium. The **Liege doctors were convinced that HBOT helped them heal difficult wounds** and save reattached limbs that would otherwise have not been healed or saved.

**HBOT helps to heal bone disorders by stimulating both the osteoclast and the osteoblasts.** (Hunt et al, 1969) (Strauss, 1987)

**Vasoconstriction.** High tissue oxygen concentrations cause blood vessels to constrict, which can lead to a 20% decrease in regional blood flow. (Marino, 1991)

In normoxic environments, tissue hypoxia may develop; however, this is not the case with $HBO_2$. **The decrease in regional blood flow is more than compensated for by the increased plasma oxygen that reaches the tissue.** The net effect is **decreased tissue inflammation without hypoxia**--a mechanism by which hyperbaric oxygen therapy is believed to improve crush injuries, thermal burns, and compartment syndrome.

**Neovascularization and epithelialization.** High tissue oxygen concentrations accelerate the development of new blood vessels. (Boerema et al, 1960)

This can be induced in both acute and chronic injuries. Regenerating epithelial cells also function more effectively in a high-oxygen environment and these effects have proven effective in treating tissue ulcers and skin grafts.

**Stimulation of fibroblasts and osteoclasts.** In a **hypoxic milieu, fibroblasts are unable to synthesize collagen, and osteoclasts are unable to lay down new bone.** Collagen deposition, wound strength, and the rate of wound healing are affected by the amount of available oxygen. Ischemic areas of wounds benefit most from the increased delivery of oxygen. $HBO_2$ increases tissue levels of oxygen, allowing for fibroblasts and osteoclasts to function appropriately. This mechanism may play a role in the treatment of osteomyelitis and slowly healing fractures.

**Immune response. When tissue oxygen tensions fall below 30 mm Hg, host responses to infection and ischemia are compromised.** (Weiss, 1994)

Studies have shown that the **local tissue resistance to infection is directly related to the level of oxygen found in the tissue.** (Hammarlund, 1995) (Jonsson et al, 1991)

High oxygen concentrations may prevent the production of certain bacterial toxins and may kill certain anaerobic organisms such as Clostridium perfringens. More important, however, **oxygen aids polymorphonuclear leukocytes** (PMN). Similar to the administration of hydrogen peroxide, oxygen is believed to aid the migration and phagocytic function of the PMN. (Hunt, Zederfeldt, Goldstick, 1969)

**Oxygen is converted within the PMN into substrates (superoxides, peroxides, and hydroxyl radicals) that are lethal to bacteria.** These effects on the immune system allow $HBO_2$ to aid the healing of soft-tissue infections and osteomyelitis.

**$HBO_2$ has also been found to inhibit PMN adherence on postcapillary venules.** (Gottrup et al, 1984)

Although this may seem like a **paradox,** this effect is beneficial because it helps limit reperfusion injury after crush injury and compartment syndrome.

**Maintaining high-energy phosphate bonds.** When circulation to a wound is compromised, resultant **ischemia lowers the concentration of adenosine triphosphate (ATP) and increases lactic acid levels.**

**ATP is necessary for ion and molecular transport across cell membranes and maintenance of cellular viability.**

**Increased oxygen delivery to the tissue with HBO$_2$ may prevent tissue damage by decreasing the tissue lactic acid level and helping maintain the ATP level.** This may help prevent tissue damage in ischemic wounds and reperfusion injuries.

Increasing pressure in HBO therapy is often expressed in multiples of atmospheric pressure absolute (ATA); 1 ATA equals 1 kg/cm$^2$ or 735.5 mm Hg.

Most HBO treatments are performed at 2 to 3 ATA. In air embolism and decompression sickness, where pressure is crucial to therapeutic effect, treatments frequently start at 6 ATA.

This additional pressure, when associated with inspiration of high levels of oxygen, substantially increases the level of oxygen dissolved into blood plasma. **This state of serum hyperoxia is the second beneficial effect of hyperbaric oxygen therapy.**

### Hyperoxia: Life without Blood

**At sea level in room air, hemoglobin is approximately 97% saturated with oxygen (19.5 vol% oxygen, of which approximately 5.8 vol% is extracted by tissue). The amount of oxygen dissolved into plasma is 0.32 vol%.**

**An increase in PO$_2$ has a negligible impact on total hemoglobin oxygen content; however, it does result in an increase in the amount of oxygen dissolved directly into plasma. With 100% inspired oxygen the amount of plasma oxygen increases to 2.09 vol%.**

**At 3 ATA plasma contains 6.8 vol% oxygen, a level equivalent to the average tissue requirements for oxygen.**

Thus, HBO treatment could and has sustained life without hemoglobin. (Boerema et al, 1960, 133)

The immune system, wound healing, and vascular tone are all affected by oxygen supply. **Oxygen <u>alone</u> has little direct antimicrobial effect, even for most anaerobes** (Tally et al, 1975); **it is, however, a crucial factor in immune function.**

Neutrophils require molecular oxygen as a substrate for microbial killing. **The oxidative burst seen in neutrophils after phagocytosis of bacteria involves a 10-to 15-fold increase in oxygen consumption.** (Badwey, Karnovsky, 1980)

Here, oxygen serves as a substrate in the formation of free radicals, which directly or indirectly initiate phagocytic killing. (Forman, Thomas, 1986)

**This endogenous antimicrobial system virtually ceases functioning under conditions of hypoxia. A tissue $PO_2$ of at least 30 mmHg of oxygen is considered necessary for normal oxidative function to occur.** (Hohn et al, 1976)

**Oxygen partial pressures below 30 mmHg are often seen in damaged and infected tissues.** Increasing the oxygen level in this tissue can allow restoration of white blood cell function and return of adequate antimicrobial action. (Knighton et al, 1984)

**The cardiovascular effects of hyperbaric oxygen include a generalized vasoconstriction and a small reduction in cardiac output.** (Risers, Tyssebotn, 1986)

This ultimately may decrease the overall blood supply to a region, but **the increase in serum oxygen content results in an overall gain in delivered oxygen.** In conditions such as burns, cerebral edema, and crush injuries, this vasoconstriction may be beneficial, reducing edema and tissue welling while maintaining tissue oxygenation. (Nulander et al, 1985)

## Complications

Usual complications of HBO therapy are a result of either barometric pressure changes or oxygen toxicity. The most common complications involve cavity trauma due to change in pressure. Any air-filled cavity that cannot equilibrate with ambient pressure, such as the middle ear when the eustachian tube is blocked, is subject to deformity and barotrauma during pressure changes in HBO therapy.

**Pneumothorax** is a rare complication of HBO treatment, usually occurring only in patients with severe lung disease.

**Air embolism**, presumably resulting from a small tear in the pulmonary vasculature, is another rare complication. One hundred percent oxygen under high pressure is neurotoxic and can lower the seizure threshold and affect central nervous system control of respiration. However, neurotoxicity is rare with the low-pressure, short-duration treatments used clinically in HBO therapy. In one series the incidence was reported as 1.3 seizures per 10 000 treatments.

Pulmonary oxygen toxic reactions can occur with 100% inspired oxygen at less than 1 ATA with prolonged exposure. **Almost all patients will show pulmonary toxicity after 6 continuous hours of inspired oxygen at 2 ATA.** (Clark, Lambertson, 1971)

No clinical HBO protocol requires this length of continuous exposure to 100% oxygen. However, HBO treatments may contribute to the pulmonary oxygen toxicity seen in critically ill patients who receive high concentrations of inspired oxygen between hyperbaric treatments.

Although a concern in premature newborns, **retrolental fibroplasia has <u>not</u> been noted in infants, children, or adults undergoing HBO therapy.** (Nichols, Lambertsen, 1969)

**Development of cataracts has been reported in patients receiving more than 150 HBO treatments.** (Plamquist, Phillipson, Barr, 1984)

## Crohn's Disease, Ulcerative Colitis and HBOT

Non-specific ulcerative colitis and Crohn's disease are difficult **chronic inflammatory** bowel diseases. Their treatment can often be frustrating for both the physician and the patient.

Crohn's disease is associated with certain disorders affecting other parts of the body such as gallstones and inadequate absorption of nutrients. **When Crohn's disease causes a flare-up of gastrointestinal symptoms, the person may also experience inflammation of the joints (arthritis).**

**I believe that this is due to the fact that both diseases are based on deficiency levels of EMODs. Rheumatoid arthritis is a disease with intense inflammation.**

Under **chronic inflammation** there are microcirculation disorders in bowel mucosa, **hypoxia (lack of oxygen)** and changes in catecholamine and other metabolic factors.

These factors are the reason to use HBO combined with conventional medical management in the treatment of this disease where medication alone has not relieved symptoms to a satisfactory degree. (Brady et al, 1989)

**$HBO_2$ limits the amount of inflammation in the bowels, lowers the CRP values, lowers Sedimentation values and lowers the WBC values. The pain is alleviated, the patient's weight improves, and bowel movements return almost to normal. The pain is relieved because hypoxia causes release of pain neurotransmitters and correction of the hypoxic conditions results in decreased pain.** Although the mechanism is not clearly understood, $HBO_2$ should be considered in treatment of Crohn's Disease not responding to conventional treatments. (Nelson et al, 1990)

When failure of $HBO_2$ treatment occurred in trial studies it became quite clear as to the **two reasons for the failures**:

1. $HBO_2$ was used at the late stages of the disease.
2. For a long time before the hyperbaric oxygenation the **hormonotherapy** was used. This refers to **steroid use, which would produce a state of immunosuppression and reduced levels of EMODs.**

**In the study published in Proceeding of the Tenth International Congress on Hyperbaric Medicine the remission of patients treated with $HBO_2$ prolonged until 4-5 years in 49% of the cases, the improvement was noted in 37%. Later none of the patients treated with HBO needed operative intervention** as compared with the patients treated only with drugs. The considerable improvement induced by HBO treatments allowed some patients to receive lower doses of drugs and in most cases to cease the hormonotherapy.

**Perchance,
if we are capable of identifying and eliminating
the "death gene," we will still
have to deal with change.
Change is the only universal constant,
other than predation and universal ignorance.**
R.M. Howes, M.D., Ph.D.
5/11/05

American doctors accept **HBOT** for use in wound healing, bone infection, carbon monoxide intoxication, and air emboli, or air bubbles in the bloodstream due to decompression sickness, open-heart surgery, and other sources.

**HBOT** can also be used for conditions such as coma resulting from head injuries, bruising of the spinal cord, stroke, and neurological disorders such as multiple sclerosis.

When adequate oxygen can't reach the damaged area, and the body's natural healing process fails to function properly.

For more than three hundred years, people have been breathing pressurized air for its therapeutic effect. One atmosphere absolute is the average atmospheric pressure exerted at sea level, or 14.7 psi.

Drugs can reduce edema but they cannot supply the brain with needed oxygen.

Studies have shown **HBOT**'s effectiveness in cases where spinal damage is associated with injuries.

During the first phase of a migraine, blood flow may be reduced by an average of 36%. Many migraine patients who receive **HBOT** find that the interval between attacks is significantly increased.

There is some evidence that **HBOT** can reverse age-related macular degeneration (**AMD**). **HBOT** was the safest and most effective treatment available for **MS**.

The Gottlieb-Neubauer theory, proposing that **MS** is caused by lack of oxygen, has been supported by research showing that **HBOT**, which overcomes a lack of oxygen, is an effective treatment method. Seventy percent of the treated **MS** patients either did not deteriorate, had their conditions stabilize, or showed small improvements.

As stated earlier, a wound's chances of becoming infected are directly related to how little oxygen there is in the affected tissues. (Hunt, 1979)

Under-oxygenation can also reduce the body's ability to heal the wound, especially since healing tissue needs even more oxygen than does healthy tissue. The creation of capillaries, the tiny blood vessels that connect arteries to veins, requires both collagen and oxygen. If either is lacking, new capillaries cannot be created, and wound healing cannot occur. Thus, a lack of oxygen in the wounded tissues interferes with the entire wound healing process. (Wells et al, 1977)

Swelling reduces the number of white blood cells and other infection fighters that can reach the affected tissues, and those cells that do find their way to the area cannot act very effectively without oxygen.

HBOT can help counteract infection indirectly by providing the white blood cells with the oxygen they need. It can also act directly by killing anaerobic organisms, stopping their multiplication, and neutralizing the toxins that some of them produce.

Oxygen is essential in the creation of granulation tissue, the pink, fleshy tissue that first grows over a healing wound. Oxygen also promotes the growth of collagen. It encourages bone repair. HBOT's effectiveness in minimizing tissue death, reducing swelling, and promoting healing has been proven in the laboratory (Strauss, M.B,).

Oxygen acts as a potent antibiotic. HBOT helps fight all microorganisms, but especially those that thrive in the absence of oxygen.

There is evidence that HBOT, because of its immune system-enchancing effects, can help the body fight these microbes. Studies suggest that HBOT works against Lyme disease by attacking the spirochete itself. Leprosy was the first infectious disease to be treated with HBOT in 1938.

HBOT can help burn patients heal faster with fewer complications.

HBOT works to heal fracture nonunion by stimulating the production of collagen.

Adding HBOT to conventional orthopedic methods shortened the process of bone regeneration and wound healing by ten to twelve days.

Radiation damage causes hypoxia, or a lack of oxygen in the body's tissues. Hyperbaric oxygen helps fight this damage by increasing the amount of oxygen within the tissues.

**HBOT can help assure that skin grafts** take hold and scars don't reveal themselves. In the case of a **pedicle graft, it is important that HBOT be employed before what little circulation that is present develops blood clots.**

**HBOT** can also help speed the healing of skin ulcers.

The use of **hyperbaric oxygen leads to the development of new capillaries, tiny blood vessels linking arteries and veins.**

**Research into HIV history also reveals the astonishing complexity of the virus and its ability to mutate and recombine with other strains -- continually producing "new and improved" versions that outpace mankind's efforts at treatment.**

**Normally, 97% of the oxygen delivered to body tissues is bound to hemoglobin, while only 3% is dissolved in the plasma. At sea level, barometric pressure is 1 ATA, or 760 mm Hg, and the partial pressure of oxygen in arterial blood ($P_aO_2$) is approximately 100 mm Hg. At rest, the tissues of the body consume about 5 mL of $O_2$ per 100 mL of blood.**

**When tissue oxygen tensions fall below 30 mm Hg, host responses to infection and ischemia are compromised. Local tissue resistance to infection is directly related to the level of oxygen found in the tissue.**

**With 100% inspired oxygen the amount of plasma oxygen increases to 2.09 vol%. At 3 ATA plasma contains 6.8 vol% oxygen, a level equivalent to the average tissue requirements for oxygen.** Thus, **HBO treatment could and has sustained life without hemoglobin.**

**The site of EMODs formation following T cell irradiation of 5 Gy has been confirmed to be apparently located in mitochondria and/or lysosomes, instead of in the nucleus.**

**As human peripheral T cells lack peroxidase activity,** these cells are considered to be easily susceptible to oxidative stress such as exogenous hydrogen peroxide.

**EMOD formations in T cells induced by hydrogen peroxide showed different distribution patterns from those induced by 5 Gy-irradiation.** (Ogawa Y.)

The work of Ogawa shows that the effect of radiation and $H_2O_2$ (EMODs) are, indeed, different in the living/breathing cell. I have said for a long time that the energetics are completely different for these two modalities and thus, it would be illogical to expect their products to be exactly the same.

The absence of a substance does not drive anything since that something is not there at all. Thus, **oxygen deficiency "allows" for pain manifestation.** This is an ingenious method to notify the body that something is wrong. This also points out the crucial need to have adequate levels of oxygen in all parts of the body at all times. It is so crucial **that the body has evolved a "pain system" to alert us of inadequate levels of oxygen.** This can occur in angina, inflammation, infections, traumatic injuries, etc.

**This is beautiful!**

A large number of **pain neurotransmitters** are involved in clinical expression of pain, including: **substance P; enkephalins; neurokinin 1, 2, and 3; serotonin; adenosine triphosphate (ATP); nitric oxide; calcitonin; vasoactive intestinal peptides; epinephrine, norepinephrine, and related sympathomimetic agents; glutamic acid, aspartic acid, and related excitatory transmitters; and GABA, glycine, and related inhibitory transmitters.**

It seems safe to predict that future work will establish that, directly and indirectly, **all those molecular species are triggered or influenced by oxygen deficit. To me, this is incredible and emphasizes the importance of oxygen to aerobic-dependent life forms.**

**I believe that this can be interpreted to mean that it is oxygen, itself or EMODs, which holds the release of pain neurotransmitters in abeyance, just as we have seen that it is EMODs which hold cancer and atherosclerosis in abeyance.**

**Over 300 molecular species have been recognized to be involved in neurotransmission. Oxygen deficit "allows" the release of substance P.** Specifically, **the carotid bodies contain SP** — in concentrations ranging from 1.4 to 1.6 ng/mg protein — **that is released in response to tissue hypoxia. The amount of SP released from the carotid bodies increases in proportion to the severity of hypoxia. The release of SP by hypoxia is a calcium-dependent process, and is primarily mediated by N- and L-type Ca2+ channels.**

Not unexpectedly in light of the oxygen/SP dynamics, **oxyradicals under certain conditions also trigger the release of substance P.**

By contrast, **antioxidants, such as ascorbic acid, inhibit the release of SP.** However, the relationships between antioxidants and SP are complex. Hence, **capsaicin increases regional perfusion and oxygen delivery, inhibiting the release of SP.**

On the other hand, **nitric oxide, through its vasodilator role, improves oxygen transport, decreases the release of SP, and mitigates some pain syndromes.**

An interesting aspect of the oxygen/substance P dynamics is revealed by the case of the **East African naked mole-rats** (Heterocephalus glaber). **This rat species lacks substance P and does not appear to suffer pain when tormented.**

The rats feel no immediate pain when cut, scraped or subjected to heat stimuli. They only feel some aches. However, **when the rats get a shot of SP, pain signaling resumes working** as in other mammals.

**Direct oxygen therapies, such as oxygen by mask and hyperbaric oxygen, have been successfully used in controlling headaches and migraine attacks.**

This may at last help explain the generalized pain and multiple pain sites experienced by the **elderly. They hurt because of hypoxia** and their bodies have a way of telling them so.

**Anginal chest pain is relieved or mitigated by the administration of oxygen, as are attacks of headache and migraine.**

---

In 2015, it occurred to me that anemia, which is associated with reduced ability to carry oxygen to the tissue and cells, could be a cofactor in "cancer allowance."

I found papers on Fanconi's syndrome which supported this notion.

The following paper also lends credence to this idea as it relates to iron deficiency anemia.

Prof Randolph M. Howes MD,PhD

# Risk of cancer in patients with iron deficiency anemia

## Abstract

## OBJECTIVE:

This study evaluated the risk of cancer among patients with iron deficiency anemia (IDA) by using a nationwide population-based data set.

## METHOD:

Patients newly diagnosed with IDA and without antecedent cancer between 2000 and 2010 were recruited from the Taiwan National Health Insurance Research Database. The **standardized incidence ratios (SIRs)** of cancer types among patients with IDA were calculated.

## RESULTS:

Patients with IDA exhibited an increased overall cancer risk (SIR: 2.15). Subgroup analysis showed that patients of both sexes and in all age groups had an increased SIR. After we excluded patients diagnosed with cancer within the first and first 5 years of IDA diagnosis, the SIRs remained significantly elevated at 1.43 and 1.30, respectively. **In addition, the risks of pancreatic (SIR: 2.31), kidney (SIR: 2.23), liver (SIR: 1.94), and bladder cancers (SIR: 1.74) remained significantly increased** after exclusion of patients diagnosed with cancer within 5 years after IDA diagnosis.

## CONCLUSION:

**The overall cancer risk was significantly elevated among patients with IDA.**

After we excluded patients diagnosed with IDA and cancer within 1 and 5 years, the SIRs remained significantly elevated compared with those of the general population.

The increased risk of cancer was not confined to gastrointestinal cancer when the SIRs of pancreatic, kidney, liver, and bladder cancers significantly increased after exclusion of patients diagnosed with IDA and cancer within the first 5 years. This finding may be caused by immune activities altered by IDA. Further study is necessary to determine the association between IDA and cancer risk. (Hung et al, 2015)

I believe that this supports the belief that lower levels of oxygen at the cellular level, leads to lower levels of EMODs, which furthers "cancer allowance." The fact that IDA allowed the formation of cancers of various tissues further supports my theory.

## Diabetes and risk of cancer in women

## The association between type 2 diabetes mellitus and women cancer: the epidemiological evidences and putative mechanisms

### Abstract

**Type 2 diabetes mellitus (T2DM), a chronic disease increasing rapidly worldwide, is well established as an important risk factor for various types of cancer.**

Although many factors impact the development of T2DM and cancer including sex, age, ethnicity, obesity, diet, physical activity levels, and environmental exposure, many epidemiological and experimental studies are gradually contributing to knowledge regarding the interrelationship between DM and cancer.

The insulin resistance, hyperinsulinemia, and chronic inflammation associated with diabetes mellitus are all associated strongly with cancer.

The changes in bioavailable ovarian steroid hormone that occur in diabetes mellitus (**the increasing levels of estrogen and androgen and the decreasing level of progesterone) are also considered potentially carcinogenic conditions for the breast, endometrium, and ovaries in women.**

**RMH Note: These are conditions which have elevated levels of the steroid antioxidants, estrogen and androgens. This leads to an EMOD insufficiency, which "allows" the development of cancer and the clustering or coexistence of various diseases.** I have written about this extensively in other tomes.

In addition, the interaction among insulin, insulin-like growth factors (IGFs), and ovarian steroid hormones, such as estrogen and progesterone, could act synergistically during cancer development. Here, we review the cancer-related mechanisms in T2DM, the epidemiological evidence linking T2DM and cancers in women, and the role of antidiabetic medication in these cancers. (Joung, Jeong, Ku, 2015)

## Physical activity and gynecologic cancer prevention

### Abstract

This reviews the findings from epidemiologic studies of the associations of physical activity with gynecologic cancers, including those of the endometrium, ovaries, and cervix, and the biological mechanisms mediating the associations.

**The epidemiologic evidence to date suggests that physical activity probably protects against endometrial cancer, with a risk reduction of about 20-30% for those with the highest levels of physical activity compared to those with the lowest levels, and that light to moderate physical activity including housework, gardening, or walking for transportation may reduce risk.**

The role of physical activity in ovarian cancer development remains uncertain, as findings from these studies have been inconsistent with **about half the studies suggesting physical activity modestly decreases risk and about half the studies suggesting no association**.

**A recent meta-analysis of studies examining recreational physical activity with ovarian cancer risk estimated a 20% reduced risk for the most active versus least active women.**

**There is mounting evidence that sedentary behaviors such as sitting time probably increase risk of endometrial and ovarian cancers.**

Overall, there is insufficient evidence to draw a conclusion on a possible role of physical activity in the development of cervical cancer, although a modest influence on risk is possible through effects on sex steroid hormones and immune function. **The biological evidence provides strong support for a protective role of physical activity on cancer of the endometrium, and moderate support for cancer of the ovaries, as these cancers have a strong hormonal etiology.**

The more established biological mechanisms that are supported by epidemiologic and experimental data involve endogenous sex hormone levels, insulin-mediated pathways, and maintenance of energy balance. In this chapter, we will discuss the evidence for an association of physical activity with gynecologic cancers including those of the endometrium, ovaries, and cervix.

Cancers of the endometrium and ovaries have a strong hormonal etiology (Risch 1998; Kaaks et al. 2002; Lukanova and Kaaks 2005), and **physical activity has been postulated as a potential modifiable risk factor for prevention of these cancers because it can influence circulating hormone levels**, energy balance, and insulin-mediated pathways that are thought to be important mediators underlying the associations.

Few studies have evaluated the association of physical activity with cervical cancer because the main causal factor is infection with certain types of human papillomavirus (HPV), although other hormonal and immune factors are also thought to play a role (Smith et al. 2003; Waggoner 2003). We review the findings from epidemiologic studies that have examined the associations of physical activity with gynecologic cancers, and the biological mechanisms that might mediate the associations. (Cust, 2011)

**RMH Note: Physical activity increases EMOD levels consistently and the increased EMODs prevent cancer development and activate EMOD induced apoptosis to kill existing cancers. Please refer to my in depth tomes on exercise and cancer.**

## Cancer, physical activity and exercise

### Abstract

This review examines the relationship between physical activity and cancer along the cancer continuum, and serves as a synthesis of systematic and meta-analytic reviews conducted to date.

**There exists a large body of epidemiologic evidence that conclude those who participate in higher levels of physical activity have a reduced likelihood of developing a variety of cancers compared to those who engage in lower levels of physical activity.**

Despite this observational evidence, the causal pathway underlying the association between participation in physical activity and cancer risk reduction **remains unclear. Physical activity is also a useful adjunct to improve the deleterious sequelae experienced during cancer treatment.**

These deleterious sequelae may include fatigue, muscular weakness, deteriorated functional capacity, and many others.

The benefits of physical activity during cancer treatment are similar to those experienced after treatment. Despite the growing volume of literature examining physical activity and cancer across the cancer continuum, a number of research gaps exist. There is little evidence on the safety of physical activity among all cancer survivors, as most trials have selectively recruited participants. The specific dose of exercise needed to optimize primary cancer prevention or symptom control during and after cancer treatment remains to be elucidated. (Brown et al, 2012)

## Physical activity and cancer prevention: etiologic evidence and biological mechanisms

### Abstract

Scientific evidence is accumulating on physical activity as a means for the primary prevention of cancer.

Nearly 170 observational epidemiologic studies of physical activity and cancer risk at a number of specific cancer sites have been conducted. **The evidence for decreased risk with increased physical activity is classified as convincing for breast and colon cancers, probable for prostate cancer, possible for lung and endometrial cancers and insufficient for cancers at all other sites.**

Despite the large number of studies conducted on physical activity and cancer, most have been hampered by incomplete assessment of physical activity and a lack of full examination of effect modification and confounding.

Several plausible hypothesized biological mechanisms exist for the association between physical activity and cancer, including changes in endogenous sexual and metabolic hormone levels and growth factors, decreased obesity and central adiposity and possibly changes in immune function. Weight control may play a particularly important role because links between excess weight and increased cancer risk have been established for several sites, and central adiposity has been particularly implicated in promoting metabolic conditions amenable to carcinogenesis.

**Based on existing evidence, some public health organizations have issued physical activity guidelines for cancer prevention, generally recommending at least 30 min of moderate-to-vigorous intensity physical activity on > or =5 d/wk.** Although most research has focused on the efficacy of physical activity in cancer prevention, **evidence is increasing that exercise also influences other aspects of the cancer experience, including cancer detection, coping, rehabilitation and survival after diagnosis.** (Friedenreich, Orenstein, 2002)

## Diabetes and cancer links

### A critical appraisal of the pathogenetic and therapeutic links

### Abstract

Diabetes and cancer represent two common, multifactorial, chronic and potentially fatal diseases, **not infrequently co-diagnosed in the same patient.**

**RMH Note: I refer to this as clustering or coexistence of diseases, which I believe is due to an overall EMOD insufficiency.**

Epidemiological data demonstrate significant increases of the cancer incidence in patients with obesity and diabetes, which is more evident for certain site-specific cancers. Although there is increasing evidence that strongly indicates an augmented risk of cancer in diabetic patients, several confounding factors complicate the ability to precisely assess the risk. Mainly in insulin-resistant states (such as in type 2 diabetes mellitus and in metabolic syndrome), direct associations between obesity-related hyperinsulinemia and increasing circulating insulin-like growth factor-1 (IGF-1) levels have been implicated as key factors in the mechanisms involved in carcinogenesis.

Whilst anti-diabetic drugs can increase the cancer risk, anti-proliferative drugs may cause diabetes or aggravate pre-existing diabetes. Additionally, an increasing number of targeted anti-cancer therapies may interfere with the pathways shared by IGF-1 and insulin receptors, showing a adverse effect on glucose metabolism through various mechanisms. Although there is a requirement for large-scale randomized evidence, the present review summarizes the majority of the

Prof Randolph M. Howes MD,PhD

epidemiological association studies between diabetes and various types of cancer, discussing the pathophysiological mechanisms that may be involved in promoting carcinogenesis in diabetes and the potential impact of different anti-diabetic therapies on cancer risk. (Gristina et al, 2015)

## Diabetes and cancer implications

## Associations, mechanisms, and implications for medical practice

## Abstract

Both diabetes mellitus and cancer are prevalent diseases worldwide. **It is evident that there is a substantial increase in cancer incidence in diabetic patients.**

**Epidemiologic studies have indicated that diabetic patients are at significantly higher risk of common cancers including pancreatic, liver, breast, colorectal, urinary tract, gastric and female reproductive cancers.**

**Mortality due to cancer is moderately increased among patients with diabetes compared with those without.**

There is increasing evidence that some cancers are associated with diabetes, but **the underlying mechanisms of this potential association have not been fully elucidated.** Insulin is a potent growth factor that promotes cell proliferation and carcinogenesis directly and/or through insulin-like growth factor 1 (IGF-1). Hyperinsulinemia leads to an increase in the bioactivity of IGF-1 by inhibiting IGF binding protein-1.

Hyperglycemia serves as a subordinate plausible explanation of carcinogenesis. High glucose may exert direct and indirect effects upon cancer cells to promote proliferation.

**RMH Note: Hyperglycemia decreases EMOD levels, thus "allowing" the development of cancer and other associated diseases.**

Also **chronic inflammation is considered as a hallmark of carcinogenesis.** The multiple drugs involved in the treatment of diabetes seem to modify the risk of cancer. Screening to detect cancer at an early stage and appropriate treatment of diabetic patients with cancer

204

are important to improve their prognosis. This paper summarizes the associations between diabetes and common cancers, interprets possible mechanisms involved, and addresses implications for medical practice. (Xu, Zhu, Shu, 2014)

**Please remember that hypoxia is a hallmark of inflammation.**

Hyperglycemia has been classically considered as a subordinate whereas hyperinsulinemia as a primary causal factor for cancer.

**Several large cohort and case-control studies have found a positive relationship between hyperglycemia and the risk of cancer.** (Giovannucci, 2001) (Muti et al, 2002) (Sayday et al, 2003) (Stattin et al, 2007) (Takahashi et al, 2011)

In a tumor-prone animal model, it was found that the number and size of liver tumors increased and **apoptosis was reduced in insulin-deficient hyperglycemic mice compared with insulin-sufficient mice**.

This phenomenon was reversed by insulin therapy.

**RMH Note: This is because hydrogen peroxide is an insulin mimetic.**

However, *in vivo* studies showed that T1DM, which is characterized by hyperglycemia, reduces the tumor growth. This finding does not support that hyperglycemia increases tumor growth, at least in the setting of insulin deficiency.

A recent research found that **tumors continue to consume high amounts of glucose, regardless of plasma glucose levels.** A recent meta-analysis confirmed this finding that improved glycemic control does not reduce cancer risk in diabetic patients. Hyperglycemia may be an independent risk factor for cancer. Further studies are needed to evaluate the relative roles of insulin and glucose.

The possible mechanisms of hyperglycemia increasing cancer risk include "indirect effect" and "direct effect". The "indirect effect" is the action that takes place at other organs and will later on influence tumor cells by inducing production of circulating growth factors (insulin/IGF-1) and inflammatory cytokines. The "direct effect" is the effect that is exerted directly upon tumor cells by increasing proliferation, inducing mutations, augmenting invasion and migration and rewiring cancer-related signaling pathways. Recently, Wnt/β-catenin signaling has been suggested as a key cancer-associated pathway and high glucose enhances

205

this signaling pathway by allowing nuclear retention and accumulation of transcriptionally active β-catenin independently of hyperinsulinemia, adipokines or inflammation. (Xu, Zhu, Shu, 2014)

---

## Hyperbaric Oxygen Effects on Sports Injuries

The following article was adapted from: (Barata et al, 2011)

**Abstract**

## Introduction

In the last decade, competitive sports have taken on a whole new meaning, where intensity has increased together with the incidence of injuries to the athletes. These sport injuries, ranging from broken bones to disrupted muscles, tendons and ligaments, may be a result of acute impact forces in contact sports or the everyday rigors of training and conditioning. (Babul et al. 2003)

Therefore, a need has emerged to discover the best and fastest treatments that will allow the injured athlete to return to competition faster than the normal course of rehabilitation, with a low risk of re-injury.

Hyperbaric oxygen therapy (HBO) is the therapeutic administration of 100% oxygen at pressures higher than 1 absolute atmosphere (ATA). It is administered by placing the patient in a multiplace or in a monoplace (one man) chamber and typically the vessels are pressurized to 1.5–3.0 ATA for periods between 60 and 120 minutes once or twice a day. (Bennett et al. 2005)

In the monoplace chamber the patient breathes the oxygen directly from the chamber but in the multiplace chamber this is done through a mask. **At 2.0 ATA, the blood oxygen content is increased 2.5% and sufficient oxygen becomes dissolved in plasma to meet tissue needs in the absence of hemoglobin-bound oxygen, increasing tissue oxygen tensions 10-fold (1000%).** (Staples and Clement, 1996)

**HBO is remarkably free of untoward side effects**.

Complications such as oxygen toxicity, middle ear barotrauma and confinement anxiety are well controlled with appropriate pre-exposure orientations. (Mekjavic et al. 2000)

HBO has been used empirically in the past, but **today information exists for its rational application**. This review aims to analyze the contribution of HBO in the rehabilitation of the different sports injuries.

## Hyperbaric oxygen therapy

Hyperbaric therapies are methods used to treat diseases or injuries using pressures higher than local atmospheric pressure inside a hyperbaric chamber. Within hyperbaric therapies, HBO is the administration of pure oxygen (100%) at pressures greater than atmospheric pressure, i.e. more than 1 ATA, for therapeutic reasons.

In order to be able to perform HBO, special facilities are required, with the capacity for withstanding pressures higher than 1 ATA, known as hyperbaric chambers, where patients breathe 100% oxygen.

In the case of single monoplace chambers (with a capacity for only one person) the oxygen is inhaled directly from the chambers' environment.

Although much less expensive to install and support, they have the major disadvantage of not being possible to access the patient during treatment. It is possible to monitor blood pressure, arterial waveform and electrocardiogram noninvasively, and to provide intravenous medications and fluids.

Mechanical ventilation is possible if chambers are equipped appropriately, although **it is not possible to suction patients during treatment**. Mechanical ventilation in the monoplace chamber is provided by a modified pressure-cycled ventilator outside of the chamber.

In multiplace chambers, the internal atmosphere is room air compressed up to 6 ATA. Attendants in this environment breathe compressed air, accruing a nitrogen load in their soft tissues, in the same way as a scuba diver breathing compressed air. These attendants need to decompress to avoid the decompression illness by using more complex decompression procedures when the treatment tables are more extended (e.g. Navy tables).

The patients, on the other hand, are breathing oxygen while at pressure. This oxygen can be administered via face mask, a hood or endotracheal tube. The advantage of such a chamber is that the patient can be attended to during treatment, but the installation and support costs are very high. These high costs preclude the widespread use of multiplace chambers.

## Biochemical, cellular and physiological effects of HBO

The level of consumption of $O_2$ by a given tissue, on the local blood stream, and the relative distance of the zone considered from the nearest arteriole and capillary determines the $O_2$ tension in this tissue. Indeed, **$O_2$ consumption causes oxygen partial pressure ($pO_2$) to fall rapidly between arterioles and vennules.**

This emphasizes the fact that in tissues there is a distribution of oxygen tensions according to a gradient. **This also occurs at the cell level such as in the mitochondrion, the terminal place of oxygen consumption, where $O_2$ concentrations range from 1.5 to 3 μM.** (Mathieu, 2006)

Before reaching the sites of utilization within the cell such as the perioxome, mitochondria and endoplasmic reticulum, **the oxygen moves down a pressure gradient from inspired to alveolar gas, arterial blood, the capillary bed, across the interstitial and intercellular fluid.**

**Under normobaric conditions, the gradient of $pO_2$ known as the 'oxygen cascade' starts at 21.2 kPa (159 mmHg) and ends up at 0.5–3 kPa (3.8–22.5 mmHg)** depending on the target tissue. (Mathieu, 2006)

**The arterial oxygen tension ($PaO_2$) is approximately 90 mmHg and the tissue oxygen tension ($PtO_2$) is approximately 55 mmHg.** (Sheridan and Shank, 1999)

**These values are markedly increased by breathing pure oxygen at greater than atmospheric pressure.**

**HBO is limited by toxic oxygen effects to a maximum pressure of 300 kPa (3 bar).** Partial pressure of carbon dioxide in the arterial blood ($PaCO_2$), water vapor pressure and respiratory quotient (RQ) do not vary significantly between 100 and 300 kPa (1 and 3 bar). Thus, for example, the inhalation of 100% oxygen at 202.6 kPa (2 ATA) provides an alveolar $PO_2$ of 1423 mmHg and, consequently, the alveolar oxygen passes the alveolar-capillary space and diffuses into the venous pulmonary capillary bed according to Fick's laws of diffusion.

## Hyperoxia and hyperoxygenation

Oxygen is transported by blood in two ways: chemically, bound to hemoglobin, and physically, dissolved in plasma.

During normal breathing in the environment we live in, hemoglobin has an oxygen saturation of 97%, representing a total oxygen content of about 19.5 ml $O_2$/100 ml of blood (or 19.5 vol%), because 1 g of 100% saturated hemoglobin carries 1.34 ml oxygen.

In these conditions the amount of oxygen dissolved in plasma is 0.32 vol%, giving a total of 19.82 vol% oxygen.

When we offer 85% oxygen through a Hudson mask or endotracheal intubation the oxygen content can reach values up to 22.2 vol%. (Jain, 2004)

**The main effect of HBO is hyperoxia.**

During this therapy, oxygen is dissolved physically in the blood plasma. At an ambient pressure of 2.8 ATA and breathing 100% oxygen, the alveolar oxygen tension ($PAO_2$) is approximately 2180 mmHg, the $PaO_2$ is at least 1800 mmHg and the tissue concentration ($PtO_2$) is at least 500 mmHg.

The oxygen content of blood is approximately ($[1.34 \times Hbg \times SaO_2]$ + $[0.0031 \times PaO_2]$), where Hbg is serum hemoglobin concentration and $SaO_2$ is arterial oxygen saturation. (Sheridan and Shank, 1999)

At a $PaO_2$ of 1800 mmHg, the dissolved fraction of oxygen in plasma ($0.0031 \times PaO_2$) is approximately 6 vol%, which means that 6 ml of oxygen will be physically dissolved in 100 ml of plasma, reaching a total volume of oxygen in the circulating blood volume equal to 26.9 vol%, equivalent to basic oxygen metabolic needs, and the $paO_2$ in the arteries can reach 2000 mmHg.

**With a normal lung function and tissue perfusion, a partial pressure of oxygen in the blood ($pO_2$) > 1000 mmHg could be reached.** (Mayer et al. 2004)

**Breathing pure oxygen at 2 ATA, the oxygen content in plasma is 10 times higher than when breathing air at sea level.**

Under normal conditions the $pO_2$ is 95 mmHg; under conditions of a hyperbaric chamber, the $pO_2$ can reach values greater than 2000 mmHg [Jain, 2004]. Consequently, during HBO, Hbg is also fully saturated on the venous side, and the result is an increased oxygen tension throughout the vascular bed.

**Since diffusion is driven by a difference in tension, oxygen will be forced further out into tissues from the vascular bed and diffuses to areas inaccessible to molecules of this gas when transported by hemoglobin.** (Mortensen, 2008) (Albuquerque, Sousa, 2007)

**After removal from the hyperbaric oxygen environment, the $PaO_2$ normalizes in minutes, but the $PtO_2$ may remain elevated for a variable period.** The rate of normalization of $PtO_2$ has not been clearly described, but is likely measured in minutes to a few hours, depending on tissue perfusion. (Sheridan and Shank, 1999)

**The physiological effects of HBO include short-term effects such as vasoconstriction and enhanced oxygen delivery, reduction of edema, phagocytosis activation and also an anti-inflammatory effect (enhanced leukocyte function). Neovascularization (angiogenesis in hypoxic soft tissues), osteoneogenesis as well as stimulation of collagen production by fibroblasts are known long-term effects. This is beneficial for wound healing and recovery from radiation injury.** (Sheridan and Shank, 1999)

## Physiological and therapeutic effects of HBO

In normal tissues, the primary action of oxygen is to cause general vasoconstriction (especially in the kidneys, skeletal muscle, brain and skin), which elicits a 'Robin Hood effect' through a reduction of blood flow to well-oxygenated tissue. (Mortensen, 2008)

HBO not only provides a significant increase in oxygen availability at the tissue level, as selective hyperoxic and not hypoxic vasoconstriction, occurring predominantly at the level of healthy tissues, with reduced blood volume and redistribution edema for peripheral tissue hypoxia, which can raise the anti-ischemic and antihypoxic effects to extremities due to this physiological mechanism. (Albuquerque, Sousa, 2007)

HBO reduces edema, partly because of vasoconstriction, partly due to improved homeostasis mechanisms. A high gradient of oxygen is a potent stimuli for angioneogenesis, which has an important contribution in the stimulation of reparative and regenerative processes in some diseases. (Mortensen, 2008)

**Also many cell and tissue functions are dependent on oxygen. Of special interest are leukocytes ability to kill bacteria, cell replication, collagen formation, and mechanisms of homeostasis, such as active membrane transport, e.g. the sodium—potassium pump. HBO has the effect of inhibiting leukocyte adhesion to the endothelium, diminishing tissue damage, which enhances leukocyte motility and improves microcirculation.** (Mortensen, 2008)

This occurs when the presence of gaseous bubbles in the venous vessels blocks the flow and induces hypoxia which causes endothelial stress followed by the release of nitric oxide (NO) which reacts with superoxide anions to form peroxynitrine. This, in turn, provokes oxidative perivascular stress and leads to the activation of leukocytes and their adhesion to the endothelium. (Antonelli et al, 2009)

Another important factor is hypoxia.

Hypoxia is the major factor stimulating angiogenesis. However, **deposition of collagen is increased by hyperoxygenation, and it is the collagen matrix that provides support for the growth of new capillary bed.** Two-hour daily treatments with HBO are apparently responsible for stimulating the oxygen in the synthesis of collagen, the remaining 22 h of real or relative hypoxia, in which the patient is not subjected to HBO, provide the stimuli for angiogenesis. Thus, the alternation of states of hypoxia and hyperoxia, observed in patients during treatment with intermittent HBO, is responsible for maximum stimulation of fibroblast activity in ischemic tissues, producing the development of the matrix of collagen, essential for neovascularization. (Jain, 2004)

**The presence of oxygen has the advantage of not only promoting an environment less hospitable to anaerobes, but also speeds the process of wound healing, whether from being required for the production of collagen matrix and subsequent angiogenesis, from the presence and beneficial effects of reactive oxygen species (ROS).** (Kunnavatana et al, 2005)

Dimitrijevich and colleagues studied the effect of HBO on human skin cells in culture and in human dermal and skin equivalents. (Dimitrijevich et al, 1999)

In that study, normal human dermal fibroblasts, keratinocytes, melanocytes, dermal equivalents and skin equivalents were exposed to HBO at pressures up to 3 ATA for up to 10 consecutive daily treatments lasting 90 minutes each. **An increase in fibroblast proliferation, collagen production and keratinocyte differentiation was observed at 1 and 2.5 ATA of HBO, but no benefit at 3 ATA.**

Kang and colleagues reported that HBO treatment up to 2.0 ATA enhances proliferation and autocrine growth factor production of normal human fibroblasts grown in a serum-free culture environment, **but showed no benefit beyond or below 2 ATA of HBO.** (Kang et al, 2004)

Therefore, a delicate balance between having enough and too much oxygen and/or atmospheric pressure is needed for fibroblast growth [Kunnavatana et al. 2005].

Another important feature to take into account is the potential antimicrobial effect of HBO.

**HBO, by reversing tissue hypoxia and cellular dysfunction, restores this defense and also increases the phagocytosis of some bacteria by working synergistically with antibiotics, and inhibiting the growth of a number of anaerobic and aerobic organisms at wound sites.** (Mader et al, 1980)

There is evidence that hyperbaric oxygen is bactericidal for Clostridium perfringens, in addition to promoting a definitive inhibitory effect on the growth of toxins in most aerobic and microaerophilic microorganisms.

**The action of HBO on anaerobes is based on the production of free radicals such as superoxide, dismutase, catalase and peroxidase. (RMH Note: this statement is incorrect.)**

More than 20 different clostridial exotoxins have been identified, and the most prevalent is alphatoxine (phospholipase C), which is haemolytic, tissue necrotizing and lethal. Other toxins, acting in synergy, promote anaemia, jaundice, renal failure, cardiotoxicity and brain dysfunction. Thetatoxine is responsible for vascular injury and consequent acceleration of tissue necrosis. **HBO blocks the production of alphatoxine and thetatoxine and inhibits bacterial growth**. (Jain, 2004)

## HBO applications in sports medicine

The healing of a sports injury has its natural recovery, and follows a fairly constant pattern irrespective of the underlying cause. Three phases have been identified in this process: the inflammatory phase, the proliferative phase and the remodelling phase. Oxygen has an important role in each of these phases. (Ishii et al, 2002)

**In the inflammatory phase, the hypoxia-induced factor-1$\alpha$,** which promotes, for example, the glycolytic system, vascularization and angiogenesis, has been shown to be important. However, if the oxygen supply could be controlled without promoting blood flow, the blood vessel permeability could be controlled to reduce swelling and consequently sharp pain.

In the proliferative phase, in musculoskeletal tissues (except cartilage), the oxygen supply to the injured area is gradually raised and is essential for the synthesis of extracellular matrix components such as fibronectin and proteoglycan.

In the remodelling phase, tissue is slowly replaced over many hours using the oxygen supply provided by the blood vessel already built into the organization of the musculoskeletal system, with the exception of the cartilage. If the damage is small, the tissue is recoverable with nearly perfect organization but, if the extent of the damage is large, a scar (consisting mainly of collagen) may replace tissue. Consequently, depending on the injury, this collagen will become deficiently hard or loose in the case of muscle or ligament repair, respectively.

The application of HBO for the treatment of sports injuries has recently been suggested in the scientific literature as a therapy modality: a primary or an adjunct treatment.

**As of 2000, although results have proven to be promising in terms of using HBO as a treatment modality in sports-related injuries, these studies have been limited due to the small sample sizes, lack of blinding and randomization problems.** (Babul, Rhodes, 2000)

Even fewer studies referring to the use of HBO in high level athletes can be found in the literature.

Ishii and colleagues reported the use of HBO as a recovery method for muscular fatigue during the Nagano Winter Olympics. In this experiment seven Olympic athletes received HBO treatment for 30–40 minutes at 1.3 ATA with a maximum of six treatments per athlete and an average of two. It was found that **all athletes benefited from the HBO treatment presenting faster recovery rates**.

**These results are concordant with those obtained by Fischer and colleagues and Haapaniemi and colleagues that suggested that lactic acid and ammonia were removed faster with HBO treatment leading to shorter recovery periods.** (Haapaniemi et al, 1995) (Fischer et al, 1988)

Also in our experience at the Matosinhos Hyperbaric Unit several situations, namely **fractures and ligament injuries, have proved to benefit from faster recovery times when HBO treatments were applied to the athletes.** (Barata et al, 2011)

### Muscle injuries

Muscle injury presents a challenging problem in traumatology and commonly occurs in sports. The injury can occur as a consequence of a direct mechanical deformation (as contusions, lacerations and strains) or due to indirect causes (such as ischemia and neurological damage). These indirect injuries can be either complete or incomplete.

In sport events in the United States, the incidence of all injuries ranges from 10% to 55%.

The majority of muscle injuries (more than 90%) are caused either by excessive strain or by contusions of the muscle. A muscle suffers a contusion when it is subjected to a sudden, heavy compressive force, such as a direct blow. In strains, however, the muscle is subjected to an excessive tensile force leading to the overstraining of the myofibers and, consequently, to their rupture near the myotendinous junction.

Muscle injuries represent a continuum from mild muscle cramp to complete muscle rupture, and in between is partial strain injury and **delayed onset muscle soreness (DOMS)**. DOMS usually occurs following unaccustomed physical activity and is accompanied by a sensation of discomfort within the skeletal muscle experienced by the novice or elite athlete. The intensity of discomfort increases within the first 24 hours following cessation of exercise, peaks between 24 and 72 hours, subsides and eventually disappears by 5–7 days post-exercise.

**Oriani and colleagues first suggested that HBO might accelerate the rate of recovery from injuries suffered in sports.** (Oriani et al. 1982)

However, the first clinical report appeared only in 1993 where results suggested a 55% reduction in lost days to injury, in professional soccer players in Scotland suffering from a variety of injuries following the application of HBO. These values were based on a physiotherapist's estimation of the time course for the injury versus the actual number of days lost with routine therapy and HBO treatment sessions.

Although promising, this study needed a control group and required a greater homogeneity of injuries as suggested by Babul and colleagues.

## Delayed onset muscle soreness (DOMS)

DOMS describes a phenomenon of muscle pain, muscle soreness or muscle stiffness that is generally felt 12–48 hours after exercise, particularly at the beginning of a new exercise program, after a change in sporting activities, or after a dramatic increase in the duration or intensity of exercise.

Staples and colleagues in an animal study, used a downhill running model to induce damage, and **observed significant changes in the myeloperoxidase levels in rats treated with hyperbaric oxygen** compared with untreated rats. It was suggested that hyperbaric oxygen could have an inhibitory effect on the inflammatory process or the ability to actually modulate the injury to the tissue.

In 1999, the same group conducted a randomized, controlled, double-blind, prospective study to determine whether intermittent exposures to hyperbaric oxygen enhanced recovery from DOMS of the quadriceps by using 66 untrained men between the ages of 18 and 35 years. After the induction of muscle soreness, the subjects were treated in a hyperbaric chamber over a 5-day period in two phases: the first phase with four groups (control, hyperbaric oxygen treatment, delayed treatment and sham treatment); and in the second phase three groups (3 days of treatment, 5 days of treatment and sham treatment). The hyperbaric exposures involved 100% oxygen for 1 hour at 2.0 ATA.

The sham treatments involved 21% oxygen for 1 hour at 1.2 ATA. In phase 1, a significant difference in recovery of eccentric torque was noted in the treatment group compared with the other groups as well as in phase 2, where there was also a significant recovery of eccentric torque for the 5-day treatment group compared with the sham group, immediately after exercise and up to 96 hours after exercise. However, **there was no significant difference in pain in either phase.**

**The results suggested that treatment with hyperbaric oxygen may enhance recovery of eccentric torque of the quadriceps muscle from delayed onset muscle soreness (DOMS).** This study had a complex protocol and the experimental design was not entirely clear (exclusion of some participants and the allocation of groups was not clarified), which makes interpretation difficult. (Bennett et al. 2005)

**Mekjavic and colleagues did not find any recovery from DOMS after HBO.**

They studied 24 healthy male subjects who were randomly assigned to a placebo group or a HBO group after being induced with DOMS in their right elbow flexors. The HBO group was exposed to 100% oxygen at 2.5 ATA and the sham group to 8% oxygen at 2.5 ATA both for 1 hour per day and during 7 days. **Over the period of 10 days there was no difference in the rate of recovery of muscle strength between the two groups or the perceived pain. Although this was a randomized, double-blind trial, this was a small study.** (Bennett et al. 2005)

Harrison and colleagues also studied the effect of HBO in 21 healthy male volunteers after inducing DOMS in the elbow flexors. The subjects were assigned to three groups: control, immediate HBO and delayed HBO. These last two groups were exposed to 2.5 ATA, for 100 min with three periods of 30 min at 100% oxygen intercalated with 5 min with 20.93% oxygen between them. The first group began the treatments with HBO after 2 hours and the second group 24 hours postexercise and both were administered daily for 4 days. The delayed HBO group were also given a sham treatment with HBO at day 0 during the same time as the following days' treatments but with 20.93% oxygen at a minimal pressure. The control group had no specific therapy. **There were no significant differences between groups in serum creatine kinase (CK) levels, isometric strength, swelling or pain, which suggested that HBO was not effective on DOMS.** This study also presented limitations such as a small sample size and just partial blinding. (Bennett et al. 2005)

Webster and colleagues wanted to determine whether HBO accelerated recovery from exercise-induced muscle damage in 12 healthy male volunteers that underwent strenuous eccentric exercise of the gastrocnemius muscle. (Webster et al. 2002)

The subjects were randomly assigned to two groups, where the first was the sham group who received HBO with atmospheric air at 1.3 ATA, and the second with 100% oxygen with 2.5 ATA, both for 60 minutes. The first treatment was 3–4 hours after damage followed by treatments after 24 and 48 hours. **There was little evidence in the recovery measured data, highlighting a faster recovery in the HBO group in the isometric torque, pain sensation and unpleasantness.** However, it was a small study with multiple outcomes and some data were not used due to difficulties in interpretation.

Babul and colleagues also conducted a randomized, double-blind study in order to find out whether HBO accelerated the rate of recovery from DOMS in the quadriceps muscle. This exercise-induced injury was produced in 16 sedentary female students that were assigned into two groups: control and HBO. The first was submitted to 21% oxygen at 1.2 ATA, and the second to 100% oxygen at 2.0 ATA for 60 minutes at 4, 24, 48 and 72 hours postinjury. **There were no significant differences between the groups in the measured outcomes.** However, this was also a small study with multiple outcomes, with a complex experimental design with two distinct phases with somewhat different therapy arms. (Bennett et al. 2005)

Germain and colleagues had the same objective as the previous study but this time the sample had 10 female and 6 male subjects that were randomly assigned into two groups: the control group that did not undergo any treatment and the HBO group that was exposed to 95% oxygen at 2.5 ATA during 100 minutes for five sessions. **There were no significant differences between the groups which lead to the conclusion that HBO did not accelerate the rate of recovery of DOMS in the quadriceps.** Once again, this was a very small and unblinded study that presented multiple outcomes. (Bennett et al. 2005)

## Muscle stretch injury

In 1998, Best and colleagues wanted to analyze whether HBO improved functional and morphologic recovery after a controlled induced muscle stretch in the tibialis anterior muscle—tendon unit. (Best et al. 1998)

They used a rabbit model of injury and the treatment group was submitted to a 5-day treatment with 95% oxygen at 2.5 ATA for 60 minutes. Then, after 7 days, this group was compared with a control group that did not undergo HBO treatment. **The results suggested that HBO administration may play a role in accelerating recovery after acute muscle stretch injury.**

## Ischemia

Another muscle injury that is often a consequence of trauma is ischemia. Normally it is accompanied by anaerobic glycolysis, the formation of lactate and depletion of high-energy phosphates within the extracellular fluid of the affected skeletal muscle tissue. When ischemia is prolonged it can result in loss of cellular homeostasis, disruption of ion gradients and breakdown of membrane phospholipids. The activation of neutrophils, the production of oxygen radicals and the release of vasoactive factors, during reperfusion, may cause further damage to local and remote tissues. However, the mechanisms of ischemia—reperfusion-induced muscle injury are not fully understood.

These authors aimed to see the effects of HBO in the skeletal muscle of rats after ischemia-induced injury and found that HBO treatment attenuated significantly the increase of lactate and glycerol levels caused by ischemia, without affecting glucose concentration, and modulating antioxidant enzyme activity in the postischemic skeletal muscle.

A similar study was performed in 1996 in which the authors concluded that **HBO had positive aspects for at least 48 hours after severe injury, by raising the levels of high-energy phosphate compounds, which indicated a stimulation of aerobic oxidation in the mitochondria.** This maintains the transport of ions and molecules across the cell membrane and optimizes the possibility of preserving the muscle cell structure.

Gregorevic and colleagues induced muscle degeneration in rats in order to see whether HBO hastens the functional recovery and myofiber regeneration of the skeletal muscle. (Gregorevic et al.2000)

The results of this study demonstrated that **the mechanism of improved functional capacity is not associated with the reestablishment of a previously compromised blood supply or with the repair of associated nerve components, as seen in ischemia, but with the pressure of oxygen inspired with a crucial role in improving the maximum force-producing capacity of the regenerating muscle fibers after this myotoxic injury**.

**In addition, there were better results following 14 days of HBO treatment at 3 ATA than at 2 ATA.**

### Ankle sprains

In 1995 a study conducted at the Temple University suggested that patients treated with HBO returned approximately 30% faster than the control group after ankle sprain. The authors stated, however, that there was a large variability in this study design due to the difficulty in quantifying the severity of sprains.

Interestingly, Borromeo and colleagues, in a randomized, double-blinded study, observed in 32 patients who had acute ankle sprains the effects of HBO in its rehabilitation. (Borromeo et al.1997)

The HBO group was submitted to 100% oxygen at 2 ATA for 90 minutes for the first session and 60 minutes for the other two. The placebo group was exposed to ambient air, at 1.1 ATA for 90 minutes, both groups for three sessions over 7 days. **The HBO group had an improvement in joint function following acute ankle sprains.** (Borromeo et al.1997)

**However, there were no significant differences between groups in the subjective pain, edema, passive or active range of motion or time to recovery.** This study included an average delay of 34 hours from the time of injury to treatment, and it had short treatment duration. (Bennett et al. 2005)

## Medical collateral ligament

Horn and colleagues in an animal study surgically lacerated medial collateral ligament of 48 rats. (Horn et al. 1999)

Half were controls without intervention and the other half were exposed to HBO at 2.8 ATA for 1.5 hours a day over 5 days. Six rats from each group were euthanized at 2, 4, 6 and 8 weeks and at 4 weeks a statistically greater force was required to cause failure of the previously divided ligaments for those exposed to HBO than in the control group. **After 4 weeks, an interesting contribution from HBO could be seen in that it promoted the return of normal stiffness of the ligament following injury to the medial collateralligament**. (Horn et al. 1999)

Ishii and colleagues induced **ligament lacerations** in the right limb of 44 rats and divided them into four groups: control group, where animals breathed room air at 1 ATA for 60 min; HBO treatment at 1.5 ATA for 30 min once a day; HBO treatment at 2 ATA for 30 min once a day; and 2 ATA for 60 min once a day. After 14 days postinjury, of the three exposures the **HBOT 2 ATA for 60 min once a day was more effective in promoting healing by enhancing extracellular matrix deposition as measured by collagen synthesis**.

**Mashitori and colleagues** removed a 2-mm segment of the medial collateral ligament in 76 rats. Half of these rats were exposed to HBO at 2.5 ATA for 2 hours for 5 days per week and the remaining rats were exposed to room air. The authors observed that **HBO promotes scar tissue formation by increasing type I procollagen gene expression, at 7 and 14 days after the injury, which contribute for the improvement of their tensile properties**.

In a randomized, controlled and double-blind study, Soolsma examined the effect of HBO at the recovery of a grade II medial ligament of the knee presented in patients within 72 hours of injury. After one group was exposed to HBO at 2 ATA for 1 hour and the control group at 1.2 ATA, room air, for 1 hour, both groups for 10 sessions, the data suggested that, **at 6 weeks, HBO had positive effects on pain and functional outcomes, such as decreased volume of edema, a better range of motion and maximum flexion improvement**, compared with the sham group. (Soolsma, 1996)

## Anterior cruciate ligament

**Yeh and colleagues** used an animal model to investigate the effects of HBO on neovascularization at the tendon-bone junction, collagen fibers of the tendon graft and the tendon graft-bony interface which is incorporated into the osseous tunnel. The authors used 40 rabbits that were divided into two groups: the control group that was maintained in cages at normal air and the HBO group that was exposed to 100% oxygen at 2.5 ATA for 2 hours, for 5 days. The authors found that the **HBO group had significantly increased the amount of trabecular bone around the tendon graft, increasing its incorporation to the bone and therefore increasing the tensile loading strength of the tendon graft.** They assumed that HBO contributes to the angiogenesis of blood vessels, improving the blood supply which leads to the observed outcomes.

**Takeyama and colleagues** studied the effects of HBO on gene expressions of procollagen and tissue inhibitor of metalloproteinase (TIMPS) in injured anterior cruciate ligaments. After surgical injury animals were divided into a control group and a group that was submitted to HBO, 2.5 ATA for 2 hours, for 5 days. It was found that even though none of the lacerated anterior cruciate ligaments (ACLs) united macroscopically, there was an increase of the gene expression of type I procollagen and of TIMPS I and 2 for the group treated with HBO. These results indicate that HBO enhances structural protein synthesis and inhibits degradative processes. Consequently **using HBO as an adjunctive therapy after primary repair of the injured ACL is likely to increase success, a situation that is confirmed by the British Medical Journal Evidence Center.** (Minhas, 2010)

## Fractures

Classical treatment with osteosynthesis and bone grafting is not always successful and the attempt to heal nonunion and complicated fractures, where the likelihood of infection is increased, is a challenge.

A Cochrane review (Bennett et al. 2005b) stated that **there is not sufficient evidence to support hyperbaric oxygenation for the treatment of promoting fracture healing or nonunion fracture as no randomized evidence was found.** During the last 10 years this issue has not been the subject of many studies.

**Okubo and colleagues** studied a rat model in which recombinant human bone morphogenetic protein-2 was implanted in the form of ly-ophilized discs, the influence of HBO. **The group treated with HBO, exposed to 2 ATA for 60 min daily, had significantly increased new bone formation compared with the control group and the cartilage was present at the outer edge of the implanted material after 7 days.**

**Komurcu and colleagues reviewed retrospectively 14 cases of infected tibial nonunion that were treated successfully.** Management included aggressive debridement and correction of defects by corticotomy and internal bone transport. The infection occurred in two patients after the operation which was successfully resolved after 20–30 sessions of HBO.

**Muhonen and colleagues** aimed to study, in a rabbit mandibular distraction osteogenesis model, the osteogenic and angiogenic response to irradiation and HBO. One group was exposed to 18 sessions of HBO until the operation that was performed 1 month after irradiation. The second group did not receive HBO and the controls underwent surgery receiving neither irradiation nor HBO. The authors concluded that previous irradiation suppresses osteoblastic activity and **HBO changes the pattern of bone-forming activity towards that of nonirradiated bone**.

**Wang and colleagues**, in a rabbit model, were able to demonstrate that **distraction segments of animals treated with HBO had increased bone mineral density and superior mechanical properties comparing to the controls and yields better results when applied during the early stage of the tibial healing process.**

## Conclusion

In the various studies, **the location of the injury seemed to have an influence on the effectiveness of treatment.** After being exposed to HBO, for example, injuries at the muscle belly seem to have less benefit than areas of reduced perfusion such as muscle—tendon junctions and ligaments.

With regards to HBO treatment, it is still necessary to determine the optimal conditions for these orthopedic indications, such as the atmosphere pressure, the duration of sessions, the frequency of sessions and the duration of treatment. Differences in the magnitude of the injury and in the time between injury and treatment may also affect outcomes.

**Injuries studies involving bones, muscles and ligaments with HBO treatment seem promising**. However, they are comparatively scarce and the quality of evidence for the efficacy of HBO is low. Orthopaedic indications for HBO will become better defined with perfection of the techniques for direct measurement of tissue oxygen tensions and intramuscular compartment pressures. Despite evidence of interesting results when treating high-performance athletes, these treatments are multifactorial and are rarely published. Therefore, there is a need for larger samples, randomized, controlled, double-blind clinical trials of human (mainly athletes) and animal models in order to identify its effects and mechanisms to determine whether it is a safe and effective therapy for sports injuries treatments.

---

## Hyperbaric oxygen in the critically ill

**Abstract**

**OBJECTIVE:**

To review aspects of hyperbaric medicine pertinent to treating critically ill patients with hyperbaric oxygen in both monoplace and multiplace chambers.

**DATA SOURCES:**

Literature review of online databases, research repositories, and clinical trial registries.

**RESULTS:**

The search of these resources produced information regarding technical considerations, feasibility, risk, and patient management. Hyperbaric oxygen is used in treating a number of disorders that occur in critically ill patients, including acute carbon monoxide poisoning, arterial gas embolism, severe decompression sickness, clostridial gas gangrene, necrotizing fasciitis, and acute crush injury. Most chambers in the United States treat outpatients with problem nonhealing wounds, and many chambers are not hospital-based. Only a few hyperbaric medicine centers have intensive care unit-level staffing, specialized equipment, a 24/7 schedule, and experience in treating critically ill patients. Not all intensive care unit-related equipment can be subjected to hyperbaric pressurization, and some equipment may increase the risk for fire inside the chamber.

## CONCLUSIONS:

Treating critically ill patients with hyperbaric oxygen requires specialized equipment and personnel with intensive care unit skills and knowledge of the physiology and risks unique to hyperbaric oxygen exposure. Like with all medical interventions, it is important to consider the risk vs. the benefit of hyperbaric oxygen for any given critical care disorder, but **hyperbaric oxygen can be delivered safely to critically ill patients**. Many critical care environments without present hyperbaric oxygen capability may wish to consider offering hyperbaric oxygen to patients with hyperbaric oxygen-approved indications. (Weaver, 2011)

### Hyperbaric medicine for the hospital-based physician

### Abstract

**Hyperbaric oxygen (HBO2) is the inhalation of 100% oxygen at pressures > 1.4 times atmospheric pressure**. Hyperbaric oxygen can be delivered in monoplace (single person) or multiplace (multiperson) chambers.

**Most clinical HBO2 exposures are between 2 and 2.4 atm abs for approximately 2 hours**.

**Hyperbaric oxygen causes the blood and tissue oxygen levels to increase**, reduces the volume of intravascular and tissue bubbles (to treat decompression sickness [DCS] and arterial gas embolism [AGE]), and accelerates wash-out of other gases, such as nitrogen or carbon monoxide (CO), which is important for DCS, AGE, and CO poisoning.

Hyperbaric oxygen favorably modulates ischemia-reperfusion injury by transiently inhibiting neutrophil-endothelial interactions, which is important for patients with DCS, AGE, CO poisoning, and potentially other acute ischemic conditions. **Because of enhanced oxygen delivery, HBO$_2$ is used for acute crush injury, ischemic flaps and** grafts, acute central retinal arterial occlusion, other acute arterial occlusions, and idiopathic sudden sensorineural hearing loss.

Hyperbaric oxygen has antimicrobial effects and is offered for patients with limb- or life-threatening infections, such as clostridial gas gangrene and necrotizing fasciitis.

The most common **US** indication for **HBO$_2$** is the treatment of ischemic wounds (i.e., diabetic lower extremity wounds, late effects of radiation, and refractory osteomyelitis). In ischemic wounds, **HBO$_2$** can deliver sufficient oxygen to the non-healing wound to stimulate angiogenesis and healing through multiple mechanisms, including increased collagen production, increased growth factor receptor numbers, upregulation of vascular endothelial growth factor, increased circulating endothelial progenitor cells, and improvement in neutrophil-mediated host defense.

Clinical trials support efficacy of **HBO$_2$** for acute **CO** poisoning, diabetic lower extremity wounds, crush injury, and radiation necrosis. Most hyperbaric chambers are associated with wound care centers and may be hospital based or nonhospital based. We review some of the disorders treated with HBO$_2$ that hospital-based clinicians may be asked to evaluate. (Weaver, 1995)

# SECTION SEVEN

## HBOT AND CANCER

The following article was adapted from: (Moen, Stuhr, 2012).

### Hyperbaric oxygen therapy and cancer—a review

**Hypoxia is a critical hallmark of solid tumors and involves enhanced cell survival, angiogenesis, glycolytic metabolism, and metastasis.**

**Hyperbaric oxygen (HBO) treatment has for centuries been used to improve or cure disorders involving hypoxia and ischemia, by enhancing the amount of dissolved oxygen in the plasma and thereby increasing $O_2$ delivery to the tissue.**

Studies on HBO and cancer have, up to recently, focused on whether enhanced oxygen acts as a cancer promoter or not. As oxygen is believed to be required for all the major processes of wound healing, one feared that the effects of HBO would be applicable to cancer tissue as well and promote cancer growth. Furthermore, one also feared that exposing patients who had been treated for cancer, to HBO, would lead to recurrence. Nevertheless, **two systematic reviews on HBO and cancer have concluded that the use of HBO in patients with malignancies is considered safe.**

**To supplement the previous reviews, we have summarized the work performed on HBO and cancer in the period 2004–2012. Based on the present as well as previous reviews, there is no evidence indicating that HBO neither acts as a stimulator of tumor growth nor as an enhancer of recurrence.**

On the other hand, **there is evidence that implies that HBO might have tumor-inhibitory effects in certain cancer subtypes**.

Pubmed was searched for articles concerning hyperbaric oxygen (HBO) and cancer for the period from 2004 to 2012, using the MeSH search terms ("hyperbaric oxygenation" and/or "hyperoxia" and "neoplasms"). A total of 28 articles were found relevant, directly involving the use of HBO as a stand-alone or as adjuvant treatment on different cancer types. We focused on growth, cell survival, angiogenesis, and metastasis observed in HBO-treated cancers the last 9 years, both as stand-alone and adjuvant treatment, and compared them to older publications involving the selected topic.

## Cancer and hypoxia

**Solid tumors often contain areas subjected to acute or chronic hypoxia**, though with variable severity in patients both within and among different tumor types. (Michiele, 2009) (Vaupel, Mayer, 2007)

**Although severe or prolonged hypoxia is deleterious, adaptation to the hypoxic microenvironment has allowed cancer cells to survive and proliferate in this hostile milieu.** (Harris, 2002)

Tumor hypoxia develops due to the structural and functional abnormalities of the tumor vasculature since **cancer growth often overrides the ability of the cancer vasculature to adapt to the increasing oxygen demand.**

Traditionally, hypoxia was thought of as a factor limiting cancer growth by reducing the ability of cells to divide. However, more recently, hypoxia has proven to be a causative factor in many pathophysiological events, including cancer progression.

**Multiple reports have demonstrated that decreased oxygen tension selects for more malignant cells and induces multiple cellular adaptations, which again sustains and fosters cancer progression and thereby induces cancer growth.**

Hypoxia is reported to result in cellular responses which improve oxygenation and viability through induction of angiogenesis, an alteration in metabolism by increased glycolysis and upregulation of genes involved in cell survival/apoptosis. (Holmquist et al, 2006)

Hypoxia has also been shown to increase genetic instability, activate invasive growth, and preserve the undifferentiated cell state. (Michiele, 2009) (Harris, 2002)

Studies have demonstrated that **hypoxia is implicated in the resistance to conventional therapy.** (Shannon et al, 2003)

**Oxygen concentration has an especially crucial role in radiation oncology and radiation resistance.** (Gray et al, 1953) (Overgaard, 2011)

**The epithelial-to-mesenchymal transition in cancer has been shown to be induced by hypoxic conditions, leading to cancers with an invasive or metastatic phenotype.** (Cannito et al, 2008) (Thiery, 2002)

Given its important role as a negative prognostics and predictive factor, **hypoxia is considered as one of the best targets in cancer treatment.**

**Hypoxia is a hallmark of solid tumors.**

The dual role of oxygen leads to the question: will lack of oxygen inhibit cancer progression, or is hyperoxygenating the tumor tissue the way to go in order to prevent cancer growth and development?

## Hyperbaric oxygen

Hyperbaric oxygen can be used to overcome hypoxia. HBO is based on administration of 100 % oxygen at higher than normal atmospheric pressure. **HBO treatment enhances the amount of dissolved oxygen in the plasma, thereby increasing $O_2$ tissue delivery independent of hemoglobin.** (Gill, Bell, 2004)

**As in normal tissue, the $pO_2$ in cancer tissue increases significantly during HBO exposure.** (Brizel et al, 1995)

Thus, **elevation of the tumor oxygen pressure has been shown to be preserved clinically for approximately 30 min after HBO exposure.** (Kinoshita et al, 1999)

HBO therapy is today accepted and routinely used for many disorders, related to both ischemia and/or hypoxia. (Gill, Bell, 2004)

HBO is considered safe and complications are rare using today's standard treatment protocols. **The Undersea and Hyperbaric Medical Society has a list of approved indications for HBO therapy, including decompression sickness, severe carbon monoxide poisoning, nonhealing wounds, and late radiation injury.**

As **oxygen is believed to be required for all the major processes involved in wound healing, including resistance to infection, activation of fibroblasts, collagen deposition, angiogenesis, and epithelization, it has been feared that HBO would have a proliferative effect in cancers.** (Hopf, Rollins, 2007)

Thus, for many decades, the focus has been to elucidate if HBO promotes cancer growth.

In the early 2000s, both Feldmeier et al. and Daruwalla et al. reviewed the literature concerning HBO and cancer. (Feldmeier et al, 2003)

The reviews included both experimental and clinical studies using different types of cancers, with and without additional therapy, and the results showed varied responses. **Nevertheless, the conclusion in both reviews was that HBO did not promote cancer growth, and that the use of HBO in patients with malignancies was considered safe.** (Feldmeier et al, 2003) (Daruwalla, Christophi, 2006)

There are extensive studies on the effect of HBO on normal tissue and wounds. Interestingly, evidence implies that cancer tissue might differ in response from normal tissue. The studies performed on HBO and cancer are complex due to a wide range of experimental designs and treatment regimes. Moen and Stuhr have summarized the literature concerning the effect of HBO on crucial hallmarks of cancer, the effect of HBO on chemo- and radiation therapy, and in addition we have clustered the different cancer type responses.

## HBO and cell survival

**Studies of prolonged hyperoxia have shown that elevated levels of reactive oxygen species (ROS) overwhelm the antioxidant defense and lead to cellular damage and possible organ dysfunction.** (Gore et al, 2010)

The tissue damage is found to be dependent on the cell type, concentration of oxygen, and the duration of the exposure. Gore et al. have summarized the molecular mechanisms behind hyperoxia-induced cell death, revealing a complex signaling system including protein kinases and receptors such as RAGE, CXCR2, TLR3, and TLR4. (Gore et al, 2010)

Studies of apoptosis in neoplasms treated with HBO are limited. **Two in vitro studies on mammary and oral cancer cells, respectively, showed no change in apoptosis after HBO**. (Sun, Chen, Hsu, 2004) (Chen et al, 2007)

On the other hand, Chen et al. observed activation of the pro-apoptotic pathway MAPK and downregulation of the anti-apoptotic ERK pathway in hematopoetic cells after HBO. (Chen et al, 2007)

Additionally, **a study of HBO using osteosarcoma cells also demonstrated induction of apoptosis.** (Kawasoe et al, 2009)

**In two different animal models, gliomas and mammary tumors, respectively, Moen and Stuhr's group has demonstrated induction of cell death after HBO treatment.** (Raa et al, 2007) (Sturh et al, 2007) (Moen et al, 2009)

Furthermore, **reduced cell proliferation, together with a significant change in histology, has also been shown after HBO treatment in DMBA-induced mammary tumors in vivo.** (Raa et al, 2007) (Sturh et al, 2007) (Moen et al, 2009)

**Granowitz et al. observed the same reduction in cell proliferation in their mammary in vitro study.** (Granowitz et al, 2005)

In addition, **two recent studies on osteosarcoma cells and nasopharyngeal carcinoma support inhibition of cell division after HBO treatment.** (Kawasoe et al, 2009) (Peng et al, 2010)

Together, this might imply that changes in oxygen concentration influence antioxidant pathways, leading to a change in cell survival signaling. However, the picture is complex, and mechanistic studies are required before any final conclusions can be drawn. (Goodman et al, 2010)

## HBO and angiogenesis

Today, **angiogenesis is proposed to be a key factor for cancer growth and metastasis.** Thus, large experimental studies and clinical trials have investigated the effect of antiangiogenic therapies in the treatment of cancers. **Since HBO in general has been shown to promote cellular and vascular proliferation in normal tissue and wounds** (although the mechanisms are not fully understood), it was assumed that it would also induce angiogenesis in cancers.

In contrary to what is expected and addressed in the literature, **HBO has been shown to induce an antiangiogenic effect in two mammary tumor models,** in addition to one glioma model.

Furthermore, **multiple studies showed no change in angiogenesis after HBO treatment.** (Shi et al, 2005) (Heys et al, 2006) (Sji et al, 2005) (Chong et al, 2004) (Schonmeyr et al, 2008) (Thom, 2011) (Tang et al, 2009) (Hampson et al, 2004)

In his review, Feldmeier et al. thoroughly discussed oxygen and tumor angiogenesis, underlining the difference between cancer tissue and wounds and **concluded that HBO is not likely to enhance tumor angiogenesis.** (Feldmeier et al, 2003)

Thom (Schonmeyr et al, 2008) commented on the fact that the influence HBO has on hypoxia-induced factor isoform expression appears to vary with different tissues and possibly with chronology (e.g., looking early or late after wounding or an ischemic insult). **There is no evidence for enhanced angiogenesis in cancerous tissue.**

## HBO and metastasis

In 1966, **Johnson and Lauchlan first raised concern that HBO might have metastatic potential.** (Johnson, Lauchlan, 1966) (Feldmeier et al, 1994)

However, **it was not possible to show a statistically significant increase in the number of patients with distant metastasis,** as the number of patients in the series was too small. Nevertheless, special attention was given to metastatic growth because the first reports suggested that HBO might be affecting this part of tumor progression. (Feldmeier et al, 1994)

Metastasis is a complex process requiring multiple steps, including local tumor cell invasion, entry into the blood or lymph vessels, and re-penetration and colonization at a distant site. Eventually, angiogenesis is also required for distant metastasis to form. (Zijl et al, 2011)

So far, only observational studies have been performed, and studies of the effect of HBO on the individual steps of the metastatic process are still lacking. (Feldmeier et al, 1994)

**None of the studies reviewed showed induced metastasis after HBO**. (Kawasoe et al, 2009) (Haroon et al, 2007) (Moen et al, 2012) (Daruwalla, Christophi, 2006) (Daruwalla et al, 2007)

Furthermore, **a recent study found HBO to induce a mesenchymal-to-epithelial transition (MET) in DMBA-induced mammary tumors, leading to a less aggressive tumor type, thus indicating that oxygen might be a key factor in MET**. (Bock et al, 2011)

**This transition should lead to cancers with a less invasive and metastatic phenotype**.

### HBO and chemotherapy

Hypoxia has been described as an important factor for chemotherapeutic resistance.

Teicher underlined that **the importance of hypoxia on the response to chemotherapy is highly drug dependent**. However, hypoxia-mediated chemoresistance has been ascribed to: (1) altered cellular metabolism reducing drug cytotoxicity; (2) **the redox state, meaning that oxygen is required to generate ROS to be maximally cytotoxic**; and (3) genetic instability, which can lead to more rapid development of drug-resistant cells. In addition to the cytotoxicity, availability of the chemotherapeutic drug in high enough dose is important to obtain a maximal effect. (Teicher, 1994)

Tumor tissue anatomy influences transport of intravenously injected substances to the cancer cells, and thus determines the efficacy of the drug.

Al-Waili et al. summarized the potential role of HBO in combination with conventional therapies. **They hypothesized that HBO could improve and help overcome chemotherapeutic resistance by increasing both tumor perfusion and cellular sensitivity.** (Al-Waili et al, 2005)

Studies on HBO as a chemotherapeutic adjuvant have shown augmented effects both in vitro and in vivo, **although the mechanism(s) are not known**.

Heys et al. studied the effect of HBO on chemotherapy in a clinical setting, using HBO as a pretreatment to improve vascularity, and thereby improve the effect of chemotherapy. However, **HBO did not increase the neovascularity**, and they correlated the lack of chemotherapeutic potentiation to this.

In a mammary tumor model, Moen et al. found that **the uptake of chemotherapy is increased for the duration of, and immediately after, HBO treatment.** (Moen et al, 2009, BMC)

**Based on this study, potentiation of chemotherapy can probably not occur unless the chemotherapeutic agent is administered during or immediately after the HBO session, when the $pO_2$ is elevated.**

Another study by Moen et al., on the same mammary tumor model, found altered genetic expression after HBO indicating a change to less tumorigenic metabolism, possibly influencing the chemotherapeutic response.

**Many have ascribed the enhanced chemotherapeutic effect after HBO to increased levels of ROS. Moen et al., however, found no change in MDA levels after HBO, indicating that in this study ROS levels cannot be the main determinant of an increased chemotherapeutic effect.** (Moen et al, 2009)

Microarray studies have made it possible to classify breast cancers at the molecular level and correlate their signatures with metastatic behavior and clinical outcome, and thereby making it easier to develop targeted therapy.

Underlining the importance of breast cancer subtyping, it is important to comment on the differences between different tumor models: **Moen et al. found an increased uptake of the chemotherapeutic drug 5-FU into DMBA-induced tumors after HBO**, while Jevne et al.

failed to find the same correlation in the 4T1 mammary tumor model. (Moen et al, 2009) (Jevne et al, 2011)

The combination of HBO and chemotherapy has also been tried in other cancer types.

Suzuki et al. suggest that HBO therapy prolongs the biological residence time of carboplatin in glioma patients. (Suzuki et al, 2009)

However, there are still uncertainties concerning the mechanisms of action of HBO on the efficacy of carboplatin. The same group found that HBO enhanced transendothelial permeability in rat brains and HBO might therefore be favorable for the uptake and therefore also the effect of carboplatin.

**Preliminary results from a small, clinical study, on nonsmall cell lung cancer, show promising results when combining hyperthermia and HBO with paclitaxel and carboplatin.**

However, they emphasize that the study lacks proper controls, and thereby the additional value of HBO to the chemohyperthermia response cannot be made.

Kawasoe et al. found, both in vitro and in vivo, that HBO enhanced the chemotherapeutic effect of carboplatin in osteosarcomas. Furthermore, **combining HBO and cisplatin significantly reduced tumor volume in a human ovarian cancer xenograft model.** (Selvendiran et al, 2010)

It is, however, important to underline that Mayer et al. list up five chemotherapeutic agents (doxorubicin, bleomycin, disulfiram, cisplatin, and mafenide acetate); all of which are strongly contradictory in combination with HBO due to potential potentiation of toxicity. (Kohshi et al, 1999)

Of the reviewed papers, only Heys et al. and Selvendiran et al. have utilized the listed chemotherapeutics in combination with HBO. (Selvendiran et al, 2010)

---

## HBO and radiotherapy

Radiotherapy in combination with HBO has been used clinically in two different applications: (1) as a therapeutic agent for treating late radiation injury and (2) **as a radiosensitizer, aiming to increase the effect of radiotherapy**.

In this review, we focus only on the latter application of HBO. (Mayer et al, 2005)

**Gray et al. proved in the 1950s that the oxygen concentration influences the effect of radiotherapy** and the influence of hypoxic modification in relation to radiotherapy has been extensively studied since then.

In 2011, **Overgaard published a meta-analysis reviewing the influence of hypoxic modification of radiotherapy in head and neck carcinoma**. Overall, **Overgaard found that out of the various hypoxic modification techniques, HBO showed the most pronounced effect, and thus will improve the results of radiotherapy**.

Nevertheless, in a recent and extensive review by Bennett et al., the authors have also reviewed the effect of radiotherapy in combination with HBO. **They concluded that there is some evidence that HBO improves local tumor control and mortality in tumors of the head and neck**; however, the outcomes seem to be related to the use of unusual fractionation schemes, and **Bennett et al. thereby conclude that the benefits of HBO should be interpreted with caution.** (Bennett et al, 2012)

**It has also been shown that adverse side effects like oxygen poisoning and severe tissue radiation injury is associated with the use of HBO in combination with radiotherapy.** (Bennett et al, 2012)

However, it is important to emphasize the importance of timing of HBO exposure in relation to the radiation.

Kohshi et al. found that to avoid hazardous side effects, irradiation should be administered immediately after and not concurrently to HBO treatment. (Kohshi et al, 1999)

**It has been shown that euoxic conditions persist for some time after HBO exposure due to postponed oxygen saturation and washout kinetics.**

Thus, a change in protocols could possibly reduce or prevent serious side effects, and thereby justify the use of HBO in radiosensitization. A conclusion regarding the use of HBO in combination with radiotherapy still remains unclear.

## HBO and cancer types   (Moen, Stuhr, 2012)

This review summarizes the work performed on HBO and cancer during the last 9 years and supports the previous findings since **none of the studies reported a cancer-promoting effect of HBO**.

However, we have changed the focus to whether HBO might have an inhibitory effect on cancer growth. The variety of responses observed in cancers after HBO treatment supports what we know today, i.e., that **no single treatment of any kind will be efficient in all types of cancers.**

However, could the treatment be efficient in some cancer types? And if so, why do we observe these differences?

## HBO and breast cancer

Breast cancer is the most frequently occurring cancer in women and comprises 22.8 % of cancer incidence in females worldwide. (Boyle, Levin, 2008)

**Granowitz et al. showed that HBO treatment alone had a strong antiproliferative effect on different mammary cancer cells in vitro.**

They suggested that HBO could be an effective therapy for breast cancer. This is supported by six different animal studies performed during the last 9 years, using clinically relevant HBO protocols. These revealed a significant inhibitory effect of HBO as a stand-alone treatment on mammary tumor growth in vivo.

**Feldmeier et al. and Daruwalla et al. reviewed three older studies on mammary tumors and HBO, all in the same C3H mouse model, where none of them found effects on tumor growth.** (Suit, Maeda, 1967) (McCredie et al, 1966) (Shewell, Thompson, 1980)

However, they did not consider an extensive study from 1964 in their reviews, where Kluft et al. reported that **HBO retarded growth of a transplanted mammary carcinoma (TM 8013) growing in C 57 black mice.** (Kluft, 1965)

As the main focus in the older studies was to confirm or reject HBO as cancer promoter, most studies focused only on cancer growth and metastasis. Nevertheless, several recent studies, showing cancer inhibitory effects, have gone into more detail. As previously mentioned, **HBO has been shown to induce an antiangiogenic effect in two mammary tumor models.**

Furthermore, **an increase in cell death and reduced cell proliferation, together with a significant change in histology, has also been shown after HBO treatment in DMBA-induced mammary tumors in vivo.**

In relation to metastasis, it has been shown that **HBO induced MET in DMBA-induced mammary tumors, leading to a less aggressive tumor type. In a 4T1 mammary tumor model, Haroon et al. found that HBO restricts the growth of large tumor cell colonies.**

Moen et al. found lung metastasis in the same tumor model after HBO, thus **HBO here did not hinder metastasis.** However, they lack comparable endpoint controls and therefore a conclusion as to whether there would be less colonies could not be drawn.

Despite a significant number of animal studies, **no clinical trials on HBO and breast cancer per se have been performed and only one small clinical study on combined treatment is available.** With this background, we conclude that the effect of HBO should be further explored in breast cancer subtypes, especially focusing on the possible effect of HBO as an adjuvant tumor therapy.

## HBO and head and neck cancer

The National Cancer Institute defines head and neck cancer as a neo-plasm that arises in the nasal cavity, sinuses, lips, mouth, salivary glands, throat, or larynx. (National Cancer Institute (2011). Available)

Only one study has been performed during recent years, where HBO has been studied in combination with radiotherapy in experimental head and neck carcinoma in mice.

They found that even though HBO did reduce the hypoxic state of the tumors, it did not have any effect on tumor growth, neither alone nor in combination with radiotherapy.

Furthermore, they did not find evidence of enhanced angiogenesis in the tumors after HBO treatment, neither when staining for CD31 nor measuring VEGF expression, supporting the notion that HBO does not induce angiogenesis in tumors.

As previously stated, Bennett et al. reviewed the effect of combining HBO with radiotherapy. Even though studies have shown beneficial re-sults on local tumor control, mortality, and local tumor recurrence, the protocols of the reviewed literature made them conclude that they could not justify the routine use of HBO in combination with radia-tion. However, as discussed in "HBO and radiotherapy," **the conclu-sion within the field of HBO and radiosensitization has not yet reached a consensus**.

## HBO and colorectal cancer

Colorectal cancer is a disease originating from the epithelial cells lining the colon or rectum of the gastrointestinal tract.

Most colorectal cancers occur due to lifestyle and increasing age with only a minority of cases associated with underlying genetic disorders.

Even though surgery can be curative if the disease is caught early, ad-ditional treatment of advanced colorectal cancer is commonly in use.

Several studies have examined the effect of HBO concomitant with oth-er therapies in colorectal cancer. **In an older clinical study, Dische**

**and Senanayake demonstrated positive results when combining HBO and radiotherapy on patients with carcinoma in the colon and the rectum.** (Dische, Senanayake, 1972)

Hjelde et al. studied the effect of hyperoxia in combination with photodynamic therapy on three different colon carcinomas in vitro. They concluded that **hyperoxia did not increase the occurrence of cell death after photodynamic therapy.** (Hjelde et al, 2005)

However, **older experimental and clinical studies have demonstrated that HBO improves the effect of photodynamic therapy.** (Maier et al, 2000) (Dong et al, 1987) (Chen et al, 2002) (Jirsa et al, 1991)

Thus, the lack of response in the study by Hjelde et al. might be ascribed to lack of hypoxic cells in the in vitro experimental setup. (Hjelde et al, 2005)

Additionally, two papers by Daruwalla et al. examine the effect of HBO in two different in vivo colon tumor models. In the first paper, the effect of HBO per se was studied. Here, **they concluded firstly that HBO did not have any tumor stimulatory effect and does not promote formation of distal metastases, and secondly that HBO therefore can safely be used in combination with other therapies.** Furthermore, they performed experiments on an in vivo model of primary colon carcinoma with HBO both alone and in combination with styrene maleic acid (SMA)–pirarubicin.

Again, they concluded that HBO alone gave no effects. However, HBO in combination with SMA–pirarubicin gave a reduction both in liver metastases and tumor growth, in addition to inducing increased levels of necrosis. Thus, **HBO as a stand-alone treatment seems to have no effect on colorectal cancer, but as a treatment adjuvant, HBO seems to be an interesting alternative** and its potential use should be explored further.

## HBO and gliomas

Gliomas are tumors originating in the glial cells in the brain or the spine. Patients with high-grade gliomas generally have poor prognosis, and the illness is rarely curable. Designing therapy is challenging due to the neoplasm's infiltrative nature, **resistance to apoptosis**, and recurrence and resistance to therapy.

In 2011, Beppu et al. reviewed the effect of HBO on gliomas. However, the review only exists in Japanese, and thus is not commented on. (Beppu et al, 2011)

In 2007, Stuhr et al. published an experimental study, examining the effect of HBO on the growth and development of rat glioma xeno-grafts per se. **They found that increased levels of $pO_2$, using both normobaric and moderate HBO, significantly reduced glioma tumor growth, possibly by increasing cell death and reducing the vascular density.**

This might indicate that HBO alone has a favorable effect on gliomas. However, it is important to underline that the experimental tumors were implanted in the neck and not in the brain, and this may well have influenced the outcome of the experiments.

Further, only three other papers in the period 2004–2012 have been published utilizing HBO on gliomas. They are all preliminary clinical studies, investigating HBO in combination with radiotherapy and chemotherapy.

**Kohshi et al. and Ogawa et al. both conclude that there is a possible advantage to combining HBO with radiotherapy,** but they also underline the need for further investigation within this field. (Kohshi et al, 2007) (Ogawa et al, 2006)

Special caution should be taken when interpreting the results from the study by Koshi et al., as anaplastic astrocytomas are included in the trial and compared with the patients with glioblastoma mulitforme.

**In a study of HBO and chemotherapy, Suzuki et al. suggest that HBO therapy prolongs the biological residence time of carboplatin.** However, the mechanisms of action of HBO on the clinical efficacy of carboplatin are still unknown.

## HBO and leukemia

Leukemia is cancer of the blood or bone marrow characterized by an abnormal increase of immature white blood cells. **Two recent in vitro experiments have shown promising results when treating leukemia cells with HBO.**

Prof Randolph M. Howes MD,PhD

In addition, Tonomura and Granowitz, in an editorial in 2007, have commented on the effect of HBO on leukemia. They concluded that since HBO promotes apoptosis in leukemia cells, it should be further exploited as a novel treatment for leukemia. (Tonomura, Granowitz, 2007)

It is, however, important to emphasize that this is based on experiments performed in cell culture, and thus needs further validation from in vivo models to exclude the possibility that this is just an in vitro phenomenon. In two older experiments, studies were performed on HBO using animal leukemia model systems. (Johnson et al, 1971) (Johnson, Kagan, Bryant, 1967)

**In neither of the in vivo experiments were differences observed in growth rate or metastasis after HBO treatment.** However, the limited number of studies might therefore call for further investigation with regard to the use of HBO in leukemia.

## HBO and prostate cancer

Cancer of the prostate gland is the second most frequent type of cancer in men worldwide, accounting for 13.6 % of all cases. Treatment of prostate cancer depends on the grade of the disease. As most prostate cancers are slow growing, some cancers are not treated at all. However, aggressive cancers are normally treated using surgery, in addition to chemotherapy, hormonal therapy, immunotherapy, and/or radiation.

Three animal studies have been published recently on HBO as stand-alone treatment of prostate cancer. **Neither Chong et al. nor Tang et al. found any change in *in vivo* tumor growth after HBO treatment.** (Tang et al, 2009, uro)

None of the pathological characteristics, such as microvessel density, differentiation status, proliferation, or apoptosis, were changed. In addition, Kalns et al. published two papers in the late 1990s where they showed that **HBO can decrease the rate of growth and increase the sensitivity to the anticancer agents taxol and doxorubicin in *in vitro* experiments, by accumulating prostate cancer cells in the chemosensitive portion of the cell cycle.** (Kalns et al, 1998) (Kalns, Piepmeier, 1999)

Further studies on in vivo prostate cancer models and the effect of HBO as an adjuvant to chemotherapy are evidently necessary before any definite conclusions can be made.

## HBO and cervical cancer and bladder cancer

Cervical cancer of the female reproductive system represents 8.8 % of cancer incidence in women and bladder cancer 3.0 % in both sexes. Based on ten clinical studies, **Daruwalla et al. stated that HBO treatment of patients with cervical and bladder cancer did not offer any improved benefit or improved outcome.** The older clinical trials, combining HBO and radiotherapy, generally showed no change in cancer growth or survival. This is presumably the reason why no new studies have been performed on the effect of HBO on these cancer types. Thus, neither cervical cancer nor bladder cancer seems to be good candidates for demonstration of an improved effect of traditional therapy in combination with HBO.

## Comments and future work

The consensus today is that research performed hitherto has failed to demonstrate that HBO has a cancer-promoting effect or that it enhances recurrence. Nevertheless, **both recent and older research studies have shown that HBO can be inhibitory and reduce cancer growth in some cancer types, like breast cancer.**

**On the other hand, cervical and bladder cancers appear to be nonresponders to HBO.**

In vitro studies have confirmed that there are discrepancies in growth fractions between different cancer cell lines following exposure to hyperoxia.

Thus, this supports the need for performing randomized studies on HBO as a stand-alone treatment or in combination with other therapies for certain cancer types or subtypes.

**The observed variety in response to HBO found during the last decades can be ascribed to both differences in types of cancers but also to the large variety in HBO treatment protocols.**

Thus, differences in response to oxygen between different cancer types should not lead to an exclusion of HBO as a form of cancer treatment or as a cancer treatment adjuvant for selected types of cancers.

Prof Randolph M. Howes MD,PhD

To clarify if tumor hypoxia is as important for cancer progression as indicated in the literature, **HBO can be used as an important research tool**. Concomitant studies of hyperoxia ("the flip of the coin") and hypoxia might be valuable and can give us additional and important information on how oxygen influences cancer growth and metastasis.

# SECTION EIGHT

## PHOTOTHERAPY

**PHOTOTHERAPY**

I have found a commonality between exercise, naked mole rats, hyperbaric oxygen therapy and phototherapy (photodynamic therapy, PDT). RMH 6-25-15

The postulated mechanism of action for many forms of chemotherapy, radiation therapy, photodynamic therapy, ozone therapy, hyperbaric oxygen therapy, intravenous mega-dose of vitamin C, the Howes singlet oxygen cancer therapy system and hydrogen peroxide therapy is the generation of electronically modified oxygen derivatives (EMODs). (Howes, 2010) (Howes R: Cancer Therapy, 2010) (Howes R: Hydrogen Peroxide: 2010) (Howes, 2005) (Howes, Farber, 2005)

**New Rules: 11 Ways to increase oxidative capacity**

1) If you do not use antioxidant supplements, don't start
2) If you use antioxidant supplements, stop
3) Exercise as much as tolerated
4) Supplemental oxygen
5) Aspirin (ASA is a good prooxidant)
6) EWOT (exercise with oxygen therapy)
7) Hyperthermia
8) Ingestion of iron (over the counter dosages)
9) Hyperbaric oxygen (HBO$_2$)
10) Vitamin D3 (a good prooxidant)
11) Artemisinin (epoxides generate prooxidants)

Prof Randolph M. Howes MD,PhD

## New Rules: others

**Hydrogen peroxide**
**Curcumin, sulphoraphane, cinnamonaldehyde**
   **(they have considerable prooxidant activity)**
**Hyperthermia**
**Methylene blue,**

### Shedding light on phototherapy

**Shedding light on a new treatment for diabetic wound healing: a review on phototherapy**

## Abstract

Impaired wound healing is a common complication associated with diabetes with complex pathophysiological underlying mechanisms and often necessitates amputation. **With the advancement in laser technology, irradiation of these wounds with low-intensity laser irradiation (LILI) or phototherapy, has shown a vast improvement in wound healing.**

**At the correct laser parameters, LILI has shown to increase migration, viability, and proliferation of diabetic cells in vitro; there is a stimulatory effect on the mitochondria with a resulting increase in adenosine triphosphate (ATP).**

In addition, LILI also has an anti-inflammatory and protective effect on these cells. In light of the ever present threat of diabetic foot ulcers, infection, and amputation, new improved therapies and the fortification of wound healing research deserves better prioritization. (Houreld, 2014)

**I believe that this can be used in combination with HBOT. I believe that phototherapy acts through mechanisms which increase excited states of oxygen, especially singlet oxygen.**

**There is a caveat, however, and it is the fact that some investigators** (Pinheiro et al, 2002) **have seen increased cancer cell proliferation with irradiation at about 630 nm laser light.**

246

**Phototherapy, also known as photobiomodulation, low-level laser therapy (LLLT)**, involves the application of light (often laser light of a specific wavelength or a light emitting diode, LED) to stimulate cellular processes.

**The effects of phototherapy are chemical and not thermal.**

Energy which is delivered to cells produces insignificant and minimal temperature changes, typically in the range of 0.1–0.5°C.

Cellular responses are the result of changes in photoacceptor molecules, or chromophores. Photoacceptors take part in cellular metabolism and are not connected to a light response, such as chlorophyll which is a photoreceptor.

Once the photon energy is absorbed, the photoacceptor assumes an electronically excited state, which in turn stimulates cellular metabolism by activating or deactivating enzymes which alter other macromolecules such as DNA and RNA.

### Photodynamic therapy: oncologic horizons

Photodynamic therapy (PDT) is a light-based intervention with a long and successful clinical track record for both oncology and non-malignancies. In cancer patients, a photosensitizing agent is intravenously, orally or topically applied and allowed time to preferentially accumulate in the tumor region. Light of the appropriate wavelength and intensity to activate the particular photosensitizer employed is then introduced to the tumor bed.

The light energy will activate the photosensitizer, which in the presence of oxygen should allow for creation of **the toxic photodynamic reaction generating reactive oxygen species. The photodynamic reaction creates a cascading series of events including initiation of apoptotic and necrotic pathways both in tumor and neovasculature, leading to permanent lesion destruction often with upregulation of the immune system.**

Cutaneous phototoxicity from unintentional sunlight exposure remains the most common morbidity from PDT. (Allison, 2014)

Prof Randolph M. Howes MD,PhD

## Photodynamic therapy (PDT): PDT Mechanisms

Some of the following was adapted from: (Allison, Moghissi, 2013)

**Abbreviations:** a photosensitizer (PS); photodynamic therapy (PDT); photodynamic reaction (PDR)

Photodynamic therapy (PDT) is an elegant light based oncologic intervention. As currently practiced, a photosensitizer (PS) is applied then activated by light of the appropriate wavelength and intensity. This creates the photodynamic reaction (PDR) which is tumor and vascular ablative.

PDT was accidentally discovered over 100 years ago by medical student Oscar Raab.

He was studying the interaction of fluorescent dyes on infusaria. Raab found that intense light applied to the dye resulted in rapid destruction of these microorganisms.

This new light based therapy was more formally described and elucidated by Raab's professors Jesionek and von Tappeiner who coined the ablative process, Photodynamische Wirkung, best translated as The PDR, and PDT was born.

By the early 1900's, patients were being successfully treated by this process for a wide variety of cancers, particularly of the skin. **Despite this early success, PDT did not achieve enough momentum and was lost for nearly 50 years when the PDR was rediscovered by Lipson and Schwartz.**

**Studies during the 1950's to 1960 revealed not only tumor ablation but the inter-related ability of photosensitizing agents to fluoresce and demarcate tumors.**

It was not until the 1970's when Dougherty, working with porphyrin compounds, accidentally **rediscovered PDT. In contrast to previous iterations, Dougherty created a commercially suitable photosensitizing drug, reliable light sources and appropriate clinical trials proving the value of PDT to the oncologic community.**

**For this Dougherty is affectionately known as "The Father of PDT."**

PS agents are natural or synthetic structures that transfer light energy. Not surprisingly, the chlorophyll derivatives from plants and bacteria are excellent PS agents. So too are dyes and porphyrins. While thousands upon thousands of structures have been identified as PS agents, perhaps two dozen have been well characterized and only about one dozen employed in clinical trials.

In the clinic, a successful PS agent has most of the following characteristics: nontoxic till activated, hydrophilic for easy systemic application, activated by a clinically useful light wavelength, and reliable generation of the PDR. It also concentrates in tumor, clears normal tissue, is eliminated from the patient relatively rapidly, is a nontoxic degradation product with ease of synthesis, pain free therapy and, just as importantly, commercial availability.

Fundamentally, specific wavelength light activates the PS which then leads to a series of photochemical reactions that ideally allow for tumor destruction without undue normal tissue injury. The active PS can also lose energy by creating a type I photochemical reaction. This Fenton reaction creates free radicals (the hydroxyl radical) which are destructive.

**However, the most important pathway for clinical PDT is the generation of a type II photochemical reaction, which is termed the PDR. Here the PS interacts with oxygen to generate singlet oxygen, which is considered to be the basis of PDT's tumor and vascular ablation ability.**

**This oxygen dependent type II PDR is a sine qua non for PDT. The half life of singlet oxygen is in the order of 40 nanoseconds which allows for destruction of a radius of 20 nanometers. Whilst a truly tiny volume, clearly it is enough for clinical success.**

**As described, singlet oxygen (an EMOD) has a radius of destruction measured in nanometers yet this allows for a significant and complex cascade of events resulting in local, regional, and systemic alteration of both tumor and immune response so that reliable tumor control is possible.**

Tumor destruction from PDT can occur by both programmed (apoptotic) pathways and non-programmed (necrosis) pathways. This is fortunate as some tumors have developed genetic mutations eliminating or minimizing apoptosis.

**Generally, when high light intensity is employed, the tumor cells are rapidly ablated by necrosis.**

This also leads to release of cytokines and toxic chemicals from, for example, the mitochondria. This leakage will then create lethal damage in cells nearby (bystander effect) as well as creating a regional and systematic reaction.

In contrast, apoptotic death may be initiated by PDT, generally when low light doses are employed. During apoptosis, the cells cease to function and undergo an orderly and programmed dissolution. No bystander effect or immune response is expected as no toxic chemicals are leaked.

Apoptotic pathways are found in both tumor and normal cells across many species including bacteria. It appears that apoptosis is a well conserved method of the organism to eliminate damaged cells. PDT appears to be able to activate this pathway.

It should be noted that PS is believed to preferentially concentrate in the rapidly dividing cells of malignancy whilst clearing preferentially from surrounding normal tissue which retains little PS. Therefore, ideally the PDR is lethal to tumors without affecting normal tissue.

Just as in tumor cells, endothelial cells of the vascular systems can concentrate PS. Several events will occur. **By disrupting the vascular walls, blood will not flow to the tumor and oxygen will become scarce (hypoxic).**

Overall, a rapid loss of blood supply in concert with direct tumor and vascular cell lysis will be a lethal event to the tumor.

Clinically, both apoptosis and necrosis occurs in the neovasculature contributing significantly to tumor cell destruction not only directly by lack of blood and hypoxia but also by release of toxic substances such as thromboxanes, platelet aggregators, and various toxic cytokines which will also prime the immune system.

One may be able to illuminate in such a fashion as to favor apoptotic versus necrotic pathways.

When PDT induces necrosis of tumors and their vasculature, an immune cascade is also initiated. **This release stimulates various white blood cells to be activated including neutrophils and macrophages which converge on the treatment region. It is felt that significant tumor cell death occurs from these activated immune cells.**

Not only does this immune reaction occur at the PDT site, it also may occur at regional and distant lymphatic tissue. These cytotoxic T cells may not only cause necrosis but may also induce apoptotic pathways whenever tumor cells are found, **even after PDT is complete.**

In short, PDR results from the interaction between a chemical PS and a specific wavelength of light in the presence of oxygen. The interaction releases cytotoxic species, notably **singlet oxygen (an EMOD).** The overall mechanism involves molecular, subcellular and vascular changes which bring about necrosis and/or apoptosis of the tumor. (Allison, Moghissi, 2013)

## Effects of low-level laser therapy on malignant cells

### Abstract

The aim of this study was to assess the effect of **635- and 670-nm laser irradiation** on H.Ep.2 cells in vitro using MTT.

In addition to our previous report on the effects of LLLT on the proliferation of laryngeal carcinoma cells in which it was found **that irradiaton H.Ep.2 cells with 670-nm laser results in increased cell proliferation,** it was decided to evaluate the effect of increased doses of laser light on these cells. The cells, obtained from SCC of the larynx, were routinely processed from defrost to the experimental condition. The cultures were kept either at 5% or 10% of FBS. Twenty-four hours after transplantation, the cells were irradiated with laser light (5-mW diode lasers; 635 and 670-nm; beam cross section approximately 1 mm) at local light doses between 0.04 and 4.8.10(4) Jm(-2). For 670 nm, significant differences in the proliferation were observed between the two concentrations of FBS (p = 0.002) and between irradiated cultures and controls (p = 0.000). **Although the results were not significant, 635-nm irradiated cells also proliferated more than nonirradiated ones.** This occurred under both conditions of nutrition. It is concluded, that **irradiation with 670-nm laser light applied at doses between 0.04 and 4.810(4) Jm(-2) could significantly increase proliferation of laryngeal cancer cells.** (Pinheiro et al, 2002)

## Cytotoxic effects of light on cancer cells

### The Cytotoxic Effects of Low Intensity Visible and Infrared Light on Human Breast Cancer (MCF7) cells

### Abstract

A concept of using low intensity light therapy (LILT) as an alternative approach to cancer treatment is at early stages of development; while the therapeutic effects of LILT as a non-invasive treatment modality for localized joint and soft tissue wound healing are widely corroborated. The LEDs-based exposure system was designed and constructed to irradiate the selected cancer and normal cells and evaluate the biological effects induced by light exposures in visible and infrared light range. In this study, human breast cancer (MCF7) cells and human epidermal melanocytes (HEM) cells (control) were exposed to selected far infrared light (3400nm, 3600nm, 3800nm, 3900nm, 4100nm and 4300nm) and visible and near infrared wavelengths (466nm, 585nm, 626nm, 810nm, 850nm and 950nm). The optical intensities of LEDs used for exposures were in the range of 15µW to 30µW. Cellular morphological changes of exposed and sham-exposed cells were evaluated using light microscopy. The cytotoxic effects of these low intensity light exposures on human cancer and normal cell lines were quantitatively determined by Lactate dehydrogenase (LDH) cytotoxic activity and PrestoBlue™ cell viability assays. **Findings reveal that far-infrared exposures were able to reduce cell viability of MCF7 cells** as measured by increased LDH release activity and PrestoBlue™ assays. Further investigation of the effects of light irradiation on different types of cancer cells, study of possible signaling pathways affected by electromagnetic radiation (EMR) and in vivo experimentation are required in order to draw a firm conclusion about the efficacy of low intensity light as an alternative non-invasive cancer treatment. (Peidaee et al, 2013)

### Low-intensity light effect on murine melanoma cells

### In vitro evaluation of low-intensity light radiation on murine melanoma (B16F10) cells

## Abstract

Changes in the energy state of biomolecules induced by electromagnetic radiation lead to changes in biological functions of irradiated biomolecules. Using the RRM approach, it was computationally predicted that far-infrared light irradiation in the range of 3500-6000 nm affects biological activity of proto-oncogene proteins. This in vitro study evaluates quantitatively and qualitatively the effects of selected far-infrared exposures in the computationally determined wavelengths on mouse melanoma B16F10 cells and Chinese hamster ovarian (CHO) cells by **MTT (thiazolyl blue tetrazolium bromide)** cell proliferation assay and confocal laser-scanning microscopy (CLSM). This paper also presents the findings obtained from irradiating B16F10 and CHO cells by the selected wavelengths in visible and near-infrared range. **The MTT (thiazolyl blue tetrazolium bromide) results show that far-infrared wavelength irradiation induces detrimental effect on cellular viability of** mouse melanoma **B16F10 cells, while that of normal CHO cells is not affected considerably.** Moreover, CLSM images demonstrate visible cellular detachment of cancer cells. The observed effects support the hypothesis that far-infrared light irradiation within the computationally determined wavelength range induces biological effect on cancer cells. From irradiation of selected visible and near-infrared wavelengths, no visible changes were detected in cellular viability of either normal or cancer cells. (Peidaee, Almansour, Pirogova, 2015)

---

**Phototherapy, also known as photobiomodulation, low-level laser therapy (LLLT)**, involves the application of light (often laser light of a specific wavelength or a light emitting diode, LED) to stimulate cellular processes.

**With the advancement in laser technology, irradiation of these wounds with low-intensity laser irradiation (LILI) or phototherapy, has shown a vast improvement in wound healing**.

**At the correct laser parameters, LILI has shown to increase migration, viability, and proliferation of diabetic cells in vitro; there is a stimulatory effect on the mitochondria with a resulting increase in adenosine triphosphate (ATP).**

**There is a caveat, however, and it is the fact that some investigators** (Pinheiro et al, 2002) **have seen increased cancer cell proliferation with irradiation at about 630 nm laser light.** It was found **that irradiation H.Ep.2 cells (laryngeal carcinoma**

253

cells) with 670-nm laser results in increased cell proliferation. Although the results were not significant, 635-nm irradiated cells also proliferated more than nonirradiated ones. This occurred under both conditions of nutrition. It is concluded, that **irradiation with 670-nm laser light applied at doses between 0.04 and 4.810 Jm(-2) could significantly increase proliferation of laryngeal cancer cells.** (Pinheiro et al, 2002)

**Findings reveal that far-infrared exposures were able to reduce cell viability of MCF7 (human breast cancer) cells.** Further investigation of the effects of light irradiation on different types of cancer cells, study of possible signaling pathways affected by electromagnetic radiation (EMR) and in vivo experimentation are required in order to draw a firm conclusion about the efficacy of low intensity light as an alternative non-invasive cancer treatment. (Peidaee et al, 2013)

**The MTT (thiazolyl blue tetrazolium bromide) results show that far-infrared wavelength irradiation induces detrimental effect on cellular viability of** mouse melanoma **B16F10 cells, while that of normal CHO cells is not affected considerably.** (Peidaee, Almansour, Pirogova, 2015)

The energy which is absorbed by the photoacceptor can be transferred to other molecules causing chemical reactions in the surrounding tissue; this gives rise to observable effects at a biological level.

**Photon energy is absorbed by the chromophores and there is an increase in adenosine triphosphate (ATP)** and cell membrane permeability, which leads to activation of secondary messengers which in turn activate a cascade of intracellular signals. There is also an increase in mitochondrial membrane potential and proton gradient.

The exact mechanisms of action following laser irradiation are not well understood, and a number of theories exist, the most studied and best understood being that of cytochrome-c oxidase (cyt $a/a_3$), the terminal enzyme in the eukaryotic mitochondrial respiratory chain (complex IV).

Cytochrome c oxidase facilitates the transfer of electrons to molecular oxygen. The end product of this complex is the production of ATP. Cytochrome c oxidase has two heme moieties (heme $a$ and heme $a_3$) and two redox-active copper sites ($Cu_A$ and $Cu_B$), and these are the possible absorbing chromophores for visible red and near infrared (NIR) light.

When photon energy is absorbed by cytochrome c oxidase, there is a change in the mitochondrial redox state and/or pumping of protons across the inner mitochondrial membrane and an increase in ATP synthesis. There is also an increase in intracellular calcium ($[Ca^{2+}]i$) which stimulates DNA and RNA synthesis.

Photoirradiation causes the reduction or oxidation of cytochrome c oxidase and is dependent on the initial redox status of the enzyme at the time of irradiation.

Hu and colleagues also found an increase in cytochrome c oxidase activity and concluded there was a cascade of reactions which altered cellular homeostasis.

**There is also an increase in the concentration of active mitochondria in irradiated cells.** Both effects lead to an increase in ATP. The effect of laser irradiation on the mitochondria at a transcriptional level was also investigated, and there is evidence that that there is an upregulation of genes involved in complexes I, IV, and V.

**Laser light is absorbed by chromophores in the cell, mitochondria in the case of visible red light. This leads to an increase in adenosine triphosphate (ATP), reactive oxygen species (ROS),** nitric oxide (NO), and intracellular calcium ($iCa^{2+}$).

**A number of studies, on various cell types, have shown positive effects of photoirradiation. Studies have been conducted on stem cells, keratinocytes, mast cells, fibroblasts, smooth muscle cells, osteoblasts, and Schwann cells** to name but a few.

Impaired diabetic wound healing has been associated with impaired cellular function, and there is a decrease in cellular migration, proliferation, NO synthesis, growth factors, and collagen synthesis. There is also an increase in proteinases that degrade the extracellular matrix and collagen (MMPs) and cells appear to be stuck in the inflammatory phase of wound healing. The increase in oxidative stress also leads to increased cell death.

**I believe that this is analogous to the effects of HBOT.**

**Laser irradiation *in vitro* has shown that these cells respond in a favorable fashion, even irradiation of diabetic cells. There is an increase in cellular migration, proliferation, viability, collagen production, ATP, mitochondria concentration, cytochrome c oxidase activity, NO, growth factors, and gene regulation.**

There is also a **decrease in MMPs, apoptosis** and proinflammatory cytokines.

The influence of wavelength was demonstrated by Gupta et al., who demonstrated that **irradiation at 635 and 810 nm had a positive effect on wound healing, while a wavelength of 730 and 980 nm had no effect**. (Gupta, Dai, Hamblin, )

This can be explained by the absorption spectrum of chromophores which absorb light at different wavelengths.

Due to its stimulatory effect and **no reported side effects**, laser therapy has been used to treat chronic wounds, including diabetic ulcers. Phototherapy has been shown to be beneficial in treating diabetic ulcers which are unresponsive to conventional treatments.

(Houreld, 2014)

---

- **Hyperbaric oxygen can enhance the effects of PDT.**

- Early observations indicate that **hypoxic or anoxic conditions almost completely reduce the antitumor effectiveness of PDT in vitro.** (Henderson and Fingar, 1987)

- **Feldmeier et al. and Daruwalla et al. reviewed three older studies on mammary tumors and HBO, all in the same C3H mouse model, where none of them found effects on tumor growth.** (Suit, Maeda, 1967) (McCredie et al, 1966) (Shewell, Thompson, 1980)

However, they did not consider an extensive study from 1964 in their reviews, where Kluft et al. reported that **HBO retarded growth of a transplanted mammary carcinoma (TM 8013) growing in C 57 black mice.** (Kluft, 1965)

### Ultrasound accelerates skin healing - especially for diabetics and the elderly

**July 16, 2015** *source: University of Bristol Research News*

Healing times for skin ulcers and bedsores can be reduced by a third with the use of low–intensity ultrasound, scientists from the Universities of Sheffield and Bristol have found. Researchers from the University of Sheffield's Department of Biomedical Science discovered the ultrasound transmits a vibration through the skin and wakes up cells in wounds helping to stimulate and accelerate the healing process. The pioneering study was published in The Journal of Investigative Dermatology.

In order to reduce the size of the foregoing material, I have summarized the most important points and placed them into a summary. This is not to repeat the material but is provided to the reader such that these important points will not be missed.

# SECTION NINE

## SUMMARY OF MY HBO TOME

**Story in a nut sack: (160 items)**

### OVERALL IMPORTANCE OF OXYGEN

**A wound's chances of becoming infected are directly related to how little oxygen there is in the affected tissues.** (Hunt, 1979)

**Under-oxygenation can also reduce the body's ability to heal the wound, especially since healing tissue needs even more oxygen than does healthy tissue.** (Niinikoski et al, 1972)

**Hypoxia is a critical hallmark of solid tumors and involves enhanced cell survival, angiogenesis, glycolytic metabolism, and metastasis**. (Moen, Stuhr, 2012)

**Hyperbaric oxygen (HBO) treatment has for centuries been used to improve or cure disorders involving hypoxia and ischemia, by enhancing the amount of dissolved oxygen in the plasma and thereby increasing $O_2$ delivery to the tissue.**

**HBOT is the best way of increasing the oxygen content of under-oxygenated tissues.** (Sheffield, 1985) (Strauss et al, 1983) (Strauss et al, 1986) (Skyhar et al, 1986) (Nylander et al, 1985)

**The use of HBOT is a very valuable way of treating difficult wounds** (Hunt and van Winkle, 1976) (Sheffield, 1985.

**The earlier and more frequently HBOT is used, the more likely it is that severely injured body parts will be saved.** (Strauss and Hart, 1984) (Strauss and Hart, 1989)

**HBOT helps to heal bone disorders by stimulating both the osteoclast and the osteoblasts.** (Hunt et al, 1969) (Strauss, 1987)

**Solid tumors often contain areas subjected to acute or chronic hypoxia,** though with variable severity in patients both within and among different tumor types. (Michiele, 2009)

**Although severe or prolonged hypoxia is deleterious, adaptation to the hypoxic microenvironment has allowed cancer cells to survive and proliferate in this hostile milieu.** (Harris, 2002)

**Multiple reports have demonstrated that decreased oxygen tension selects for more malignant cells and induces multiple cellular adaptations, which again sustains and fosters cancer progression and thereby induces cancer growth.** (Moen, Stuhr, 2012)

Studies have demonstrated that **hypoxia is implicated in the resistance to conventional therapy.** (Shannon et al, 2003)

**Gray et al. proved in the 1950s that the oxygen concentration influences the effect of radiotherapy.**

**Oxygen concentration has an especially crucial role in radiation oncology and radiation resistance.** (Gray et al, 1953) (Overgaard, 2011)

**The epithelial-to-mesenchymal transition in cancer has been shown to be induced by hypoxic conditions, leading to cancers with an invasive or metastatic phenotype.** (Cannito et al, 2008) (Thiery, 2002)

**As in normal tissue, the $pO_2$ in cancer tissue increases significantly during HBO exposure.** (Brizel et al, 1995)

**The conclusion in two reviews was that HBO did not promote cancer growth, and that the use of HBO in patients with malignancies was considered safe.** (Feldmeier et al, 2003) (Daruwalla, Christophi, 2006)

The work performed on HBO and cancer during the last 9 years supports the previous findings since **none of the studies reported a cancer-promoting effect of HBO**.

**Studies of prolonged hyperoxia have shown that elevated levels of reactive oxygen species (ROS) overwhelm the antioxidant defense and lead to cellular damage and possible organ dysfunction.** (Gore et al, 2010)

Teicher underlined that **the importance of hypoxia on the response to chemotherapy is highly drug dependent.** However, hypoxia-mediated chemoresistance has been ascribed to: (1) altered cellular metabolism reducing drug cytotoxicity; (2) **the redox state, meaning that oxygen is required to generate ROS to be maximally cytotoxic**; and (3) genetic instability, which can lead to more rapid development of drug-resistant cells. In addition to the cytotoxicity, availability of the chemotherapeutic drug in high enough dose is important to obtain a maximal effect. (Teicher, 1994)

**Oxygen is a prerequisite for successful wound healing due to the increased demand for reparative processes such as cell proliferation, bacterial defense, angiogenesis and collagen synthesis. Many experimental and clinical observations have shown wound healing to be impaired under hypoxia.** (Schreml et al, 2010)

Neutrophils require molecular oxygen as a substrate for microbial killing. **The oxidative burst seen in neutrophils after phagocytosis of bacteria involves a 10-to 15-fold increase in oxygen consumption.** (Badwey, Karnovsky, 1980)

Here, in the neutrophil, **oxygen serves as a substrate in the formation of free radicals, which directly or indirectly initiate phagocytic killing.** (Forman, Thomas, 1986)

**Direct oxygen therapies, such as oxygen by mask and hyperbaric oxygen, have been successfully used in controlling anginal chest pain, headaches and migraine attacks.**

Prof Randolph M. Howes MD, PhD

## EMOD ROLE IN HBOT

It is understood that ROS (EMOD) signaling is fundamental to HBOT but the exact manner in which HBOT modulates ROS signaling pathways in the wound and protects ischemic tissue from oxidative stress remains unclear. (Thom, 2009)

- Principal mechanisms of HBO$_2$ are based on intracellular generation of reactive species of oxygen (ROS, EMODs) and nitrogen (RNS). (Thom, 2011)

This has highlighted some of the beneficial actions of HBO$_2$ and the data that indicate oxidative stress brought about by hyperoxia can have therapeutic effects. (Thom, 2011)

- It is well accepted that breathing greater than 1 ATA O$_2$ will increase production of reactive oxygen species (ROS, EMODs). (ATA, 1977) (Thom, 1989)

- The presence of oxygen has the advantage of not only promoting an environment less hospitable to anaerobes, but also speeds the process of wound healing, whether from being required for the production of collagen matrix and subsequent angiogenesis, from the presence and beneficial effects of reactive oxygen species (ROS). (Kunnavatana et al, 2005)

Examination of blood from persons undergoing hyperbaric oxygen (HBO) exposure, by low temperature electron spin resonance (ESR) spectroscopy, demonstrated a marked increase in the magnitude of a signal with properties consistent with a free radical. It is postulated that HBO exposure increases ascorbate radical levels in blood, which is likely to reflect increased ascorbate turnover in human red blood cells. (Narkowicz, Vial, McCartney, 1993)

Hyperbaric oxygen, tissue levels may approach 1200 mmHg, in which increased production of superoxide, peroxide and other oxygen radicals occurs. (Delaney, Montgomery, 2001)

Increased oxygen delivery to the tissue with HBO$_2$ may prevent tissue damage by decreasing the tissue lactic acid level and helping maintain the ATP level. This may help prevent tissue damage in ischemic wounds and reperfusion injuries.

- **When subjects are breathing HBO$_2$, the cumulative effects of EMODs are well recognized because of their role in CNS O$_2$ toxicity; yet, adverse reactions to HBO$_2$ are rare.** (Demchenko et al, 2003) (Demchenko et al, 2001) (Tibbles and Edelsberg, 1996) (Torbati et al, 1992) (Torbati et al, 1989)

- **Hyperbaric oxygen therapy (HBOT) increases the production of ROIs (reactive oxygen intermediates, EMODs) throughout the body, leaving no safe harbor for the virus to hide outside the genome.** (Baugh, 2000)

---

## HBOT FACTS AND POSITIVE EFFECTS

- **HBO, by reversing tissue hypoxia and cellular dysfunction, restores this defense and also increases the phagocytosis of some bacteria by working synergistically with antibiotics, and inhibiting the growth of a number of anaerobic and aerobic organisms at wound sites.** (Mader et al, 1980)

- **HBO blocks the production of alphatoxine and thetatoxine and inhibits bacterial growth.** (Jain, 2004)

Because exposure to hyperoxia in clinical HBO$_2$ protocols is rather brief, **studies show that antioxidant defenses are adequate so that biochemical stresses related to increases in reactive species are reversible.** (Narkowicz, Vial, McCartney, 1993) (Dennog et al, 1999) (Dennog et al, 1996) (Rothfuss, Radermacher, Speit, 2001)

**At 1 ATA, the amount of oxygen dissolved into plasma is 0.32 vol%. At 3 ATA plasma contains 6.8 vol% oxygen, a level equivalent to the average tissue requirements for oxygen.**

**HBOT can help counteract infection indirectly by providing the white blood cells with the oxygen** they need. It can also act directly by **killing anaerobic organisms**, stopping their multiplication, and neutralizing the toxins that some of them produce.

Most HBO treatments are performed at 2 to 3 ATA. In air embolism and decompression sickness, where pressure is crucial to therapeutic effect, treatments frequently start at 6 ATA. This additional pressure, when associated with inspiration of high levels of oxygen, substantially increases the level of oxygen dissolved into blood plasma. **This state of serum hyperoxia is the second beneficial effect of hyperbaric oxygen therapy**.

- **HBOT, if readily available, appears effective for the management of acute, difficult to heal wounds**. (Eskes et al, 2011)

- **The physiological effects of HBO include short-term effects such as vasoconstriction and enhanced oxygen delivery, reduction of edema, phagocytosis activation and also an anti-inflammatory effect (enhanced leukocyte function). Neovascularization (angiogenesis in hypoxic soft tissues), osteoneogenesis as well as stimulation of collagen production by fibroblasts are known long-term effects. This is beneficial for wound healing and recovery from radiation injury**. (Sheridan and Shank, 1999)

- **Also many cell and tissue functions are dependent on oxygen. Of special interest are leukocytes ability to kill bacteria, cell replication, collagen formation, and mechanisms of homeostasis, such as active membrane transport, e.g. the sodium—potassium pump. HBO has the effect of inhibiting leukocyte adhesion to the endothelium, diminishing tissue damage, which enhances leukocyte motility and improves microcirculation**. (Mortensen, 2008)

- **American doctors accept HBOT for use in wound healing, bone infection, carbon monoxide intoxication, and air emboli, or air bubbles in the bloodstream due to decompression sickness, open-heart surgery, and other sources**.

- **Hyperbaric oxygen can be delivered safely to critically ill patients**. Many critical care environments without present hyperbaric oxygen capability may wish to consider offering hyperbaric oxygen to patients with hyperbaric oxygen-approved indications. (Weaver, 2011)

- **Because of enhanced oxygen delivery, HBO$_2$ is used for acute crush injury, ischemic flaps and grafts, acute central retinal arterial occlusion, other acute arterial occlusions, and idiopathic sudden sensorineural hearing loss**.

**Hyperbaric oxygen has antimicrobial effects and is offered for patients with limb- or life-threatening infections, such as clostridial gas gangrene and necrotizing fasciitis**.

The most common **US** indication for **HBO$_2$** is the treatment of ischemic wounds (eg, diabetic lower extremity wounds, late effects of radiation, and refractory osteomyelitis). In ischemic wounds, **HBO$_2$** can deliver sufficient oxygen to the nonhealing wound to stimulate angiogenesis and healing through multiple mechanisms, including increased collagen production, increased growth factor receptor numbers, upregulation of vascular endothelial growth factor, increased circulating endothelial progenitor cells, and improvement in neutrophil-mediated host defense.

Clinical trials support efficacy of **HBO$_2$** for acute **CO** poisoning, diabetic lower extremity wounds, crush injury, and radiation necrosis. (Weaver, 1995)

- **HBOT** can also be used for conditions such as coma resulting from head injuries, bruising of the spinal cord, stroke and neurological disorders such as multiple sclerosis.

- There is a strong scientific basis for oxygen treatment as prophylaxis against infection, to facilitate wound closure, and to prevent amputation in wounded patients. Oxygen supports biochemical metabolism and cellular function, and has roles in combating infection and facilitating the wound healing cascade. (Eisenbud, 2012)

- **HBOT** increases growth factors and local wound signaling, while also promoting a central stem cell release of endothelial progenitor cells from the bone marrow via nitric oxide pathways.

The clinical data continue to accumulate in support of **HBOT** to help hasten wound healing, and reduce the amputation rate in diabetic ulcers. In appropriate patients, **HBOT** is an effective, noninvasive, adjunct modality that can be used to hasten chronic wound healing. (Goldstein, 2013)

- Hyperoxia has effects of a number of cell signaling events that converge to influence cell recruitment/chemotaxis and gene regulation/protein synthesis responses which mediate wound healing. (Fosen, Thom, 2014)

- **HBO$_2$** has also been found to inhibit **PMN** adherence on postcapillary venules. (Gottrup et alo, 1984)

- **HBOT** is an effective treatment for patients with chronic wounds, due to a variety of causes. However, **HBOT** is less effective in patients with Diabetes Mellitus than in patients with venous stasis because hemodialysis, which is more common in patients with DM, has negative effects on wound healing. (Ueno et al, 2014)

- In review, **oxidative stress responses triggered by HBO$_2$** improve outcome from a wide variety of post-ischemic/inflammatory insults. **HBO$_2$** also improves ischemic tolerance when used in a prophylactic manner. Augmented synthesis of reactive species (**EMODs**) temporarily inhibits adherence/sequestration of neutrophils by inhibiting $\beta_2$ integrin function and in many tissues **HBO$_2$** will induce antioxidant enzymes and anti-inflammatory proteins.

- **HBOT** not only increased antioxidant enzyme expression, such as Cu/Zn-superoxide dismutase, catalase, and glutathione peroxidase, but also significantly decreased pro-oxidant enzyme levels, such as **iNOS** and gp91-phox, thereby decreasing net oxygen radical production by means of negative feedback. (**RMH Note: I take issue with the way this is stated**)

- **Hyperbaric oxygen therapy (HBOT)** increases the production of **ROIs** throughout the body, leaving no safe harbor for the virus to hide outside the genome. (Baugh, 2000)

- **HIV** viral load was decreased in the infected cells, and few viruses entered uninfected peripheral blood mononuclear cells (**PBMCs**) exposed to HBO. The results of this study support the theory that **HBO** has an antiviral effect. (Reillo, Altieri, 1996)

- **HBO**-treated ischemic wounds also manifested reduced phosphorylation of extracellular signal–regulated kinases 1/2, c-Jun N-terminal kinase, and c-Jun, indicating downregulation of mitogen-activated protein kinases (**MAPKs**).

- **HBOT** decreased the expression of several **MMPs** while simultaneously increasing tissue inhibitor of MMP (tissue inhibitor of metalloproteinase 2).

- **HBOT** corrected the dysfunction of **ROS**-related signals in ischemic wounds, changing the molecular pattern to closely resemble the acute non-ischemic wounds. (Zhang, Gould, 2014)

- **HBOT acts via the ROS/MAPK/MMP signaling axis to reduce tissue degeneration and improve ischemic wound healing.** (Zhang, Gould, 2014)

- **HBOT provides a stimulus that promotes endogenous antioxidants to establish a therapeutic balance of oxidants and antioxidants, decreasing net oxygen radical production by means of negative feedback.** The effect of HBOT on the ROS/MAPK/MMP axis alters the MMP/TIMP balance to increase extracellular matrix deposition. (Zhang, Gould, 2014)

- **Hyperbaric oxygen treatment (HBOT) is an effective adjunct for wound healing that has both systemic and local effects.** (Kessler et al, 2003)

- **At the tissue level, HBOT modulates cytokine release, accelerates microbial oxidative killing, reduces apoptosis, and modulates leukocyte activation and adhesion.** (Jon, 2000)

- **Hyperbaric oxygen (HBO) increases bone marrow–derived endothelial progenitor cell mobilization.** (Zhang, Gould, 2014)

- **HBOT-induced MMP9 is known to be an important mediator for endothelial progenitor cell migration at the systemic level.** (Liu and Velazquez, 2008)

- **HBOT is indicated for treating compromised flaps and grafts and to enhance healing in selected problem wounds, i.e., delayed effects of radiation and refractory diabetic wounds.** (Zhang, Gould, 2014)

- **We have demonstrated a synergistic effect of systemic hyperbaric oxygen and growth factors that has been substantiated by Hunt's group.** (Tandara, Mistoe, 2003)

- A French trial (n = 36 patients) reported that **significantly more crush wounds healed with HBOT than with sham HBOT.** (Eskes et al, 2011)

- **There were significantly fewer additional surgical procedures required with HBOT (RR 1.60, 95% CI 1.03-2.50), and there was significantly less tissue necrosis.** (Eskes et al, 2011)

- In one of two American trials (n = 141) **burn wounds healed significantly quicker with HBOT (P < 0.005) than with routine burn care.** (Eskes et al, 2011)

- A British trial (n = 48) compared HBOT with usual care. **HBOT resulted in a significantly higher percentage of healthy graft area in split skin grafts.** (Eskes et al, 2011)

- **HBOT, if readily available, appears effective for the management of acute, difficult to heal wounds.** (Eskes et al, 2011)

- **Animal trials have documented wound healing benefits of HBO$_2$.** (Marx et al, 1990) (Gallagher et al, 2007) (Zhang et al, 2008) (Goldstein et al, 2006)

- **In animal models, stem/progenitor cells (SPCs) mobilized by HBO$_2$ home to wounds and accelerate healing.** (Gu et al, 2008)

- **HBO$_2$-mediated oxidative stress at sites of neovascularization will stimulate stem/progenitor cells (SPCs) growth factor production.** (Hunt et al, 2007) (Milovanova et al, 2008)

- **Pluripotent mesenchymal stem cells were shown *in vitro* to be stimulated by HBO$_2$ to synthesize placental growth factor. This too is an EMOD-dependent phenomenon and will significantly increase cell migratory and tube formation functions.** (Shyu et al, 2008)

- **HBO$_2$ also stimulates synthesis of basic fibroblast growth factor (bFGF) and transforming growth factor $\beta$1 by human dermal fibroblasts, angiopoietin-2 by human umbilical vein endothelial cells, bFGF and hepatocyte growth factor in ischemic limbs, and it up-regulates platelet derived growth factor (PDGF) receptor in wounds.** (Kang et al, 2004 (Lin et al, 2002) (Asano et al, 2007) (Bonomo et al, 1998)

- **Administration of HBO$_2$ prior to and for three days following skin grafting led to a significant 29% improvement in graft survival.** (Perrins, Cantab, 1967)

- **Clinical studies have documented significant survival enhancement with HBO$_2$ for extremity re-implantation and free tissue transfer, and following crush injury.** (Bouachour et al, 1996) (Waterhouse et al, 1993)

- **HBOT can improve oxygen supply to the injured brain, reduce the swelling associated with low oxygen levels and reduce the volume of brain that will ultimately perish.**

- **The use of HBO was found to significantly decrease the incidence of postoperative infections in neuromuscular scoliosis patients. Hyperbaric oxygen has a possibility to reduce the rate of post-surgical deep infections in complex spine deformity in high risk neuromuscular patients.** (Inanmaz et al, 2014)

- **$HBO_2$ is used to treat refractory diabetic lower extremity wounds and delayed radiation injuries.** They share several elements including depletion of epithelial and stromal cells, chronic inflammation, fibrosis, an imbalance or abnormalities in extracellular matrix components and remodeling processes, and impaired keratinocyte functions. (Thom, 2011)

- Another meta-analysis concluded that **only four patients needed to be treated with $HBO_2$ to prevent one amputation.** (Kranke et al, 2004)

- **For patients with diabetic foot ulcers (DFU) complicated by surgical infection, HBOT reduces chance of amputation (7 studies) and improves chance of healing (6 studies).** (Goldman, 2009)

- **IGF-1 increased significantly in the healed group. We believe that HBOT is effective in the treatment of diabetic foot ulcers, with an elevation of IGF-1.** (Aydin et al, 2013)

- **HBOT is associated with remission of about 85% of cases of refractory lower extremity osteomyelitis.** (Goldman, 2009)

- **There is a moderate level of evidence that HBOT promotes healing of arterial ulcers, calciphylactic and refractory vasculitic ulcers, as well as refractory osteomyelitis.** (Goldman, 2009)

- **There is a low to moderate level of evidence that HBOT promotes successful "take" of compromised flaps and grafts.** (Goldman, 2009)

- **The benefit of $HBO_2$ for radiation injury also has been shown in randomized trials and its utilization supported by independent evidence-based reviews.** (Bennett et al, 2008) (Clarke et al, 2008) (Marx, Johnson, Kline, 1985)

- **Clinical trials have shown that $HBO_2$ can reduce coronary artery re-stenosis after balloon angioplasty/stenting,** (Sharifi et al, 2004) (Sharifi et al, 2002) **decrease muscle loss after**

**thrombolytic treatment for myocardial infarction,** (Dekleva et al, 2004) (Shandling et al, 1997) (Stavitsky et al, 1998) **improve hepatic survival after transplantation and lead to more rapid return of donor liver function** (Mazariegos et al, 1999) (Suehiro et al, 2008and **reduced the incidence of encephalopathy seen after cardio-pulmonary bypass and following carbon monoxide poisoning.** (Alex et al, 2005) (Weaver et al, 2002)

- **When animals or humans are exposed to HBO$_2$ at 2.8 to 3.0 ATA for at least 45 minutes, the ability of circulating neutro-phils to adhere to target tissues is temporarily inhibited.** (Kalns et al, 2002) (Labouche et al, 1999) (Thom, 1993) (Zamboni et al, 1993)

- It also appears that **benefits of HBO$_2$ in decompression sick-ness are related to the temporary inhibition of neutrophil $\beta_2$ integrins,** in addition to the Boyle's Law-mediated reduction in bubble volume as discussed in the introduction. (Martin, Thom, 2002)

- **Exposure to HBO$_2$ inhibits neutrophil $\beta_2$ integrin function because hyperoxia increases synthesis of reactive species derived from iNOS and myeloperoxidase,** leading to excessive S-nitrosylation of cytoskeletal $\beta$ actin. (Thom, Bhopale, 2008)

- **HBO$_2$ does not reduce neutrophil viability and functions such as degranulation, phagocytosis and oxidative burst in response to chemoattractants remain intact.** (Juttner et al, 2003) (Thom, Mendiguren, Hardy et al, 1997)

- Probably the most compelling evidence that HBO$_2$ does not cause immunocompromise comes from **studies in sepsis models, where HBO$_2$ has a beneficial effect.** (Buras et al, 2006) (Ross, McAllister, 1965) (Thom, Lauermann, Hart, 1986)

- **A separate anti-inflammatory pathway for HBO$_2$ involves impaired pro-inflammatory cytokine production by mono-cyte-macrophages.** This action has been shown in animal models and human beings. (Benson et al, 2003) (Lahat et al, 1995) (Weisz et al, 1997)

- **HBO$_2$ limits the amount of inflammation in the bowels, low-ers the CRP values, lowers Sedimentation values and lowers the WBC values. The pain is alleviated, the patient's weight improves, and bowel movements return almost to normal. The pain is relieved because hypoxia causes release of pain neurotransmitters and correction of the hypoxic conditions results in decreased pain.** Although the mechanism is not clearly understood, HBO$_2$ should be considered in treatment of Crohn's Disease not responding to conventional treatments. (Nelson et al, 1990)

- **In the study published in Proceeding of the Tenth International Congress on Hyperbaric Medicine the remission of patients treated with HBO$_2$ prolonged until 4-5 years in 49% of the cases, the improvement was noted in 37%. Later, none of the patients treated with HBO needed operative intervention for inflammatory bowel disease.**

- **HBO$_2$ has been shown in numerous models to augment ischemic tolerance of brain, spinal cord, liver, heart and skeletal muscle by mechanisms involving induction of antioxidant enzymes and anti-inflammatory proteins.** (Gregorevic, Lynch, Williams, 2001) (Hirata et al, 2007) (Kim et al, 2001) (Nie et al, 2006) (Yu et al, 2005)

- In several models, **exposure to HBO$_2$ ameliorates post-ischemic injuries by decreasing HIF-1 expression.** (Calvert et al, 2006) (Li et al, 2005)

- **Pathological changes in association with isolated O$_2$-mediated seizures have not been found in studies with guinea pigs, rabbits and humans.** (Clark, 2008)

- **At all doses, cognitive function of the irradiated rats breathing 100% O(2) was improved over that of the irradiated rats breathing air.** These data suggest that astronauts are not at greater risk of developing cognitive impairment when exposed to space radiation while breathing 100% O(2) during an EVA. (Wheeler et al, 2014)

- **Hyperbaric oxygen (HBO) treatment of cholesterol-fed rabbits dramatically reduces the development of arterial lesions despite having little or no effect on plasma or individual lipoprotein cholesterol concentrations.** (Delaney, Montgomery, 2001)

- Similarly, in regression studies, **HBO treatment has no effect on the rate of plasma (or lipoprotein) cholesterol decline but significantly accelerates aortic lesion regression** compared with no treatment. (Kudchodkar et al, 2000)

- **There is some evidence that HBOT can reverse age-related macular degeneration (AMD),** the leading cause of severe visual loss in people over the age of fifty. (Bojic et al, 2015)

- Ishii and colleagues reported the use of HBO as a recovery method for muscular fatigue during the Nagano Winter Olympics. In this experiment seven Olympic athletes received HBO treatment for 30–40 minutes at 1.3 ATA with a maximum of six treatments per athlete and an average of two. It was found that **all athletes benefited from the HBO treatment presenting faster recovery rates.**

- **These results are concordant with those obtained by Fischer and colleagues and Haapaniemi and colleagues that suggested that lactic acid and ammonia were removed faster with HBO treatment leading to shorter recovery periods.** (Haapaniemi et al, 1995) (Fischer et al, 1988)

- Also in observations at the Matosinhos Hyperbaric Unit several situations, namely **fractures and ligament injuries, have proved to benefit from faster recovery times when HBO treatments were applied to the athletes.** (Barata et al, 2011)

- **The results suggested that treatment with hyperbaric oxygen may enhance recovery of eccentric torque of the quadriceps muscle from delayed onset muscle soreness (DOMS).** (Bennett et al. 2005)

- **The HBO group had an improvement in joint function following acute ankle sprains.** (Borromeo et al.1997)

- **After 4 weeks, an interesting contribution from HBO could be seen in that it promoted the return of normal stiffness of the ligament following injury to the medial collateral ligament.** (Horn et al. 1999)

- **At 6 weeks, HBO had positive effects on pain and functional outcomes on short term recovery from grade II medial collateral ligament injuries, such as decreased volume of edema, a better range of motion and maximum flexion improvement,** compared with the sham group. (Soolsma, 1996) RCT

- **Using HBO as an adjunctive therapy after primary repair of the injured anterior cruciate ligament (ACL) is likely to increase success, a situation that is confirmed by the British Medical Journal Evidence Center.** (Minhas, 2010)

- **Okubo and colleagues** used a rat model study, in which recombinant human bone morphogenetic protein-2 was implanted in the form of lyophilized discs to measure the influence of HBO. **The group treated with HBO, exposed to 2 ATA for 60 min daily, had significantly** increased new bone formation compared with the control group and the cartilage was present at the outer edge of the implanted material after 7 days.

- **Komurcu and colleagues reviewed retrospectively 14 cases of infected tibial nonunion that were treated successfully.**

- **Wang and colleagues**, in a rabbit model, were able to demonstrate that **distraction segments of animals treated with HBO had increased bone mineral density and superior mechanical properties comparing to the controls and yields better results when applied during the early stage of the tibial healing process.**

- **Injuries studies involving bones, muscles and ligaments with HBO treatment seem promising.** (Barata et al, 2011)

- **HBO promotes scar tissue formation by increasing type I procollagen gene expression, at 7 and 14 days after the injury, which contribute for the improvement of their tensile properties.** (Mashitori and colleagues)

- **Two systematic reviews on HBO and cancer have concluded that the use of HBO in patients with malignancies is considered safe.** (Moen, Stuhr, 2012)

- **We have summarized the work performed on HBO and cancer in the period 2004–2012. Based on the present as well as previous reviews, there is no evidence indicating that HBO neither acts as a stimulator of tumor growth nor as an enhancer of recurrence.** (Moen, Stuhr, 2012)

- On the other hand, **there is evidence that implies that HBO might have tumor-inhibitory effects in certain cancer subtypes.** (Moen, Stuhr, 2012)

- **A study of HBO using osteosarcoma cells also demonstrated induction of apoptosis.** (Kawasoe et al, 2009)

- **In two different animal models, gliomas and mammary tumors, respectively, Moen and Stuhr's group has demonstrated induction of cell death after HBO treatment.** (Raa et al, 2007) (Sturh et al, 2007) (Moen et al, 2009)

- **Reduced cell proliferation, together with a significant change in histology, has also been shown after HBO treatment in**

Prof Randolph M. Howes MD,PhD

**DMBA-induced mammary tumors in vivo.** (Raa et al, 2007) (Sturh et al, 2007) (Moen et al, 2009)

- **Two recent studies on osteosarcoma cells and nasopharyngeal carcinoma support inhibition of cell division after HBO treatment.** (Kawasoe et al, 2009) (Peng et al, 2010)

- **HBO has been shown to induce an antiangiogenic effect in two mammary tumor models,** in addition to one glioma model. Furthermore, **multiple studies showed no change in angiogenesis after HBO treatment.** (Shi et al, 2005) (Heys et al, 2006) (Chong et al, 2004) (Schonmeyr et al, 2008) (Thom, 2011) (Tang et al, 2009) (Tang et al, 2004) (Hampson et al, 2004)

- **HBO is not likely to enhance tumor angiogenesis.** (Feldmeier et al, 2003)

- **None of the studies reviewed showed induced metastasis after HBO.** (Kawasoe et al, 2009) (Haroon et al, 2007) (Moen et al, 2012) (Daruwalla, Christophi, 2006) (Daruwalla et al, 2007)

- **A recent study found HBO to induce a mesenchymal-to-epithelial transition (MET) in DMBA-induced mammary tumors, leading to a less aggressive tumor type, thus indicating that oxygen might be a key factor in MET.** (Bock et al, 2011)

- In a mammary tumor model, Moen et al. found that **the uptake of chemotherapy is increased for the duration of, and immediately after, HBO treatment.** (Moen et al, 2009)

- **Moen et al. found an increased uptake of the chemotherapeutic drug 5-FU into DMBA-induced tumors after HBO,** while Jevne et al. failed to find the same correlation in the 4T1 mammary tumor model. (Moen et al, 2009) (Jevne et al, 2011)

- Kawasoe et al. found, both in vitro and in vivo, that HBO enhanced the chemotherapeutic effect of carboplatin in osteosarcomas. Furthermore, **combining HBO and cisplatin significantly reduced tumor volume in a human ovarian cancer xenograft model.** (Selvendiran et al, 2010)

- In 2011, **Overgaard published a meta-analysis reviewing the influence of hypoxic modification of radiotherapy in head and neck carcinoma.** Overall, **Overgaard found that out of the various hypoxic modification techniques, HBO showed the** most pronounced effect, and thus will improve the results of radiotherapy.

- Granowitz et al. showed that HBO treatment alone had a strong antiproliferative effect on different mammary cancer cells in vitro.

- An increase in cell death and reduced cell proliferation, together with a significant change in histology, has also been shown after HBO treatment in DMBA-induced mammary tumors in vivo. (Mayer et al, 2005)

- In relation to metastasis, it has been shown that HBO induced MET in DMBA-induced mammary tumors, leading to a less aggressive tumor type. In a 4T1 mammary tumor model, Haroon et al. found that HBO restricts the growth of large tumor cell colonies. (Mayer et al, 2005)

- In an older clinical study, Dische and Senanayake demonstrated positive results when combining HBO and radiotherapy on patients with carcinoma in the colon and the rectum. (Dische, Senanayake, 1972)

- Older experimental and clinical studies have demonstrated that HBO improves the effect of photodynamic therapy. (Maier et al, 2000) (Dong et al, 1987) (Maier et al, 2000), EJCS) (Chen et al, 2002) (Jirsa et al, 1991)

- Additionally, two papers by Daruwalla et al. examine the effect of HBO in two different in vivo colon tumor models. In the first paper, the effect of HBO per se was studied. Here, they concluded firstly that HBO did not have any tumor stimulatory effect and does not promote formation of distal metastases, and secondly that HBO therefore can safely be used in combination with other therapies.

- In 2007, Stuhr et al. published an experimental study, examining the effect of HBO on the growth and development of rat glioma xenografts per se. They found that increased levels of $pO_2$, using both normobaric and moderate HBO, significantly reduced glioma tumor growth, possibly by increasing cell death and reducing the vascular density.

- Kohshi et al. and Ogawa et al. both conclude that there is a possible advantage to combining HBO with radiotherapy, but they also underline the need for further investigation within this field. (Kohshi et al, 2007) (Ogawa et al, 2006)

**- Two recent in vitro experiments have shown promising results when treating leukemia cells with HBO.**

In addition, Tonomura and Granowitz, in an editorial in 2007, have commented on the effect of HBO on leukemia. They concluded that since HBO promotes apoptosis in leukemia cells, it should be further exploited as a novel treatment for leukemia. (Tonomura, Granowitz, 2007)

**- Both recent and older research studies have shown that HBO can be inhibitory and reduce cancer growth in some cancer types, like breast cancer.** (Moen, Stuhr, 2012)

---

## NEGATIVE STATEMENTS REGARDING HBOT

**There is clearly a potential for negative effects. The risks for $O_2$ toxicity depend on the concentration and intracellular localization of reactive species.**

**- As of 2000, although results have proven to be promising in terms of using HBO as a treatment modality in sports-related injuries, these studies have been limited due to the small sample sizes, lack of blinding and randomization problems.** (Babul, Rhodes, 2000)

**- There is a lack of high quality, valid research evidence regarding the effects of HBOT on wound healing.** Whilst **two small trials suggested that HBOT may improve the outcomes of skin grafting and trauma** these trials were at risk of bias. Further evaluation by means of high quality RCTs is needed. (Eskes et al, 2010)

- In a Chinese trial (n = 145) HBOT did not significantly improve flap survival in patients with limb skin defects. (Eskes et al, 2011)

**- There are also some potential adverse effects of the therapy, including damage to the ears, sinuses and lungs from the effects of the pressure and oxygen poisoning.** (Bennett, Trytko, Jonker, 2012)

- **In people with traumatic brain injury, while the addition of HBOT may reduce the risk of death and improve the final Glasgow Coma Scale (GCS), there is little evidence that the survivors have a good outcome. The routine application of HBOT to these patients cannot be justified from this review.** (Bennett, Trytko, Jonker, 2012)

- This intervention has been demonstrated to enhance pulmonary $O_2$ tolerance. **CNS $O_2$ toxicity is manifested as a grand mal seizure. This occurs at an incidence of approximately 1 to 4 in 10,000 patient treatments.** (Hart, Strauss, 1987) (Davis, Dunn, Heimbach, 1988) (Plafki et al, 2000)

- **Progressive myopia has been reported in patients who undergo prolonged daily therapy, but this typically reverses within 6 weeks after termination of treatments.** (Lyne, 1978)

- Development of nuclear cataracts has been reported with excessive treatments that exceed a total of 150 to 200 hours, and the change does not spontaneously reverse. (Palmquist, Philipson, Barr, 1984)

- A Cochrane review (Bennett et al. 2005b) stated that **there is not sufficient evidence to support hyperbaric oxygenation for the treatment of promoting fracture healing or nonunion fracture as no randomized evidence was found.**

- **It has also been shown that adverse side effects like oxygen poisoning and severe tissue radiation injury is associated with the use of HBO in combination with radiotherapy.** (Bennett et al, 2012)

- **Neither Chong et al. nor Tang et al. found any change in *in vivo* tumor growth after HBO treatment.** (Tang et al, 2009)

- **Daruwalla et al. stated that HBO treatment of patients with cervical and bladder cancer did not offer any improved benefit or improved outcome.**

- **Many have ascribed the enhanced chemotherapeutic effect after HBO to increased levels of ROS. Moen et al., however, found no change in MDA levels after HBO, indicating that in this study ROS levels cannot be the main determinant of an increased chemotherapeutic effect.** (Moen et al, 2009)

# SECTION TEN

## CONDENSED HBOT SUMMARY

To further reduce the burden on the reader, I have condensed the above summary as follows:

### LISTING SUMMARY (92 items)

### HBOT FACTS AND POSITIVE EFFECTS

- used in wound healing, bone infection, carbon monoxide intoxication, and air emboli, or air bubbles in the bloodstream due to decompression sickness, and open-heart surgery.

- reverses tissue hypoxia and cellular dysfunction,

- Injuries studies involving bones, muscles and ligaments with HBO treatment seem promising.

- used for acute crush injury,

- ischemic flaps and grafts,

- acute central retinal arterial occlusion, other acute arterial occlusions,

- and idiopathic sudden sensorineural hearing loss.

- can be delivered safely to critically ill patients.

- an effective adjunct for wound healing that has both systemic and local effects.

- **At the tissue level, HBOT** modulates: cytokine release, accelerates microbial oxidative killing,
   reduces apoptosis (in normal cells),
   and modulates leukocyte activation and adhesion

- treatment of ischemic wounds (eg, diabetic lower extremity wounds, late effects of radiation, and refractory osteomyelitis).

- only four patients needed to be treated with **HBO$_2$** to prevent one amputation.

- **HBOT** is associated with remission of about 85% of cases of refractory lower extremity osteomyelitis.

- **HBOT** promotes healing of arterial ulcers, calciphylactic and refractory vasculitic ulcers, as well as refractory osteomyelitis.

- **For patients with diabetic foot ulcers (DFU)** complicated by surgical infection, **HBOT** reduces chance of amputation (7 studies) and improves chance of healing (6 studies).

- treat **CO** poisoning, diabetic lower extremity wounds, crush injury, and radiation necrosis.

- treat coma resulting from head injuries, bruising of the spinal cord, stroke and neurological disorders such as multiple sclerosis.

- treatment as prophylaxis against infection, to facilitate wound closure, and to prevent amputation in wounded patients.

- inhibits **PMN** adherence on postcapillary venules.

- improve outcome from a wide variety of post-ischemic/inflammatory insults.

- improves ischemic tolerance when used in a prophylactic manner.

- inhibits adherence/sequestration of neutrophils by inhibiting $\beta_2$ integrin function.

- **HBO$_2$** inhibits neutrophil $\beta_2$ integrin function because hyperoxia increases synthesis of reactive species derived from **iNOS** and myeloperoxidase.

- induces antioxidant enzymes and anti-inflammatory proteins.

- increased antioxidant enzyme expression, such as Cu/Zn-superoxide dismutase, catalase, and glutathione peroxidase,

- also significantly decreased pro-oxidant enzyme levels, such as iNOS and gp91-phox, thereby decreasing net oxygen radical production by means of negative feedback.

- increases the production of ROIs (EMODs) throughout the body, leaving no safe harbor for the virus to hide outside the genome.

- HIV viral load was decreased in the infected cells, and few viruses entered uninfected peripheral blood mononuclear cells (PBMCs).

- HBO has an antiviral effect.

- can deliver sufficient oxygen to the nonhealing wound to stimulate angiogenesis and healing through multiple mechanisms, including increased collagen production, increased growth factor receptor numbers, upregulation of vascular endothelial growth factor, increased circulating endothelial progenitor cells, and improvement in neutrophil-mediated host defense.

- restores this defense and also increases the phagocytosis of some bacteria by working synergistically with antibiotics,

- and inhibits the growth of a number of anaerobic and aerobic organisms at wound sites.

- blocks the production of alphatoxine and thetatoxine and inhibits bacterial growth.

- offered for patients with limb- or life-threatening infections, such as clostridial gas gangrene and necrotizing fasciitis.

- counteract infection indirectly by providing the white blood cells with the oxygen.

- acts directly by **killing anaerobic organisms**, stopping their multiplication, and neutralizing the toxins that some of them produce.

- substantially increases the level of oxygen dissolved into blood plasma. **This state of serum hyperoxia is the second beneficial effect of hyperbaric oxygen therapy.**

- **appears effective for the management of acute, difficult to heal wounds.**

- **short-term effects such as vasoconstriction and enhanced oxygen delivery,**

- **reduction of edema,**

- **phagocytosis activation and also an anti-inflammatory effect (enhanced leukocyte function).**

- **Neovascularization (angiogenesis in hypoxic soft tissues),**

- **osteoneogenesis as well as stimulation of collagen production by fibroblasts.**

- **inhibiting leukocyte adhesion to the endothelium,**

- **diminishing tissue damage, which enhances leukocyte motility and improves microcirculation.**

- **corrected the dysfunction of ROS-related signals in ischemic wounds, changing the molecular pattern to closely resemble the acute non-ischemic wounds.**

- **HBO$_2$-mediated oxidative stress at sites of neovascularization will stimulate stem/progenitor cells (SPCs) growth factor production.**

- **acts via the ROS/MAPK/MMP signaling axis to reduce tissue degeneration and improve ischemic wound healing.**

- **increases bone marrow–derived endothelial progenitor cell mobilization.**

- **indicated for treating compromised flaps and grafts and to enhance healing in selected problem wounds, i.e., delayed effects of radiation and refractory diabetic wounds.**

- **resulted in a significantly higher percentage of healthy graft area in split skin grafts.**

- **HBOT** promotes successful "take" of compromised flaps and grafts.

- **Administration of HBO$_2$ prior to and for three days following skin grafting led to a significant 29% improvement in graft survival.**

- significantly more crush wounds healed with **HBOT** than with sham **HBOT**.

- Clinical studies have documented significant survival enhancement with **HBO$_2$** for extremity re-implantation and free tissue transfer, and following crush injury.

- burn wounds healed significantly quicker with **HBOT** (**P < 0.005**) than with routine burn care.

- stem/progenitor cells (**SPCs**) mobilized by **HBO$_2$** home to wounds and accelerate healing.

- Pluripotent mesenchymal stem cells were shown *in vitro* to be stimulated by **HBO$_2$** to synthesize placental growth factor.

- stimulates synthesis of basic fibroblast growth factor (**bFGF**) and transforming growth factor $\beta 1$ by human dermal fibroblasts, angiopoietin-2 by human umbilical vein endothelial cells, bFGF and hepatocyte growth factor in ischemic limbs, and it up-regulates platelet derived growth factor (**PDGF**) receptor in wounds.

- improves oxygen supply to the injured brain,
  reduce the swelling associated with low oxygen levels
  and reduce the volume of brain that will ultimately perish.

- **HBO$_2$** can reduce coronary artery re-stenosis after balloon angioplasty/stenting,
  - and decrease muscle loss after thrombolytic treatment for myocardial infarction.
  - improve hepatic survival after transplantation and lead to more rapid return of donor liver function
  - reduced the incidence of encephalopathy seen after cardiopulmonary bypass and following carbon monoxide poisoning.

- significantly decreased the incidence of postoperative infections in neuromuscular scoliosis patients.

- **HBO$_2$ limits the amount of inflammation (Crohn's disease) in the bowels,**
    - **lowers the CRP values (an indicator of inflammation),**
    - **lowers Sedimentation values and lowers the WBC values.**
    - **The pain is alleviated,**
    - **the patient's weight improves,**
    - **and bowel movements return almost to normal.**

- **augments ischemic tolerance of brain, spinal cord, liver, heart and skeletal muscle by mechanisms involving induction of antioxidant enzymes and anti-inflammatory proteins.**

- **ameliorates post-ischemic injuries by decreasing HIF-1 expression.**

- **significantly accelerates aortic lesion regression.**

- **There is some evidence that HBOT can reverse age-related macular degeneration (AMD).**

- **all athletes benefited from the HBO treatment presenting faster recovery rates.**

- **lactic acid and ammonia were removed faster with HBO treatment leading to shorter recovery periods.**

- **fractures and ligament injuries, have proved to benefit from faster recovery times when HBO treatments were applied to the athletes.**

- **treatment with hyperbaric oxygen may enhance recovery of eccentric torque of the quadriceps muscle from delayed onset muscle soreness (DOMS).**

- **HBO group had an improvement in joint function following acute ankle sprains.**

- HBO **promoted the return of normal stiffness of the ligament following injury to the medial collateral ligament.**

- **14 cases of infected tibial nonunion were treated successfully.**

- **promotes scar tissue formation by increasing type I procollagen gene expression.**

- **HBO might have tumor-inhibitory effects in certain cancer subtypes.**

- **A study of HBO using osteosarcoma cells demonstrated induction of apoptosis.**

- **In two different animal models, gliomas and mammary tumors, respectively, Moen and Stuhr's group has demonstrated induction of cell death after HBO treatment.**

- **Reduced cell proliferation, together with a significant change in histology, has also been shown after HBO treatment in DMBA-induced mammary tumors in vivo.**

- **HBO has been shown to induce an antiangiogenic effect in two mammary tumor models and multiple studies showed no change in angiogenesis after HBO treatment.**

- **None of the studies reviewed showed induced metastasis after HBO.**

- **the uptake of chemotherapy is increased for the duration of, and immediately after, HBO treatment.**

- **combining HBO and cisplatin significantly reduced tumor volume in a human ovarian cancer xenograft model.**

- **HBO showed the most pronounced effect in head and neck cancer and thus will improve the results of radiotherapy.**

- **Granowitz et al. showed that HBO treatment alone had a strong antiproliferative effect on different mammary cancer cells in vitro.**

- **An increase in cell death and reduced cell proliferation, together with a significant change in histology, has also been shown after HBO treatment in DMBA-induced mammary tumors in vivo.**

- **Dische and Senanayake demonstrated positive results when combining HBO and radiotherapy on patients with carcinoma in the colon and the rectum.**

- **HBO improves the effect of photodynamic therapy.**

- increased levels of $pO_2$, using both normobaric and moderate **HBO**, significantly reduced glioma tumor growth, possibly by increasing cell death and reducing the vascular density.

- **Kohshi et al.** and **Ogawa et al.** both conclude that there is a possible advantage to combining **HBO** with radiotherapy.

- Two recent in vitro experiments have shown promising results when treating leukemia cells with **HBO**.

- Both recent and older research studies have shown that **HBO** can be inhibitory and reduce cancer growth in some cancer types, like breast cancer.

## My closing thoughts on HBOT

My summary of the above findings is that **HBOT** has great future potential for clinical application in the treatment of a wide range of diseases. In a sense, **HBOT** is still in its infancy but its studied past reveals its effectiveness in correcting ailments which responded poorly or did not respond at all to traditional medical practices.

I eagerly await investigations into its likely effect on the aging process, let alone, its future potential in reducing the ravages of cancer and heart disease.

Once again, I am more than impressed with the critical and salutary role of a singular molecular entity, oxygen. I have arduously searched for the points of overlap and convergence in the various disciplines which have studied oxygen, such as phototherapy, photodynamic therapy, **HBOT**, chemotherapy, radiation therapy, sonotherapy, etc. and I have found many such points of commonality.

In short, there is no doubting the crucial role of oxygen and its **EMOD** progeny in protecting and maintaining the overall healthspan and lifespan of man. **HBOT** has **EMODs** as part of its integral mechanisms.

# References

(Acs et al, 2003) (Acs, G., Zhang, P.J., McGrath, C.M., Acs, P., McBroom, J., Mohyeldin, A., Liu, S., Lu, H. and Verma, A. Hypoxia-inducible erythro-poietin signaling in squamous dysplasia and squamous cell carcinoma of the uterine cervix and its potential role in cervical carcinogenesis and tumor progression. Am J Path 2003; 162: 1789-1806)

(Acker, 1994) (Acker H. Mechanisms and meaning of cellular oxygen sensing in the organism. Respir Physiol 95: 1-10, 1994)

(Adams, Sutton, Mader, 1987) (Adams, K.R., Sutton, E.E. and Mader, J.T. In vitro potentiation of tobramycin under hyperoxic conditions. Undersea Biomed Res 1987; 14(suppl): 37)

(Adams, Mader, 1987) (Adams, K.R. and Mader, J.T. Aminoglycoside Poetentiation with adjunctive hyperbaric oxygen therapy in experi-mental Pseudomonas aeruginosa osteomyelitis. Undersea Biomed Res 1987; 14(suppl): 37)

(Al-Waili et al, 2005) (Al-Waili NS, Betler G, Beale J, Hamilton RW, Lee BY, Lucas P. Hyperbaric oxygen and malignancies: a potential role in radiotherapy, chemotherapy, tumor surgery and phototherapy. MedSciMonit. 2005;11:RA279–RA289)

(Albuquerque, Sousa, 2007) (Albuquerque J.G., Sousa J.G. (2007) Oxigenoterapia hiperbárica (OTHB). Perspectiva histórica, efeitos fi-siológicos e aplicações clínicas. Rev Soc Poruguesa Med Interna 14: 219–227)

(Alex et al, 2005) (Alex J, Laden G, Cale A, et al. Pretreatment with hyperbaric oxygen and its effect on neuropsychometric dysfunction and systemic inflammatory response after cardiopulmonary bypass: a prospective randomized double-blind trial. J Thorac Cardiovasc Surg. 2005;130:1623–1630)

(Allison, 2014) (Allison RR. Photodynamic therapy: oncologic horizons. Future Oncol. 2014 Jan;10(1):123-4)

(Allison, Moghissi, 2013) (Ron R. Allison and Keyvan Moghissi. Photodynamic Therapy (PDT): PDT Mechanisms. Clin Endosc. 2013 Jan; 46(1): 24–29)

(Alvarez et al, 2003) (Alvarez S, Valdez LB, Zaobornyj T, Boveris A. Oxygen dependence of mitochondrial nitric oxide synthase activity. Biochem Biophys Res Commun. 2003;305:771–775)

(Ames, Gold, 1991) (Ames, B. N., Gold, L. S. 1991. Endogenous mutagens and the causes of aging and cancer. Murat. Res. 250:3-16)

(Antonelli et al, 2009) (Antonelli C., Franchi F., Della Marta M.E., Carinci A., Sbrana G., Tanasi P., et al. (2009) Guiding principles in choosing a therapeutic table for DCI hyperbaric therapy. Minerva Anestesiologica 75: 151–161)

(Araki, Nashimoto, Takano, 1988) (Araki, R., Nashimoto, I. and Takano, T. The effect of hyperbaric oxygen on cerebral hemoglobin oxygenation and dissociation rate of carboxyhemoglobin in anesthetized rats: spectroscopic approach. Adv Ex Med Biol 1988; 222: 375-381)

(Asano et al, 2007) (Asano T, Kaneko E, Shinozaki S, et al. Hyperbaric oxygen induces basic fibroblast growth factor and hepatocyte growth factor expression and enhances blood perfusion and muscle regeneration in mouse ischemic hind limbs. Circ J.2007;71:405–411)

(ATA, 1977) (ATA by intermittent $O_2$ exposure. J Appl Physiol. 1977;42:593–599)

(Artu et al, 1976) (Artu, F., Philippon, B., Gau, F., Berger, M. and Deleuze R. Cerebral blood flow, cerebral metabolism and cerebrospinal fluid biochemistry in brain-injured patients after exposure to hyperbaric oxygen. Eur Neurol 1976; 14: 351-364)

(Arzinger-Jonasch et al, 1978) (Arzinger-Jonasch, H., Sandner, K. and Bittner, H. Die widkung hyperbaren sauerstoffs auf brandwunden unterschiedlicher tiefe im tierexperiment. [The effect of hyperbaric oxygen on burn wounds of different depths in animal experiments]. Z Exp Chir Transplant Kunstliche Organe 1978; 11: 6-10)

(Astrup et al, 1981) (Astrup, J., Siesjo, B.K. and Symon, L. The state of penumbra in the ischemic brain: viable and lethal threshold in cerebral ischemia. Stroke 1981; 12: 723-725)

(Austin, 1993) (Austin, F. Maintenance of infective Borrelia burgdorferi Sh-2-82 in four percent oxygen/five percent carbon dioxide in vitro. Cardio J of Microbiol 1993; 39(12): 1103-1110)

(Aydin et al, 2013) (Aydin F, Kaya A, Karapinar L, Kumbaraci M, Imerci A, Karapinar H, Karakuzu C, Incesu M. IGF-I Increases with Hyperbaric Oxygen Therapy and Promotes Wound Healing in Diabetic Foot Ulcers. J Diabetes Res. 2013;2013:567834)

(Babul et al. 2003) (Babul S., Rhodes E. (2000) The Role of Hyperbaric Oxygen Therapy in Sports Medicine. Sports Med 30: 395–03)

(Babul, Rhodes, 2000) (Babul S., Rhodes E. (2000) The Role of Hyperbaric Oxygen Therapy in Sports Medicine. Sports Med 30: 395–03)

(Badwey, Karnovsky, 1980) (Badwey, J.A and Karnovsky, M.L. Active oxygen species and the functions of phagocytic leukocytes. Ann Rev Biochem 1980; 49: 695-726)

(Bakker, 1988) (Bakker, D.J. Clostridial myonecrosis. In Davis, J.C. and Hunt, T.K. (Eds): Problem Wounds: The Role of Oxygen. New York: Elsevier, 1988; pp. 153-172)

(Balaban et al, 2005) (Balaban, R.S., Nemoto, S., Finkel, T., 2005. Mitochondria, oxidants, and aging. Cell 120, 483–495)

(Barata et al, 2011) (Pedro Barata, Mariana Cervaens, Rita Resende, Óscar Camacho, and Frankim Marques. Hyperbaric Oxygen Effects on Sports Injuries. Ther Adv Musculoskelet Dis. 2011 Apr; 3(2): 111–121)

(Barton, Furrer, 2003) (Barton, M. and Furrer, J. Cardiovascular consequences of the obesity pandemic: need for action. Exp Opin Invest Drugs 2003; 12: 1757-1759)

(Bass, 1970) (Bass, B.H. The treatment of varicose leg ulcers by hyperbaric oxygen. Postgrad Med J 1970; 46: 407-408)

(Bauer et al, 2001) (J Bauer, K Maier, O Linderkamp, and R Hentschel. Effect of Caffeine on Oxygen Consumption and Metabolic Rate in Very Low Birth Weight Infants With Idiopathic Apnea. Peditatrics Vol. 107 No. 4 April 2001, pp. 660-663)

(Baugh, 2000) (Baugh MA. HIV: reactive oxygen species, enveloped viruses and hyperbaric oxygen. Med Hypotheses. 2000 Sep;55(3):232-8)

(Badwey, Karnovsky, 1980) (Badwey, J.A and Karnovsky, M.L. Active oxygen species and the functions of phagocytic leukocytes. Ann Rev Biochem 1980; 49: 695-726)

(Beckman, Ames, 1998) (Beckman, K.B., Ames, B.N., 1998. The free radical theory of aging matures. Physiol. Rev. 78, 547–581)

(Beckman & Koppenol, 1996) (Beckman JS, Koppenol WH. Nitric oxide superoxide and peroxynitrite: the good the bad and the ugly. Am J Physiol. 1996;271:C1424–1437)

(Bennett et al. 2005) (Bennett M., Best T., Babul-Wellar S., Taunton J. (2005a) Hyperbaric oxygen therapy for delayed onset muscle soreness and closed soft tissue injury. Cochrane Database Syst Rev 19: 1–39)

(Bennett et al. 2005b) (Bennett M.H., Stanford R.E., Turner R. (2005b) Hyperbaric oxygen therapy for promoting fracture healing and treating fracture non-union. Cochrane Database Syst Rev 1: CD004712DOI)

(Bennett et al, 2008) (Bennett M, Feldmeier J, Hampson N, et al. Hyperbaric oxygen therapy for late radiation tissue injury (Cochrane review) The Cochrane Library. 2008;(Issue 1)

(Bennett et al, 2012) (Bennett MH, Feldmeier J, Smee R, Milross C. Hyperbaric oxygenation for tumour sensitisation to radiotherapy. Cochrane Database Syst Rev. 2012;4:CD005007)

(Bennett, Trytko, Jonker, 2012) (Bennett MH, Trytko B, Jonker B. Hyperbaric oxygen therapy for the adjunctive treatment of traumatic brain injury. Cochrane Database Syst Rev. 2012 Dec 12;12:CD004609)

(Beppu et al, 2002) (Beppu T, Kamada K, Yoshida Y, Arai H, Ogasawara K, Ogawa A. Change of oxygen pressure in glioblastoma tissue under various conditions. J Neurooncol. 2002;58:47–52)

(Beppu et al, 2011) (Beppu T, Tanaka K, Kohshi K. Hyperbaric oxygenation for treatment of glioma. Gan To Kagaku Ryoho. 2011;38:933–936)

(Bernard, 1878) (Bernard, C. 1878. Lecons sur les Phenomenes de La Vie Communs aux Animaux et aux Vegetaux. Vol. I. Paris: Bailliere)

(Benson et al, 2003) (Benson RM, Minter LM, Osborne BA, et al. Hyperbaric oxygen inhibits stimulus-induced proinflammatory cytokine synthesis by human blood-derived monocyte-macrophages. Clin Exp Immunol. 2003;134:57–62)

(Best et al. 1998) (Best T., Loitz-Ramage B., Corr D., Vanderby R.J. (1998) Hyperbaric oxygen in the treatment of acute muscle stretch injuries: Results in an animal model. Am J Sports Med 26: 367–372)

(Bock et al, 2011) (Bock K, Mazzone M, Carmeliet P. Antiangiogenic therapy, hypoxia, and metastasis: risky liaisons, or not? Nat Rev Clin Oncol. 2011;8:393–404)

(Boden, 1948) (Boden, G. Radiation myelitis of the cervical spinal cord. Br J Radiol 1948; 21: 464)

(Boerema et al, 1960, 133) (Boerema, I., Meyne, N.G., Brummelkamp, W.K., et al. Life without blood: a study of the influence of high atmospheric pressure and hypothermia on dilution of blood. J Cardiovasc Surg 1960; 1: 133-146)

(Boerema et al, 1960) (Boerema I, Meyne NG, Brummelkamp WK, et al: Life without blood: a study of the influence of high atmospheric pressure and hypothermia on dilution of the blood. J Cardiovasc Surg 1960;1:161-164)

(Boerema, 1961) (Boerema, I. An operating room for high oxygen pressure. Surgery 1961; 47: 291-298)

(Bojic et al, 2015) (Bojic, L., Gosovic, S., Kovacecic, H. and Denoble, P. Hyperbaric Oxygenation in the Treatment of Macular Degeneration. Split, Yugoslavia: Split Naval Medical Institute. 2015. pp 1-4)

(Bonomo et al, 1998) (Bonomo SR, Davidson JD, Yu Y, et al. Hyperbaric oxygen as a signal transducer: upregulation of platelet derived growth factor-beta receptor in the presence of $HBO_2$ and PDGF. Undersea Hyperb Med. 1998;25:211–216)

(Borromeo et al, 1997) (Borromeo C.N., Ryan J.L., Marchetto P.A., Peterson R., Bove A.A. (1997) Hyperbaric oxygen therapy for acute ankle sprains. Am J Sports Med 25: 619–625)

(Bouachour et al, 1996) (Bouachour G, Cronier P, Gouello JP, et al. Hyperbaric oxygen therapy in the management of crush injuries: a randomized double-blind placebo-controlled clinical trial. J Trauma. 1996;41:333–339)

(Boveris et al, 1972) (Boveris, A., N. Oshino, and B. Chance. The cellular production of hydrogen peroxide. Biochem. J. 128: 617-630, 1972)

(Boveris, Chance, 1973) (Boveris, A. and Chance, B. The mitochondrial generation of hydrogen peroxide: General properties and effect of hyperbaric oxygen. Biochem J 1973; 134: 707-716)

(Boyle, Levin, 2008) (Boyle P., Levin B. (eds) (2008) World cancer report. IARC, Lyon)

(Brady et al, 1989) (Brady CE et al. healing of severe perineal and cutaneous Crohn's disease with hyperbaric oxygenation. Gastronenterology 1989;97:756-60)

(Braunwald, 2001) (Braunwald, E. Coronary blood flow and myocardial ischemia. Heart disease: a textbook of cardiovascular medicine. 2001; W.B. Saunders Company. Philadelphia, PA 1161-1183)

(Brizel et al, 1995) (Brizel DM, Lin S, Johnson JL, Brooks J, Dewhirst MW, Piantadosi CA. The mechanisms by which hyperbaric oxygen and carbogen improve tumor oxygenation. Br J Cancer. 1995;72:1120–1124)

(Brown et al, 2012) (Brown JC, Winters-Stone K, Lee A, Schmitz KH. Cancer, physical activity, and exercise. Compr Physiol. 2012 Oct;2(4):2775-809)

(Buras et al, 2006) (Buras J, Holt D, Orlow D, et al. Hyperbaric oxygen protects from sepsis mortality via an interleukin-10-dependent mechanism. Crit Care Med.2006;34:2624–2629)

(Burgdorfer, 1996) (Burgdorfer W. National Institutes of Health, Rocky Mountain Laboratory. Personal letter 10 September, 1996)

Burt, Kapp, Smith, 1987) (Burt, J.T., Kapp, J.P. and Smith, R.R. Hyperbaric oxygen and cerebral infarction in the gerbil. Surg Gynecol 1987; 28: 265)

(Cadenas & Davies, 2000) (Cadenas E, Davies KJ. Mitochondrial free radical generation oxidative stress and aging. Free Radic Biol Med. 2000;29:222–230)

(Calvert et al, 2006) (Calvert J, Cahill J, Yamaguchi-Okada M, et al. Oxygen treatment after experimental hypoxia-ischemia in neonatal rats alters the expression of HIF-1a and its downstream target genes. J Appl Physiol. 2006;101:853–865)

(Cannito et al, 2008) (Cannito S, Novo E, Compagnone A, Valfre di Bonzo L, Busletta C, Zamara E, Paternostro C, Povero D, Bandino A, Bozzo F, Cravanzola C, Bravoco V, Colombatto S, Parola M. Redox mechanisms switch on hypoxia-dependent epithelial-mesenchymal transition in cancer cells. Carcinogenesis. 2008;29:2267–2278)

(Carmekiet, 2000) (Carmeliet P. Mechanisms of angiogenesis and arteriogenesis. Nat Med. 2000; 6:389–395)

(Casarett, Bruce, 1980) (Casarett, L.J. and Bruce, M. C. Origin and scope of toxicology. In: Doull J, Klaassen, C.D., and Amdur, M.O., editors. Casarett and Doull's toxicology. 2nd ed. New York: Macmillan, 1980:6)

(Champion, Mcsherry, Goulian, 1967) (Champion, W.M., McSherry, C.K. and Goulian, D. Effect of hyperbaric oxygen on the survival of the pedicled skin flaps. J Surg Res 1967; 7(12)

(Chance et al, 1979) (Chance, B., H. Sies, and A. Boveris. Hydroperoxide metabolism in mammalian organs. Physiol. Rev. 59: 527-605, 1979)

(Chapman et al, 1991) (Chapman, J.D., Stobbe, C.C., Arnfield, M.R., Santus, R., Lee, L. and McPhee, M.S. Oxygen dependency of tumor cell killing in vitro by light-activated Photofrin II. Radiat Res 1991; 126: 73-79)

(Chattaway, 1989) (Chattaway, SJ.S. What's new in the pathogenesis of multiple sclerosis? A review. J Roy Soc Med 1989; 82: 159-162)

(Chen et al, 2002) (Chen Q, Huang Z, Chen H, Shapiro H, Beckers J, Hetzel FW. Improvement of tumor response by manipulation of tumor oxygenation during photodynamic therapy. Photochem Photobiol. 2002;76:197–203)

(Chen et al, 2007) (Chen YC, Chen SY, Ho PS, Lin CH, Cheng YY, Wang JK, Sytwu HK. Apoptosis of T-leukemia and B-myeloma cancer cells induced by hyperbaric oxygen increased phosphorylation of p38 MAPK. Leuk Res. 2007;31:805–815)

(Chong et al, 2004) (Chong KT, Hampson NB, Bostwick DG, Vessella RL, Corman JM. Hyperbaric oxygen does not accelerate latent in vivo prostate cancer: implications for the treatment of radiation-induced haemorrhagic cystitis. BJU Int. 2004;94:1275–1278)

(Circu, Aw, 2008) (Circu ML, Aw TY. Glutathione and apoptosis. Free Rad Res. 2008;42:689–706)

(Clark, 2008) (Clark J. Oxygen toxicity. In: Neuman TS, Thom SR, editors. Physiology and Medicine of Hyperbaric Oxygen Therapy. Philadelphia: Saunders; 2008. pp. 527–563)

(Clarke et al, 2008) (Clarke R, Tenorio C, Hussey J, et al. Hyperbaric oxygen treatment of chronic radiation proctitis:A randomized and controlled double blind crossover trial with long-term follow-up. Int J Rad Oncol Biol Phys.2008;72:134–143)

(Clark, Lambertson, 1971) (Clark, J.M., and Lambertson, C.J. Pulmonary oxygen toxicity: a review. Pharmacol Rev 1971; 23: 37-133)

(Coburn et al, 1986) (Coburn, R. F., Eppinger, R., Scott, D. P. 1986. Oxygen-dependent tension in vascular smooth muscle. Does the endothelium play a role? Circ. Res. 58:34. 1-47)

(Coburn, Marers, 1974) (Coburn, R. F. , Mayers, L. B. 1974. Myoglobin $O_2$ tension determined from measurements of carboxyhemoglobin in skeletal muscle. Am. J. Physiol. 220:66-74)

(Corkill et al, 1985) (Corkill, G., Dhousen, K., Hein, H. et al. Videodensimetric estimation of the protective effect of hyperbaric oxygen in the ischemic gerbil brain. Surg Neurol 1985; 24: 406)

(Crapo et al, 1983) (Crapo JD, Freeman BA, Barry BE, Turrens JF, Young SL. Mechanisms of hyperoxic injury to the pulmonary microcirculation. Physiologist.1983;26:170–176)

(Cust, 2011) (Cust AE. Physical activity and gynecologic cancer prevention. Recent Results Cancer Res. 2011;186:159-85)

(Daruwalla, Christophi, 2006) (Daruwalla J, Christophi C. Hyperbaric oxygen therapy for malignancy: a review. World J Surg. 2006;30:2112–2131)

(Daruwalla et al, 2007) (Daruwalla J, Greish K, Nikfarjam M, Millar I, Malcontenti-Wilson C, Iyer AK, Christophi C. Evaluation of the effect of SMA-pirarubicin micelles on colorectal cancer liver metastases and of hyperbaric oxygen in CBA mice. J Drug Target. 2007;15:487–495)

(Davidson, 1989) (Davidson, D.L.W. Hyperbaric oxygen therapy in the treatment of multiple sclerosis. Report from Action for Research into Multiple Sclerosis, London, England 1989)

(Davis et al, 1986) (Davis, J.C., Heckman, J.D., Delee, J.C. and Buckwold, F.J. Chronic non-hematogenous osteomyelitis treated with adjuvant hyperbaric oxygen. J Bone Joint Surg 1986; 68: 1210-1217)

(Davies, 1995) (Davies, K.J. Oxidative stress: the paradox of aerobic life. Biochem Soc Symp 1995; 61: 1-31)

(Davis, Dunn, Heimbach, 1988) (Davis JC, Dunn JM, Heimbach RD. Hyperbaric medicine: patient selection, treatment procedures, and side-effects. In: Davis JC, Hunt TK, editors. Problem Wounds. New York: Elsevier; 1988. pp. 225–235)

(Davis, Hunt, 1977) (Davis, J.C. and Hunt, T.K. Refractory osteomyelitis of the extremities and the axial skeleton. In Davis, J.C. and Hunt, T.K. (Eds): Hyperbaric Oxygen Therapy. Bethesda, Maryland: Undersea Medical Society, 1977; pp. 217-227)

(Dawber, 1980) (Dawber, T.R. The Framingham Study. Boston: Harvard University Press, 1980; pp. 62-75)

(DeChatelet, 1975) (DeChatelet, L.R. Oxidative bactericidal mechanisms of polymorphonuclear leukocytes. J Infect Dis 1975; 131: 295-303)

(Dekleva et al, 2004) (Dekleva M, Neskovic A, Vlahovic A, et al. Adjunctive effect of hyperbaric oxygen treatment after thrombolysis on left ventricular function in patients with acute myocardial infarction. Am Heart J. 2004; 148:E14)

(Delaney, Montgomery, 2001) (Delaney, J. and Montgomery, D. How can hyperbaric oxygen contribute to treatment? The Physician and Sportsmedicine, Vol. 29, No. 3, March 2001)

(Demchenko et al, 2001) (Demchenko IT, Boso AE, Whorton AR, and Piantadosi CA. Nitric oxide production is enhanced in rat brain before oxygen-induced convulsions. Brain Res 917: 253-261, 2001)

(Demchenko et al, 2003) (Demchenko IT, Atochin DN, Boso AE, Astern J, Huang PL, and Piantadosi CA. Oxygen seizure latency and peroxynitrite formation in mice lacking neuronal or endothelial nitric oxide synthases. Neurosci Lett 344: 53-56, 2003)

(Demello, 1970) (Demello, F.J., Hashinmoto, T., Hitchcock, C.R. and Haglin, J.J. The effect of hyperbaric oxygen on the germination and toxin production of Clostridium perfringens spores: In Wada, J. and Iwa, J.T. (Eds): Proceedings of the Fourth International Congress of Hyperbaric Medicine. Baltimore: The Williams & Wilkins Col, 1970; p. 276)

(Dennog et al, 1996) (Dennog C, Hartmann A, Frey G, et al. Detection of DNA damage after hyperbaric oxygen (HBO) therapy. Mutagenesis. 1996; 11:605–609)

(Dennog et al, 1999) (Dennog C, Gedik C, Wood S, et al. Analysis of oxidative DNA damage and HPRT mutations in humans after hyperbaric oxygen treatment. Mutation Res. 1999;431:351–359)

(DeVolder et al, 1990) (DeVolder, A.G., Goffinet, A.M., Bol, A. et al. Brain glucose metabolism in post-anoxic syndrome. Arch Neurol 1990; 47: 197-204)

(Dimitrijevich et al, 1999) (Dimitrijevich S.D., Paranjape S., Wilson J.R., Gracy R.W., Mills J.G. (1999) Effect of hyperbaric oxygen on human skin cells in culture and in human dermal and skin equivalents. Wound Repair Regen 7: 53–64)

(Dinkel, Bochner, Pampuro, 1986) (Dinkel, R., Bochner, K. and Pampuro, M. Socio-economic importance of vein disorders. Health Econ. LTD, Health Service Consultants, Basle, Switzerland. Ninth World Congress of Phlebology, Kyoto, Japan, 22-26 September, 1986)

(Dische, Senanayake, 1972) (Dische S, Senanayake F. Radiotherapy using hyperbaric oxygen in the palliation of carcinoma of colon and rectum. Clin Radiol. 1972;23:512–518. doi: 10.1016/S0009-9260(72)80032-1)

(Dong et al, 1987) (Dong GC, Hu SX, Zhao GY, Gao SZ, Wu LR. Experimental study on cytotoxic effects of hyperbaric oxygen and photodynamic therapy on mouse transplanted tumor. Chin Med J (Engl) 1987;100:697–702)

(Dripps, Comroe, 1947) (Dripps and Comroe (Dripps RD and Comroe JH Jr. The effect of the inhalation of high and low oxygen concentration on respiration, pulse rate, ballistocardiogram and arterial oxygen saturation (oximeter) of normal individuals. J Physiol 149: 277-291, 1947)

(Droge, 2001) (Droge W. Free radicals in the physiological control of cell function. Physiol Rev 82: 47-95, 2001)

(Duenas, 1969) (Duenas, F.C. Die fruhdiagnose, therapie and forschung in der lerabekamfung. [The diagnosis, therapy and investigation of leprosy]. Das Offentliche Gesundheitswese 1969; 12: 667-671)

(Dulak, Jozkowicz, 2003) (Dulak J, Jozkowicz A. Regulation of vascular endothelial growth factor synthesis by nitric oxide: facts and controversies. Antioxid Redox Signal.2003;5:123–132)

(Duzgun et al, 2008) (Duzgun AP, Satir AZ, Ozozan O, et al. Effect of hyperbaric oxygen therapy on healing of diabetic foot ulcers. J. Foot & Ankle Surg. 2008;47:515–519)

(Eisenbud, 2012) (Eisenbud DE. Oxygen in wound healing: nutrient, antibiotic, signaling molecule, and therapeutic agent. Clin Plast Surg. 2012 Jul;39(3):293-310)

(Ellis, Mandal, 1971) (Ellis, M.E. and Mandal, B.K. Hyperbaric oxygen treatment: 10 years' experience of a regional infectious disease unit. J Infect Dis 1971; 6: 187-190)

(Eskes et al, 2010) (Eskes A, Ubbink DT, Lubbers M, Lucas C, Vermeulen H. Hyperbaric oxygen therapy for treating acute surgical and traumatic wounds. Cochrane Database Syst Rev. 2010 Oct 6;(10):CD008059)

(Evans et al, 1976) (Evans, B.E., Jacobson, H.H., Pierce, E.C., Friedman, E.W. and Schwartz, A.E. Chronic osteomyelitis of mandible. NY State J Med 1976; 76(6): 966-967)

(Eskes et al, 2011) (Eskes AM, Ubbink DT, Lubbers MJ, Lucas C, Vermeulen H. Hyperbaric oxygen therapy: solution for difficult to heal acute wounds? Systematic review. World J Surg. 2011 Mar;35(3):535-42)

(Feldmeier et al, 1994) (Feldmeier JJ, Heimbach RD, Davolt DA, Brakora MJ, Sheffield PJ, Porter AT. Does hyperbaric oxygen have a cancer-causing or -promoting effect? A review of the pertinent literature. Undersea Hyperb Med. 1994;21:467–475)

(Feldmeier et al, 2003) (Feldmeier J, Carl U, Hartmann K, Sminia P. Hyperbaric oxygen: does it promote growth or recurrence of malignancy? Undersea Hyperb Med. 2003;30:1–18)

(Fife, Freeman, 1997) (Fife, W.P. and Freeman, D.M. Preliminary Clinical Study on the Use of Hyperbaric Oxygen Therapy for the Treatment of Lyme Disease. College Station, Texas: Texas A&M University Hyperbaric Laboratory, 1997 (submitted for publication)

(Finkel, Holbrook, 2000) (Finkel, T., Holbrook, N.J., 2000. Oxidants, oxidative stress and the biology of ageing. Nature 408, 239–247)

(Fischer et al, 1988) (Fischer, B., Jain, K.K., Braun, E. and Lehrl, S. Handbook of Hyperbaric Oxygen Therapy. Berlin: Springer-Verlag, 1988)

(Fischer et al, 1988) (Fischer et al, (1988) Handbook of Oxygen Therapy, Springer Verlag: Berlin, pp. 251–260)

(Fischer, 1969) (Fisher, B.H. Hyperbaric oxygen for skin ulcers. Roche Med Image Commentary, 1969)

(Forman et al, 2003) (Signal Transduction by reactive Oxygen and Nitrogen Species: Pathways and Chemical Principles. Edited by H.J. Forman, J. Fukuto and M. Torres, Kluwer Academic Publishers, 2003)

(Forman, Azzi, 1997) (Forman, H. J., and A. Azzi. On the virtual existence of superoxide anion in mitochondria: thoughts regarding its role in pathophysiology. FASEB J. 11: 374-375, 1997)

(Forman, Thomas, 1986) (Forman, H.J. and Thomas, M.J. Oxidant production and bactericidal activity of phagocytes. Ann Rev Physiol 1986; 48: 669-680)

(Forster, Estabrook, 1993) (Foster RE, Estabrook RW. Is oxygen an essential nutrient? Annu. Rev. Nutr. 1993. 13-383-403)

(Fosen, Thom, 2014) (Fosen KM, Thom SR. Hyperbaric oxygen, vasculogenic stem cells, and wound healing. Antioxid Redox Signal. 2014 Oct 10;21(11):1634-47)

(Fredenucci, 1982) (Fredenucci, P. Arteriopathies et O.H.B. Medecine du Dud-Est 6300-6306, 1982)

(Fredenucci, 1983) (Fredenucci, P. Oygenotherapie hyperbare en patholgie vasculaire. 19 annees d'expeience. [Nineteen years of experience with hyperbaric oxygenation and vascular pathology]. IXth Congress of European Undersea Biomedical Society, Barcelona, September, 1983)

(Fredrich, 2003) (Fredrich MJ. Studying cancer in 3 dimensions. JAMA. 2003;290(15):1977-1979)

(Fridovich, 2004) (Fridovich I. Mitochondria: are they the seat of senescence? Aging Cell. 2004;3:13–16)

(Friedenreich, Orenstein, 2002) (Friedenreich CM, Orenstein MR. Physical activity and cancer prevention: etiologic evidence and biological mechanisms. J Nutr. 2002 Nov;132(11 Suppl):3456S-3464S)

(Friedman et al, 2006) (Friedman HIF, Fitzmaurice M, Lefaivre JF, et al. An evidence-based appraisal of the use of hyperbaric oxygen on flaps and grafts. Plast Reconstr Surg. 2006;117 Suppl:175S–190S)

(Fyles et al, 2002) (Fyles, A., Milosevic, M. and Hedley, D., et al. Tumor hypoxia has independent predictor impact only in patients with node-negative cervix cancer. J Clin Oncol 2002; 20: 680-687)

(Gallagher et al, 2007) (Gallagher KA, Liu ZJ, Xiao M, et al. Diabetic impairments in NO-mediated endothelial progenitor cell mobilization and homing are reversed by hyperoxia and SDF-1 alpha. J Clin Invest. 2007;117:1249–1259)

(Gerad et al, 1967) (Gerad, R., Fredenucci, P., Barthelemy, L., Bourde, J., Lamy, J., Jouve, A. and Appaix, A. L'oxygene hyperbare dans le traitement des arteriopathies. [Hyperbaric oxygen in the treatment of arteriopathologies]. Arch Mal Coeur 1967; 4: 472-483)

(Gerschman et al, 1954) (Gerschman R, Gilbert DL, Nye SW, Dwyer P, Fenn WO. Oxygen poisioning and X-irradiation: a mechanism in common. Science.1954;119:623–626)

(Gerweck, Richards, Jennings, 1981) (Gerweck, L.E., Richards, B. and Jennings, M. The influence of variable oxygen concentration on the response of cells to heat or X irradiation. Radiat Res. 1981; 85:314-320)

(Gesell, 2008) (Gesell Le. Hyperbaric oxygen therapy indications. 12th ed. Durham, NC: Undersea and Hyperbaric Medical Society; 2008)

(Giaccia, 1996) (Giaccia, A.J. Hypoxic stress proteins: Survival of the fittest. Semin Radiat Oncol 1996; 6: 45-58)

(Gill, Bell, 2004) (Gill AL, Bell CNA. Hyperbaric oxygen: its uses, mechanisms of action and outcomes.QJM. 2004;97:385–395)

(Giordano, 2005) (Giordano, F.J. Oxygen, oxidative stress, hypoxia and heart failure. J Clin Invest. 115:500-508 (2005)

(Giovannucci, 2001) (Giovannucci E. Insulin, insulin-like growth factors and colon cancer:a review of the evidence.J Nutr.2001;131:3109S–3120S)

(Glassburn, Brady, Plenk, 1977) (Glassburn, J.R., Brady, L.W. and Plenk, H.P. Hyperbaric oxygen in radiation therapy. Cancer 1977; 39: 751-765)

(Goldhaber, 1996) (Goldhaber, J.I. Free radicals enhance Na+/Ca2+ exchange in ventricular myocytes. Am J Physiol 1996; 271: H823-H833)

(Goldman, 2009) (Goldman RJ. Hyperbaric oxygen therapy for wound healing and limb salvage:a systematic review.PM R.2009 May;1(5):471-89)

(Goldstein et al, 2006) (Goldstein LJ, Gallagher KA, Bauer SM, et al. Endothelial progenitor cell release into circulation is triggered by hyperoxia-induced increases in bone marrow nitric oxide. Stem Cells. 2006;24:2309–2318)

(Goldstein, 2013) (Goldstein LJ. Hyperbaric oxygen for chronic wounds. Dermatol Ther. 2013 May-Jun;26(3):207-14)

(Godman et al, 2010) (Godman CA, Joshi R, Giardina C, Perdrizet G, Hightower LE. Hyperbaric oxygen treatment induces antioxidant gene expression. Ann N Y Acad Sci. 2010;1197:178–183)

(Gordeeva et al, 2003) (Gordeeva, A.V., Zvyagilskaya, R.A. and Labas, Y.A. Cross-talk between reactive oxygen species and calcium in living cells. Biochemistry (Moscow), Oct. 2003, vol. 68, no. 10, pp. 1077-1080)

(Gore et al, 2010) (Gore A, Muralidhar M, Espey MG, Degenhardt K, Mantell LL. Hyperoxia sensing: from molecular mechanisms to significance in disease. J Immunotoxicol. 2010;7:239–254)

(Gotlieb et al, 1964) (Gottlieb, S.F., Rose, N.R., Maurizi, J. and Lamphier, E.H. Oxygen inhibition of growth of Mycobacterium tuberculosis. J Bacteriol 1964; 87: 838-843)

(Gottlieb, Pakman, 1968) (Gottlieb, S.F. and Pakman, L.M. Effect of high oxygen tensions on the growth of selected, aerobic, gram-negative bacteria. J Bacteriol 1968; 95: 1003-1010)

(Gottlieb et al, 1974) (Gottlieb, Solsky, Aubrey, Nedelkoff, 1974) (Gottlieb, S.F., Solosky, J.A., Aubrey, R. and Nedelkoff, D.D. Synergistic action of increased oxygen tensions and PABA-folic acid antagonists on bacterial growth. Aerosp Med 1974; 45: 829-833)

(Gottlieb, 1989) (Gottlieb, S.F. Proposed criteria for evaluating disease entities for inclusion in accepted indications category for hyperbaric oxygen treatment. J Hyper Med 1989; 4: 33-37)

(Gottliev, Neubauer, 1988) (Gottlieb, S.R. and Neubauer, R.A. Multiple sclerosis: its etiology, pathogenesis, and therapeutics with emphasis on the controversial use of HBO. J Hyper Med 1988; 5: 143-164)

(Gottrup et al, 1984) (Gottrup F, Firmin R, Hunt TK, et al. The dynamic properties of tissue oxygen in healing flaps. Surgery 1984; 95(5): 527-536)

(Gray et al, 1953) (Gray LH, Conger AD, Ebert M, Hornsey S, Scott OC. The concentration of oxygen dissolved in tissues at the time of irradiation as a factor in radiotherapy. Br J Radiol. 1953;26:638–648)

(Green et al, 2002) (Green, D., Cheetham C, et al. Effect of lower limb exercise on forearm vascular function: contribution of nitric oxide. Am J Physiol 2002; 283: H899-H907)

(Greenlee et al, 2001) (Greenlee, R.T., Hill-Harmon, M.B., Murray, T. and Thun, M. Cancer statistics, 2001. CA - Cancer J Clin 2001; 51: 15-36)

(Greenwood, Gilchrist, 1973) (Greenwood, T.W. and Gilchrist, A.G. Hyperbaric oxygen and wound healing in post-irradiation head and neck surgery. Br J Surg 1973; 50: 394)

(Gregorevic et al.2000) (Gregorevic P., Lynch G.S., Williams D.A. (2000) Hyperbaric oxygen improves contractile function of regenerating rat skeletal muscle after myotoxic injury. J Appl Physiol 89: 1477–1482)

(Gregorevic, Lynch, Williams, 2001) (Gregorevic P, Lynch GS, Williams DA. Hyperbaric oxygen modulates antioxidant enzyme activity in rat skeletal muscles. Eur J Appl Physiol.2001;86:24–27)

(Grieb et al, 19985) (Grieb, P., Pape, P. C., Forster, R. E., Goodwin, C. W., Nioka, S. , Labbatte, L. 1985. Oxygen exchanges between blood and resting skeletal muscle: a shunt-sink hypothesis. Adv. Exp. Med. Bioi. 191:309-22)

(Gristina et al, 2015) (Gristina V, Cupri MG, Torchio M, Mezzogori C, Cacciabue L, Danova M. Diabetes and cancer: A critical appraisal of the pathogenetic and therapeutic links. Biomed Rep. 2015 Mar;3(2):131-136)

(Grossman, 1978) (Grossman, A.R. Hyperbaric oxygen in the treatment of burns. Ann Plast Surg 1978; 1 / 2: 163-171)

(Gu et al, 2008) (Gu GJ, Li YP, Peng ZY, et al. Mechanism of ischemic tolerance induced by hyperbaric oxygen preconditioning involves up-regulation of hypoxia-inducible factor-1 alpha and erythropoietin in rats. J Appl Physiol.2008;104:1185–1191)

(Guerra et al, 1996) (Guerra, L., Cerbai, E., Gessi, S., Borea, P.A. and Mugelli, A. The effect of oxygen free radicals on calcium current and dihydrophyridine binding sites in guinea pigs ventricular myocytes. Br J Pharmacol 1996; 118:1278-1284)

(Gupta, Dai, Hamblin, ) (Gupta A, Dai T, Hamblin MR. Effect of red and near-infrared wavelengths on low-level laser (light) therapy-induced healing in partial-thickness dermal abrasion in mice. Lasers in Medical Science. 2014 Jan;29(1):257-65)

Prof Randolph M. Howes MD,PhD

(Haapaniemi et al, 1995) (Haapaniemi T., Sirsjo A., Nylander G., Larsson J. (1995) Hyperbaric oxygen treatment attenuates glutathione depletion and improves metabolic restitution in post-ischemic skeletal muscle. Free Radic Res 23: 91–101)

(Haapaniemi et al, 1996) (Haapaniemi T, Nylander G, Sirsjo A. Hyperbaric oxygen reduces ischemia-induced skeletal muscle injury. Plast Reconstr Surg 1996;97:602-7)

(Hall, 1994) (Hall, E.J. editor. Radiobiology for the radiologist 4th ed. Philadelphia, PA Lippincott; 1994)

(Hall, 2000) (Hall, E.J. Radiobiology for the Radiologist. Philadelphia, PA Lippincott Williams & Wilkins, 2000)

(Hamblin, 1968) (Hamblin, D.L. Hyperbaric oxygen: its effect on experimental staphylococcal osteomyelitis in rats. J Bone Joint Surg 1968; 50: 1129-1141)

(Hamilton, 1990) (Hamilton, G. A. 1990. Mechanisms of biological oxidation reactions involving oxygen and reduced oxygen derivatives. See Ref. 26, pp. 3-19)

(Hammarlund, 1995) (Hammarlund C: The physiologic effects of hyperbaric oxygenation, in Whelan HT, Kindwall EP (Eds): Hyperbaric Medicine Practice, Ed 2. Flagstaff, Arizona, Best Pub Co, 1995, pp 37-68)

(Hampson et al, 2004) (Hampson NB, Bostwick DG, Vessella RL, Corman JM. Hyperbaric oxygen does not accelerate latent in vivo prostate cancer: implications for the treatment of radiation-induced haemorrhagic cystitis. BJU Int. 2004;94:1275–1278)

Hansford et al. 1997) (Hansford, R. G., B. A. Hogue, and V. Mildaziene. Dependence of $H_2O_2$ formation by rat heart mitochondria on substrate availability and donor age. J. Bioenerg. Biomembr. 29: 89-95, 1997)

(Harman, 1956) (Harman, D. Aging: a theory based on free radical and radiation chemistry. J. Gerontol. 2: 298-300, 1956)

(Harman, 1981) (Harman, D.. The aging process. Proc. Natl. Acad. Sci. USA 78: 7124-7128, 1981)

(Harman, 1987) (Harman, D. H.. Free radical theory of aging: effects of antioxidants on mitochondrial function. Age 10: 58-61, 1987)

(Haroon et al, 2007) (Haroon AT, Patel M, Al-Mehdi AB. Lung metastatic load limitation with hyperbaric oxygen. Undersea Hyperb Med. 2007;34:83–90)

(Harrelson, Hills, 1970) (Harrelson, J.M. and Hills, B.A. Changes in bone marrow pressure in response to hyperbaric exposure. Aerosp Med 1970; 41: 1018-1021)

(Harris, 2002) (Harris AL. Hypoxia—a key regulatory factor in tumor growth. Nat Rev Cancer.2002;2:38–47)

(Hart et al, 1974) (Hart, G.B., O'Reilly, R.R., Broussard, N.D., et al. Treatment of burns with hyperbaric oxygen. Surg Gynecol Obstet 1974; 139: 693-696)

(Hart, Lamb, Strauss, 1983) (Hart, G.B., Lamb, R.C. and Strauss, M.B. Gas gangrene I. A. collective review. II. A 15-year experience with hyperbaric oxygen. J Trauma 1983; 23: 991-1000)

(Hart, Strauss, 1986) (Hart, G.B. and Strauss, M.B. Hyperbaric oxygen in the management of radiation injury. In Schmutz, J. (ed): Proceedings of the First Swiss Symposium on Hyperbaric Medicine. Basel, Switzerland: Foundation for Hyperbaric Medicine, 1986; pp. 31-51)

(Hart, Strauss, 1987) (Hart GB, Strauss MB. Central nervous system oxygen toxicity in a clinical setting. In: Bove AA, Bachrack AJ, Greenbaum LJ, editors. Undersea and Hyperbaric Physiology IX. Bethesda: Undersea and Hyperbaric Med. Soc; 1987. pp. 695–699)

(Hattori et al, 2001) (Hattori K, Dias S, Heissig B, et al. Vascular endothelial growth factor and angiopoietin-1 stimulate postnatal hematopoiesis by recruitment of vasculogenic and hematopoietic stem cells. J. Exp. Med. 2001;193:1005–1014)

(Henderson, Fingar, 1987) (Henderson, B.W. and Fingar, V.H. Relationship of tumor hypoxia and response to photodynamic treatment in an experimental mouse tumor. Cancer Res 1987; 47: 3110-3114)

(Hensley et al, 2000) (Hensley, K., Robinson, K.A., Gabbita, S.P., Salsman, S. and Floyd, R.A. Reactive oxygen species cell signaling and cell injury. Free Rad Biol Med 2000; 28: 1445-1462)

(Herbig, 1981) (Herbig, G. H. 1981.The Origin and astronomical history of terrestrial oxygen. See Ref. 35, pp. 65-73)

(Heys et al, 2006) (Heys SD, Smith IC, Ross JA, Gilbert FJ, Brooks J, Semple S, Miller ID, Hutcheon A, Sarkar T, Eremin O. A pilot study with long term follow up of hyperbaric oxygen pretreatment in patients with locally advanced breast cancer undergoing neo-adjuvant chemotherapy. Undersea Hyperb Med. 2006;33:33–43)

(Hirata et al, 2007) (Hirata T, Cui Y, Funakoshi T, et al. The temporal profile of genomic responses and protein synthesis in ischemic tolerance of the rat brain induced by repeated hyperbaric oxygen. Brain Res. 2007;1130:214–222)

(Hjelde et al, 2005) (Hjelde A, Gederaas OA, Krokan HE, Brubakk AO. Lack of effect of hyperoxia on photodynamic therapy and lipid peroxidation in three different cancer cell lines. Med Sci Monit. 2005;11:BR351–BR356)

(Hockel et al, 1996) (Hockel, M., Schlenger, K.,Aral, B., Mitze, M., Schaffer, U. and Vaupel, P. Association between tumor hypoxia and malignant progression in advanced cancer of the uterine cervix. Cancer Res 1996; 56: 4509-4515)

(Hockel et al, 1999) (Hockel, M., Schlenger, K., Hockel, S. and Vaupel, P. Hypoxic cervical cancers with low apoptotic index are highly aggressive. Cancer Res 1999; 59: 4525-4528)

(Hockel, Vaupel, 2001) (Hockel, M. and Vaupel, P. Tumor hypoxia: Definitions and current clinical, biologic and molecular aspects. J Natl Cancer Instit 2001; 93(4): 266-276)

(Hohn et al, 1976) (Hohn D.C., MacKay, R.D., Halliday, B. and Hunt, T.K. The effect of $O_2$ tension on the microbicidal function of leukocytes in wounds and in vitro. Surg Forum 1976; 27: 18-20)

(Hohn, 1977) (Hohn, D.C. Oxygen and leukocyte microbial killing. Davis, J.C., Hunt, T.K. Eds. Hyperbaric Oxygen Therapy, Bethesda, Undersea Med Soc 1977; 101-110)

(Hohn, 1980) (Hohn, D.C. Host resistance of Infection: established and emerging concepts. In Hunt, T.K. (Ed): Wound Healing and wound Infection: Theory and Surgical Practice. New York: Appleton-Century-Crofts, 1980; pp. 264-280)

(Holbach, Wassmann, Kolberg, 1974) (Holbach, K.H., Wassmann, H. and Kolberg, T. Berbesserte reversibilatat des traumatischen mittelhirn-syndrome bei anwendung der hyperbaren oxygenierung. [Improved reversal of traumatic-brain syndrome by application of hyperbaric oxygen] Acta Neurochir 1974; 30-247-256)

(Holmquist et al, 2006) (Holmquist L, Lofstedt T, Pahlman S. Effect of hypoxia on the tumor phenotype: the neuroblastoma and breast cancer models. Adv Exp Med Biol. 2006;587:179–193)

(Hopewell, 1979) (Hopewell, J.W. Hyperbaric oxygenation after irradiation and its effect on the production of radiation myelitis. Int J Radiat Oncol Bio Phys 1979; 5: 1917)

(Hopf et al, 2005) (Hopf HW, Gibson JJ, Angeles AP, et al. Hyperoxia and angiogenesis. Wound Repair Regen. 2005;13:558–564)

(Hopf, Rollins, 2007) (Hopf HW, Rollins MD. Wounds: an overview of the role of oxygen. Antioxid Redox Signal. 2007;9:1183–1192)

(Horn et al. 1999) (Horn P.C., Webster D.A., Amin H.M., Mascia M.F., Werner F.W., Fortino M.D. (1999) The effect of hyperbaric oxygen on medial collateral ligament healing in a rat model. Clin Orthopaed Rel Res 360: 238–242)

(Houreld, 2014) (Houreld NN. Shedding light on a new treatment for diabetic wound healing: a review on phototherapy. ScientificWorld Journal. 2014 Jan 6;2014:398412)

(Howes, Steele, 1971) (Howes, R. M. and Steele, R. H., Microsomal chemiluminescence induced by NADPH and its relation to lipid peroxidation, Res. Commun. Chem. Path. Pharmacol., July-Sept. 1971, 2; 4 & 5:619-626)

(Howes, Steele, 1972) (Howes, R.M. and Steele, R.H., Microsomal chemiluminescence induced by NADPH and its relation to aryl-hydroxylations, Res Commun. Chem. Path. Pharmacol., March 1972, 3; 2:349-357)

(Howes, Steele, 1976) (Howes, R.M., Steele, R.H. and Hoopes, J.E., Peroxide induced Chemiluminescence in an in vitro proline hydroxylation system, 1976, 8; 1:77-84)

(Howes et al, 1976) (Howes, R. M., Allen, R.C., Su, C.T. and Hoopes, J.E., Altered polymorphonuclear leukocyte bioenergetics in patients with thermal injury, the Surgical Forum, 1976, 27:558-560)

(Howes et al, 1977) (Howes, R.M., Steele, R.H. and Hoopes, J.E., The role of Electronic excitation states in collagen biosynthesis, Persp. In Biol. And Med., Summer 1977, 20; 4:539-544)

(Howes, 2004, UTOPIA) (Howes, R. M. U.T.O.P.I.A. - Unified Theory of Oxygen Participation in Aerobiosis. © 2004. Free Radical Publishing Co. Kentwood, LA, available at www.iwillfindthecure.org)

(Howes, 2005, Med Sci) (Howes R. M. The Medical and Scientific Significance of Oxygen Free Radical Metabolism. © 2005. Free Radical Publishing Co. Kentwood, LA. USA. available at www.iwillfindthecure. org)

(Howes, 2005) (Howes, R.M. Tumoricidal Activity of An Injectable Singlet Oxygen System Generated From Physiological Agents: The Howes Singlet Oxygen Cancer Therapy System). In The Medical and Scientific Significance of Oxygen Free Radical Metabolism. © 2005. Free Radical Publishing Co. Kentwood, LA. pp. 893-912)

(Howes, Farber, 2005) (Howes, R.M. and Farber, G. Tumoricidal Activity of the Howes Singlet Oxygen Delivery System in Human Basal Cell Carcinoma. In The Medical and Scientific Significance of Oxygen Free Radical Metabolism. © 2005. Free Radical Publishing Co. Kentwood, LA. pp. 883-892)

(Howes, 2006, Diabetes) (Howes, R. M. Diabetes and Oxygen Free Radical Sophistry, © 2006;Free Radical Publishing Co. USA. Free Radical Publishing Co. USA. 366 pages) available at www.iwillfindthecure.org)

(Howes, 2006, H2O2) (Howes, R. M. Hydrogen Peroxide Monograph 1: Scientific, Medical and Biochemical Overview. © 2006; Free Radical Publishing Co. USA. 200 pages) available at www.iwillfindthecure.org.)

(Howes, 2006, CVD) (Howes, R. M. Cardiovascular Disease and Oxygen Free Radical Mythology, © 2006; Free Radical Publishing Co. USA. 308 pages) available at www.iwillfindthecure.org)

(Howes, 2006, AOX A,C,E) (Howes, R. M. Monograph 2: Antioxidant vitamins A, C & E: Equivocal Scientific Studies, © 2006; Free Radical Publishing Co. USA. 171 pages) available at www.iwillfindthecure.org)

(Howes, 2006, fantasy) (Howes, R.M.: "The Free Radical Fantasy," The Annals of New York Academy of Sciences, 2006, Vol. 1067, pp. 22-26)

(Howes, 2007, #75) (Howes M.D., PhD., R. (2007). The Consequent Downfall of the Free Radical Theory. PHILICA.COM Article number 75)

(Howes, 2008, ROSI) (Howes, R. M. Reactive Oxygen Species Insufficiency (ROSI)as the Basis for Disease Allowance and Coexistence:

Extraordinary Support for an Extraordinary Theory. Vol I, II & III. © 2008; 1564 pages) available at www.iwillfindthecure.org)

(Howes R: Hydrogen Peroxide: 2010) (Hydrogen Peroxide: A Health, Homeostatic and Protective Essentiality, CreateSpace and Free Radical Publishing, © 2014)

(Howes, 2011, Anti-aging) (Howes, R.M. Anti-Aging Anti-oxidant Scams, CreateSpace and Free Radical Publishing, © 2011)

(Howes RM, 2015, Naked mole rats) (Howes, RM. Cancer and Longevity: Naked Mole Rats, Exercise, and EMODs (ROS). CreateSpace and Free Radical Publishing, © 2015)

(Huang et al, 2004) (Huang, Y., et al. Cardia myocyte-specific HIF-1 alpha deletion alters vascularization, energy availability, calcium flux and contractility in the normoxic heart. FASEB j 2004; 18: 1138-1140)

(Hung et al, 2015) (Hung N, Shen CC, Hu YW, Hu LY, Yeh CM, Teng CJ, Kuan AS, Chen SC, Chen TJ, Liu CJ. Risk of cancer in patients with iron deficiency anemia: a nationwide population-based study. PLoS One. 2015 Mar 17;10(3):e0119647)

(Hunt, Pai, 1972) (Hunt, T.K. and Pai, M.P. The effect of varying ambient oxygen tensions on wound metabolism and collagen synthesis. Surg Gynecol Obstet 1972; 135: 561-567)

(Hunt, Zederfeldt, Goldstick, 1969) (Hunt, T.K., Zederfeldt, B. and Goldstick, T.K. Oxygen and healing. Am J Surg 1969; 118(4): 521-525)

(Hunt, Niinikoske, Zederfeldt, et al, 1977) (Hunt, T.K., Niinikoski, J., Zederfeldt, B.H. et al. Oxygen in wound healing enhancement: cellular effects of oxygen. In Davis, J.C. and Hunt, T.K. (Eds): Hyperbaric Oxygen Therapy. Bethesda, Maryland: Undersea Medial Society, 1977; pp. 111-122)

(Hunt, 1979) (Hunt, T.K. Disorders of repair and their management. In Hunt T.K. and Dunphy J.E. (Eds): Fundamentals of Wound Management. New York: Appleton-Century-Crofts, 1979; pp. 68-168)

(Hunt et al, 2007) (Hunt T, Aslam R, Beckert S, et al. Aerobically derived lactate stimulates revascularization and tissue repair via redox mechanisms. Antioxid Redox Signal. 2007;9:1115–1124)

(Hunt, Cononlly et al, 1979) (Hunt, T.K., Conolly, W.B., Aronson, S.B., et al. Anaerobic metabolism and wound healing: an hypothesis for the initiation and cessation of collagen synthesis in wounds. Am J Surg 1979; 135: 328-332)

(Hunt, van Winkle, 1976) (Hunt, T.K. and van Winkle, W. Wound healing: normal repair. In Dunphy, J.E. (ed): Fundamental of Wound Management in Surgery. South Plainfield, New Jersey: Chirurgecom, Inc., 1976; pp. 1-68)

(Hunt, Zederfeldt, Goldstick, 1969) (Hunt, T.K., Zederfeldt, T.B. and Goldstick, T.K. Oxygen and healing. Am J Surg 1969; 118: 521)

(Imlay, Fricovich, 1991) (Imlay, J. A., and I. Fridovich. Assay of metabolic superoxide production in Escherichia coli. J. Biol. Chem. 266: 6957-6965, 1991)

(Inanmaz et al, 2014) (Inanmaz ME, Kose KC, Isik C, Atmaca H, Basar H. Can hyperbaric oxygen be used to prevent deep infections in neuro-muscular scoliosis surgery? BMC Surg. 2014 Oct 27;14:85)

(Ishii et al, 2002) (Ishii Y., Ushida T., Tateishi T., Shimojo H., Miyanaga Y. (2002) Effects of different exposures of hyperbaric oxygen on ligament healing in rats. J Orthopaed Res 20: 353–356)

(Jafri et al, 2001) (Jafri, M.S., Dudycha, S.J. and O'Rourke, B. Cardiac energy metabolism: models of cellular respiration. Ann Res Biomed Eng 2001; 3: 57-81)

(Jain et al, 1990) (Jain, K.K., ed. Textbook of Hyperbaric Medicine. Toronto: Hogrefe & Huber, 1990)

(Jain, 1995) (Jain, K.K. Textbook of Hyperbaric Medicine. Toronto: Hogrefe & Huber, 1995; pp. 317-341)

(Jain, 1995, 446) (Jain, K.K. Textbook of Hyperbaric Medicine. Toronto: Hogrefe & Huber, 1995; pp. 446-463)

(Jain, 2004) (Jain K.K. (2004) Textbook of Hyperbaric Medicine. Military Medicine)

(Jevne et al, 2011) (Jevne CMI, Salvesen G, Reed RK, Stuhr LEB. A reduction in the interstitial fluid pressure per se, does not enhance the uptake of the small molecule weight compound 5-fluorouracil into 4T1 mammary tumours. Drug Ther Stud. 2011;1:10–14)

(Jirsa et al, 1991) (Jirsa M, Jr, Pouckova P, Dolezal J, Pospisil J, Jirsa M. Hyperbaric oxygen and photodynamic therapy in tumour-bearing nude mice. Eur J Cancer. 1991;27:109)

(Jon, 2000) (Jon B (2000) Basic mechanism of hyperbaric oxygen in the treatment of ischemia-reperfusion injury. Int Anesthesiol Clin 38:91–109)

(Jones, 1984) (Jones, H.P. The role of oxygen and its derivatives in bacterial killing and inflammation. In Gottlieb, S.F., Longmuir, I.S. and Totter, J.R. (eds): Oxygen: An In-Depth Study of its Pathophysiology. Bethesda, Maryland: Undersea Medical Society, 1984; pp. 493-516)

(Johnson, Lauchlan, 1966) (Johnson R, Lauchlan SC (1966) Epidermoid carcinoma of the cervix treated by 60Co therapy and hyperbaric oxygen. In: Proceedings Int Cong of Hyperb Med, pp. 648–652)

(Johnson et al, 1971) (Johnson RJ, Wiseman N, Lauchlan SC. The effect of hyperbaric oxygen on tumour metastases in mice. Clin Radiol. 1971;22:538–540)

(Johnson, Kagan, Bryant, 1967) (Johnson RE, Kagan AR, Bryant TL. Hyperbaric oxygen effect on experimental tumor growth. Radiology. 1967;88:775–777)

(Jonsson et al, 1991) (Jonsson K, Jensen JA, Goodson WH III, et al: Tissue oxygenation, anemia, and perfusion in relation to wound healing in surgical patients. Ann Surg 1991;214(5):605-613)

(Joung, Jeong, Ku, 2015) (Joung KH, Jeong JW, Ku BJ. The association between type 2 diabetes mellitus and women cancer: the epidemiological evidences and putative mechanisms. Biomed Res Int. 2015;2015:920618)

(Juttner et al, 2003) (Juttner B, Scheinichen D, Bartsch S, et al. Lack of toxic side effects in neutrophils following hyperbaric oxygen. Undersea and Hyperbaric Med.2003;30:305–311)

(Kaiser et al, 1985) (Kaiser, W., Berger, A., Leith, H. and Heymann, H. Hyperbaric oxygenation in burns. Handchir Mikrochir Plast Chir 1985; 17: 326-330)

(Kalns et al, 1998) (Kalns J, Krock L, Piepmeier E., Jr The effect of hyperbaric oxygen on growth and chemosensitivity of metastatic prostate cancer. Anticancer Res. 1998;18:363–367)

(Kalns, Piepmeier, 1999) (Kalns JE, Piepmeier EH. Exposure to hyperbaric oxygen induces cell cycle perturbation in prostate cancer cells. In Vitro Cell Dev Biol Anim. 1999;35:98–101)

(Kalns et al, 2002) (Kalns J, Lane J, Delgado A, et al. Hyperbaric oxygen exposure temporarily reduces Mac-1 mediated functions of human neutrophils. Immunol Lett. 2002;83:125–131)

(Kamen, 1963) (Kamen, M. P. 1963. Primary Processes in Photosynthesis. New York: Academic)

(Kang et al, 2004) (Kang TS, Gorti GK, Quan SY, et al. Effect of hyperbaric oxygen on the growth factor profile of fibroblasts. Arch Facial Plast Surg. 2004;6:31–35)

(Kato, 1987) (Kako, K. 1987. Free radical effects on membrane protein in myocardial ischemia/reperfusion injury. J. Mol. Cell. Cardiol. 19:209-11)

(Kawasoe et al, 2009) (Kawasoe Y, Yokouchi M, Ueno Y, Iwaya H, Yoshida H, Komiya S. Hyperbaric oxygen as a chemotherapy adjuvant in the treatment of osteosarcoma. Oncol Rep.2009;22:1045–1050)

(Keck, Gottlief, Conley, 1980) (Keck, P.E., Gottlief, S.F. and Conley, J. Interaction of increased pressure of oxygen and sulfonamides on the in vitro and in vivo growth of pathogenic bacteria. Undersea Biomed Res 1980; 7: 95-106)

(Kemp, Go, Jones, 2008) (Kemp M, Go YM, Jones DP. Nonequilibrium thermodynamics of thiol/disulfide redox systems: a perspective on redox systems in biology. Fr. Radic. Biol. Med. 2008;44:921–937)

(Kessler et al, 2003) (Kessler L, Bilbault P, Ortega F et al. (2003) Hyperbaric oxygenation accelerates the healing rate of nonischemic chronic diabetic foot ulcers: a prospective randomized study. Diabetes Care 26:2378–2382)

(Ketchum et al, 1967) (Ketchum, S.A., Zubrin, J.R., Thomas, A.N., et al. Effect of HBO on small first, second and third degree burns. Surg Forum 1967; 18: 65-67)

(Ketchum, Thomas, Hall, 1969) (Ketchum, S.A., III, Thomas, A.N. and Hall, A.D. Angiographic studies of the effects of hyperbaric oxygen on burn wound revascularization. In Wada, J. and Iwa, T. (Eds): Proceedings of the Fourth International Congress on Hyperbaric Medicine. Baltimore: Williams and Wilkins, 1969; pp. 388-394)

(Kim et al, 2001) (Kim C, Choi H, Chun Y, et al. Hyperbaric oxygenation pretreatment induces catalase and reduces infarct size in ischemic rat myocardium. Pflugers Arch. 2001;442:519–525)

(Kindwall, 1979) (Kindwall, E.P. Hyperbaric Medicine Procedures. Milwaukee, Wisconsin: St. Luke's Hospital, 1979; p. 17)

(Kindwall, Goldmann, 1984) (Kindwall, EP. And Goldmann, R.W. Hyperbaric Medicine Procedures. Milwaukee, Wisconsin: St. Luke's Hospital, 1984; p. 85)

(Kinoshita et al, 1999) (Kinoshita Y, Kohshi K, Kunugita N, Tosaki T, Yokota A. Preservation of tumor oxygen after hyperbaric oxygenation monitored by magnetic resonance imaging. Br J Cancer. 2000;82:88–92)

(Kivisaari, Niinikoski, 1975) (Kivisaari, J. and Niinikoski, J. Effects of hyperbaric oxygenation and prolonged hypoxia on the healing of open wounds. Acta Chirurg Scand 1975; 141: 14-19)

(Kivisaari, Niinikoski, 1973) (Kivisaari, J. and Niinikoski, J. Use of silastic tube and capillary sampling technique in the measurement of tissue $PO^2$ and $PCO^2$. Am J Surg 1973; 125: 623-627)

(Kluft, 1965) (Kluft O. Hyperbaric oxygen in experimental cancer in mice. Amsterdam: Universiteit van Amsterdam; 1965)

(Knighton et al, 1984) (Knighton, D.R., Halliday, B. and Hunt, T.K. Oxygen as an antibiotic: the effect of inspired oxygen on infection. Arch Surg 1984; 119: 199-204)

(Knighton, Silver, Hunt, 1981) (Knighton, D.R., Silver, I.A. and Hunt, T.K. Regulation of wound healing angiogenesis effect of oxygen gradients and inspired oxygen concentration. Surgery 1981; 90: 262-270)

(Koppenol, 1988) (Koppenol, W. H. 1988. The paradox of oxygen: thermodynamics versus toxicity. In Oxidases and Related Redox Systems, Progress in Clinical and Biological Research, ed. T. E. King, H. S. Mason. M. Morrison. pp. 93-109. New York: Liss)

(Koppenol et al, 1992) (Koppenol WH, Moreno JJ, Pryor WA, et al. Peroxynitrite, a cloaked oxidant formed by nitric oxide and superoxide. Chem.Res.Toxicol.1992;5:834–842)

(Kohshi et al, 1999) (Kohshi K, Kinoshita Y, Imada H, Kunugita N, Abe H, Terashima H, Tokui N, Uemura S. Effects of radiotherapy after hyperbaric oxygenation on malignant gliomas. Br J Cancer. 1999;80:236–241)

(Kohshi et al, 2007) (Kohshi K, Yamamoto H, Nakahara A, Katoh T, Takagi M. Fractionated stereotactic radiotherapy using gamma unit after hyperbaric oxygenation on recurrent high-grade gliomas. J Neurooncol. 2007;82:297–303. doi: 10.1007/s11060-006-9283-1)

(Kranke et al, 2004) (Kranke P, Bennett M, Roeckl-Wiedmann I, et al. Hyperbaric oxygen therapy for chronic wounds. Cochrane Database Syst Rev. 2004 CD004123)

(Kudchodkaar et al, 2000) (Kudchodkar, B.J., Wilson, J., Lacko, A. and Dory, L. Hyperbaric oxygen reduces the progression and accelerates the regression of atherosclerosis in rabbits. Arterioscler Thromb Vasc Biol 2000; 20(6): 1637-1643)

(Kulagin et al, 1981) (Kulagin, L.M., Varguzina, V.I., Kirsanove, L.N., et al. Regenerative potentials of tissue under HBO conditions depending on the character of the injury. In Yefun, S.N. (ed): Abstracts of Seventh International Congress of HBO Medicine, Moscow, USSR Academy of Sciences, 1981; pp. 326-327)

(Kunnavatana et al, 2005) (Kunnavatana S.S., Quan S.Y., Koch R.J. (2005) Combined effect of hyberbaric oxygen and N-acetylcysteine on fibroblast proliferation. Arch Otolaryngol Head Neck Surg 131: 809–814)

(Kwon et al, 2003) (Kwon, S.H., Pimentel, D.R., Remondino, A., Sawyer, D.B. and Colucci, W.S. $H_2O_2$ regulates cardiac myocyte phenotype via concentration-dependent activation of distinct kinase pathways. J Mol Cell Cardiol 2003; 35: 615-621)

(Labouche et al, 1999) (Labrouche S, Javorschi S, Leroy D, et al. Influence of hyperbaric oxygen on leukocyte functions and haemostasis in normal volunteer divers. Thromb Res. 1999;96:309–315)

(Lahat et al, 1995) (Lahat N, Bitterman H, Yaniv N, Kinarty A, Bitterman N. Exposure to hyperbaric oxygen induces tumor necrosis factor-alpha (TNF-alpha) secretion from rat macrophages. Clin Exp Immunol. 1995;102:655–659)

(Lavoisier, 1777) (Lavoisier, A.-L. 1777. Experiences sur la respiration des animaux et sur les changements qui arrivent a l' air en passant par leur poumon. Mem. Acad. Sci., p. 185. Republished 1862 in Oeuvres de Lavoisier, Memoires de Chimie et de Physique. 2: 174-83. Paris: Imp. Imperiale)

(Le et al, 2003) (Le, Q.T., Sutphin, P.D., Raychaudhuri, S., Ching, S., Yu, T., Terris, D.J., Lin, H.S., Lum, B., Pinto, H.A., Koong, A.C. and Giaccia, A.J.

Identification of osteopontin as a prognostic plasma marker for head and neck squamous cell carcinomas. Clinc Cancer Res 2003; 9: 59-67)

(Lee, Koo, Min, 2004) (Lee, J., Koo, N. and Min, D.B. Reactive oxygen species, aging and antioxidative neutraceuticals. Comprehensive Reviews in Food Science and Food Safety. 2004, Vol. 3, pp. 21-33)

(Lesko, Epstein, Mitchell. 1990) (Lesko SM, Epstein MF, Mitchell AA Recent patterns of drug use in newborn intensive care. J Pediatr 1990; 116:985-990)

(Li et al, 2005) (Li Y, Zhou C, Calvert J, et al. Multiple effects of hyperbaric oxygen on the expression of HIF-1a and apoptotic genes in a global ischemia-hypotension rat model. Exp Neurol. 2005;191:198–210)

(Lin et al, 2002) (Lin S, Shyu KG, Lee CC, et al. Hyperbaric oxygen selectively induces angiopoietin-2 in human umbilical vein endothelial cells. Biochem Biophys Res Commun. 2002;296:710–715)

(Liu and Velazquez, 2008) (Liu ZJ, Velazquez OC (2008) Hyperoxia, endothelial progenitor cell mobilization, and diabetic wound healing. Antioxid Redox Signal 10:1869–1882)

(Londahl et al, 2010) (Londahl M, Katzman P, Nilsson A, et al. Hyperbaric oxygen therapy facilitates healing of chronic foot ulcers in patients with diabetes. Diab Care.2010;33:998–1003)

(Loschen et al, 1973) (Loschen, G., Assim, A. and Richter, C. Superoxide radicals as precursors of mitochondrial hydrogen peroxide. FEBS Lett 1973; 33: 84-88)

(Luk, Baker, Fellows, 1978) (Luk, K.H., Baker, D.G. and Fellows, C.F. Hyperbaric oxygen after radiation and its effect on the production of radiation myelitis. Int J Radiat Oncol bi Phys 1978; 4: 457-3459)

(Lyne, 1978) (Lyne AJ. Ocular effects of hyperbaric oxygen. Trans. Ophthalmol. Soc. U.K. 1978;98:66–68)

(Madamanchi et al, 2005) (Madamanchi, N.R., Vendrov, A. and Runge, M.S. Oxidative stress and vascular disease. Arterio Throm Vas Biol 2005; 25: 29)

(Mader et al, 1980) (Mader J.T., Brown G.L., Guckian J.C., Wells C.H., Reinarz J.A. (1980) A mechanism for the amelioration by hyperbaric oxygen of experimental staphylococcal osteomyelitis in rabbits. J Infectious Dis 142: 915–922)

(Maier et al, 2000) (Maier A, Anegg U, Fell B, Rehak P, Ratzenhofer B, Tomaselli F, Sankin O, Pinter H, Smolle-Juttner FM, Friehs GB. Hyperbaric oxygen and photodynamic therapy in the treatment of advanced carcinoma of the cardia and the esophagus. Lasers Surg Med.2000;26:308–315)

(Maier et al, 2000, EJCS) (Maier A, Tomaselli F, Anegg U, Rehak P, Fell B, Luznik S, Pinter H, Smolle-Juttner FM. Combined photodynamic therapy and hyperbaric oxygenation in carcinoma of the esophagus and the esophago-gastric junction. Eur J Cardiothorac Surg. 2000;18:649–654)

(Mainous, 1977) (Mainous, E.G. Hyperbaric oxygen in maxillofacial osteomyelitis, osteoradionecrosis and osteogenesis enhancement. In Davis, J.C. and Hunt, T.K. (Eds): Hyperbaric Oxygen Therapy. Bethesda, Maryland: Undersea Medical Society, 1977; pp. 191-203)

(Mainous, 1982) (Mainous, E.G. Osteogenesis enhancement utilizing hyperbaric oxygen therapy. HBO Review 1982; 3: 181-185)

(Mainous, Boyne, Hart, 1973) (Mainous, E.G., Boyne, P.J. and Hart, G.B. Hyperbaric oxygen treatment of mandibular osteomyelitis: Report of three cases. J Am Dent Assoc 1973; 87: 1426-1430)

(Manheim et al, 1969) (Manheim, S.D., Voleti, C., Ludwig, A. and Jacobson, J.H. Hyperbaric oxygen in the treatment of actinomycosis. JAMA 1969; 210(3): 552-553)

(Marino, 1991) (Marino PL: Oxygen transport, in Marino PL (ed): The ICU Book, ed 1. Philadelphia, Lea & Febiger, 1991, pp 14-24)

(Martin, Thom, 2002) (Martin JD, Thom SR. Vascular leukocyte sequestration in decompression sickness and prophylactic hyperbaric oxygen therapy in rats. Aviat Space Environ Med. 2002;73:565–569)

(Marx et al, 1990) (Marx RE, Ehler WJ, Tayapongsak P, et al. Relationship of oxygen dose to angiogenesis induction in irradiated tissue. Am.J.Surg. 1990;160:519–524)

(Marx, Johnson, 1988) (Marx, R.E. and Johnson, R.P. Problem wounds in oral and maxillofacial surgery: the role of hyperbaric oxygen. In Davis, J.C. and Hunt, T.K. (Eds): Problem Wounds: The Role of Oxygen. New York: Elsevier, 1988; pp. 65-123)

(Marx, Johnson, Kline, 1985) (Marx, R.E., Johnson, R.P. and Kline, S.N. Prevention of osteoradionecrosis: a randomized prospective clinical trail of hyperbaric oxygen versus penicillin. J Am Dent Assn 1985; 111: 49-54)

(Mathieu, 2006) (Mathieu De. Handbook on Hyperbaric Medicine. Netherlands: Springer, Dordrecht; 2006)

(Mayer et al. 2004) (Mayer R., Hamilton-Farrell M.R., Kleij A.J.v.d., Schmutz J., Granström G., Sicko Z., et al. (2004) Hyperbaric oxygen and radiotherapy. Strahlenther Onkol 181: 113–123)

(Mayer et al, 2005) (Mayer R, Hamilton-Farrell MR, Kleij AJ, Schmutz J, Granstrom G, Sicko Z, Melamed Y, Carl UM, Hartmann KA, Jansen EC, Ditri L, Sminia P. Hyperbaric oxygen and radiotherapy. Strahlenther Onkol. 2005;181:113–123)

(Mazariegos et al, 1999) (Mazariegos G, O'Toole K, Mieles L, et al. Hyperbaric oxygen therapy for hepatic artery thrombosis after liver transplantation in children. Liver Transpl Surg. 1999;5:429–436)

(Mazzeo, Tanaka, 2001) (Mazzeo, R.S. and Tanaka, H. Exercise prescription for the elderly: current recommendations. Sports Med 2001; 31: 809-818)

(McBride et al, 1991) (McBride, T., Preston, B. and Loeb, L. Mutagenic spectrum resulting from DNA damage by oxygen radicals. Biochemistry 30: 207-212, 1991)

(McCredie et al, 1966) (McCredie JA, Inch WR, Kruuv J, Watson TA. Effects of hyperbaric oxygen on growth and metastases of the C3HBA tumor in the mouse. Cancer. 1966;19:1537–1542)

(McDonald, 1985) (McDonald, W.I. The mystery of the origin of multiple sclerosis. J Neurol Neurosurg Psychiatry 1985; 49: 113-123)

(Mekjavic et al. 2000) (Mekjavic I.B., Exner J.A., Tesch P.A., Eiken O. (2000) Hyperbaric oxygen therapy does not affect recovery from delayed on-set muscle soreness. Med Sci Sports Exercise 32: 558–563)

(Michiele, 2009) (Michieli P. Hypoxia, angiogenesis and cancer therapy: to breathe or not to breathe?Cell Cycle. 2009;8:3291–3296)

(Milovanova et al, 2008) (Milovanova T, Bhopale VM, Sorokina EM, et al. Lactate stimulates vasculogenic stem cells via the thioredoxin system and engages an autocrine activation loop involving hypoxia inducible factor-1. Mol Biol Cell.2008;28:6248–6261)

(Minhas, 2010) (Minhas R. (2010) Best Practice, BMJ Evidence Center. Available at:http://group.bmj.com/products/evidence-centre/best-practice)

Prof Randolph M. Howes MD,PhD

(Mitchell, 1977) (Mitchell P. Vectorial chemiosmotic processes. Annu Rev Biochem.1977;46:996–1005)

(Moen et al, 2009) (Moen I, Oyan AM, Kalland KH, Tronstad KJ, Akslen LA, Chekenya M, Sakariassen PO, Reed RK, Stuhr LE. Hyperoxic treatment induces mesenchymal-to-epithelial transition in a rat adenocarcinoma model. PLoS One. 2009;4:e6381)

(Moen et al, 2009, BMC) (Moen I, Tronstad KJ, Kolmannskog O, Salvesen GS, Reed RK, Stuhr LE. Hyperoxia increases the uptake of 5-fluorouracil in mammary tumors independently of changes in interstitial fluid pressure and tumor stroma. BMC Cancer. 2009;9:446)

(Moen et al, 2012) (Moen I, Jevne C, Wang J, Kalland KH, Chekenya M, Akslen LA, Sleire L, Enger PO, Reed RK, Oyan AM, Stuhr LE. Gene expression in tumor cells and stroma in dsRed 4T1 tumors in eGFP-expressing mice with and without enhanced oxygenation. BMC Cancer.2012;12:21)

(Moen, Stuhr, 2012) (Moen, I and Stuhr, LE. Hyperbaric oxygen therapy and cancer—a review. Target Oncol. 2012 Dec; 7(4): 233–242. Published online 2012 Oct 2) doi: 10.1007/s11523-012-0233-x. http://www.ncbi.nlm.nih.gov/pmc/articles/PMC3510426/)

(Moore et al, 1966) (Moore, G.F., Fuson, R.L., Margolis, G. et al. An evaluation of the protective effect of hyperbaric oxygenation on the central nervous system during circulatory arrest. J Thorac Cardiovasc Surg 1966; 52: 618)

(Morgami et al, 1969) (Mogami, H., Hayakawa, T., Kanal, N. et al. Clinical application of hyperbaric oxygenation in the treatment of acute cerebral damage. J Neurosurg 1969; 31: 636-643)

(Morrey et al, 1979) (Morrey, B.F., Dunn, J.M., Heimbach, R.D. and Davis, J. Hyperbaric oxygen and chronic osteomyelitis. Clin Orthop 1979; 144: 121-127)

(Mortensen, 2008) (Mortensen C. (2008) Hyperbaric oxygen therapy. Curr Anaesth Crit Care 19: 333–337)

(Mulkey et al, 2003) (Mulkey DK, Henderson RA III, Putnam RW, and Dean JB. Hyperbaric oxygen and chemical oxidants stimulate $CO_2/H^+$-sensitive neurons in rat brain stem slices. J Appl Physiol 95: 910-921, 2003)

(Muti et al, 2002) ( Muti P, Quattrin T, Grant BJ, Krogh V, Micheli A, Schünemann HJ, Ram M, Freudenheim JL, Sieri S, Trevisan M, et al. Fasting glucose is a risk factor for breast cancer: a prospective study. Cancer Epidemiol Biomarkers Prev. 2002;11:1361–1368)

(Narkowicz, Vial, McCartney, 1993) (Narkowicz CK, Vial JH, McCartney PW. Hyperbaric oxygen therapy increases free radical levels in the blood of humans. Free Radic Res Commun. 1993;19(2):71-80)

(Nelson et al, 1990) (Nelson EW, et al. Closure of refractory perineal Crohn's lesion; integration of hyperbaric oxygenation into case management. Digestive Diseases and Sciences 1990;35:1561-1565)

(Neubauer, Kagan, Gottliev, 1989) (Neubauer, R.A., Kagan, R.L. and Gottlieb, S.F. Use of hyperbaric oxygen for the treatment of aseptic bone necrosis. J Hyper Med 1989; 4: 69-76)

(Neubauer, End, 1980) (Neubauer, R.A. and End, E. Hyperbaric oxygenation as an adjunct therapy in strokes due to thrombosis. Stroke 1980; 11: 297-300)

(Neubauer, Walker, 1998) (Hyperbaric Oxygen therapy. Richard A. Neubauer, M.D. and Morton Walker, DPM. Avery [a member of Putnam Inc.] 1998)

(Neuman, Thom, 2008) (Neuman TS, Thom SRe. Physiology and Medicine of Hyperbaric Oxygen Therapy. Philadelphia, PA: Saunders-Elsevier; 2008)

(Nichols, Lambertsen, 1969) (Nichols, C.W. and Lambertsen, C.J. Effects of high oxygen pressures on the eye. N Engl J Med 1969; 291: 25-30)

(Nie et al, 2006) (Nie H, Xiong L, Lao N, et al. Hyperbaric oxygen preconditioning induces tolerance against spinal cord ischemia by upregulation of antioxidant enzymes in rabbits. J Cereb Blood Flow Metab. 2006;26:666–674)

(Niinikoski, 1969) (Niinikoski, J. Effect of oxygen supply on wound healing and formation of experimental granulation tissue. Acta Physiol Scand 1969; 334: 1-72)

(Niinikoske, Hunt, 1972) (Niinikoski, J. and Hunt, T.K. Oxygen tensions in healing bone. Surg Gynecol Obstet 1972; 134: 746-750)

(Niinikoski, Hunt, Zederfeldt, 1972) (Niinikoski, J., Hunt, T.K. and Zederfeldt, B. Oxygen supply in healing tissue. Am J Surg 1972; 123: 247-253)

(Nohl et al, 1996) (Nohl, H., L. Gille, K. Schonheit, and Y. Liu. Conditions allowing redox-cycling ubisemiquinone in mitochondria to establish a direct redox couple with molecular oxygen. Free Radical Biol. Med. 20: 207-213, 1996)

(Norden, Kleti, 1980) (Norden, C.W. and Kleti, E. Experimental osteomyelitis caused by Pseudomonas aeruginosa. J Infect Dis 1980; 141: 71-75)

(Nordsmark, Overgaard, 2000)(Nordsmark, M. and Overgaard, J. A confirmatory prognostic study on oxygenation status and loco-regional control in advanced head and neck squamous cell carcinoma treated by radiation therapy. Radiother Oncol 2000; 57: 39-43)

(Nulander et al, 1985) (Nylander, G., Lewis, D., Nordstrom, H. and Larsson, J. Reduction of postischemic edema with hyperbaric oxygen. Plast Reconstr Surg 1985; 76: 596-601)

(Nylander et al, 1985) (Nylander, G., Lewis, D., Nordstrom, H. and Larson, J. Reduction of postischemic edema with hyperbaric oxygen. Plast Reconstr Surg 1985; 76: 595-603)

(Nylander, et al, 1986) (Nylander, G., Lewis, D., Nordstrom, H. and Larson, J. Reduction of post-ischemic edema with hyperbaric oxygen. Plast Reconstr Surg 1985: 76: 595-603)

(Ogawa et al, 2006) (Ogawa K, Yoshii Y, Inoue O, Toita T, Saito A, Kakinohana Y, Adachi G, Iraha S, Tamaki W, Sugimoto K, Hyodo A, Murayama S. Phase II trial of radiotherapy after hyperbaric oxygenation with chemotherapy for high-grade gliomas. Brit J of Cancer.2006;95:862–868)

(Olejniczak, 1969) (Olejniczak, S. Employment of low hyperbaric therapy in management of leg ulcers. Mich Med, 1969)

(Oriani et al. 1982) (Oriani G., Barnini C., Marroni G. (1982) Hyperbaric oxygen therapy in the treatment of various orthopedic disorders. Minerva Medica 73: 2983–2988)

(Overgaard, 2011) (Overgaard J. Hypoxic modification of radiotherapy in squamous cell carcinoma of the head and neck—a systematic review and meta-analysis. Radiother Oncol. 2011;100:22–32)

(Ozorio, Costa, 1938) (Ozorio de Almeida, A. and Costa, H.M. Treatment of leprosy by oxygen at high pressure associated with methylene blue. Revist de Leprologia 1938; 6: 237-265)

(Palmquist, Philipson, Barr, 1984) (Palmquist BM, Philipson BO, Barr PO. Nuclear cataract and myopia during hyperbaric oxygen therapy. Br. J. Ophthalmol. 1984;68:113–117)

(Parbhakar, 2000) (Prabhakar NR. Oxygen sensing by the carotid body chemoreceptors. J Appl Physiol 88: 2287-2295, 2000)

(Pasteur, 1861) (Pasteur, L. 1861. Animalicules infusoires vivant sans gaz oxygene libre. et determinant des fermentations. C. R. Acad. Sci. 52:344-47)

(Peidaee et al, 2013) (Peidaee P, Almansour N, Shukla R, Pirogova E. The Cytotoxic Effects of Low Intensity Visible and Infrared Light on Human Breast Cancer (MCF7) cells. Comput Struct Biotechnol J. 2013 Oct 20;6:e201303015)

(Peidaee, Almansour, Pirogova, 2015) (Peidaee P, Almansour NM, Pirogova E. In vitro evaluation of low-intensity light radiation on murine melanoma (B16F10) cells. Med Biol Eng Comput. 2015 May 23)

(Peirce, 1969) (Peirce, E.C. Pathophysiology, apparatus and methods including the special techniques of hypothermia and hyperbaric oxygen. In Peirce, E.C. (Ed): Extra-corporeal Circulation for Open-Heart Surgery. Springfield, Illinois: Charles C. Thomas, 1969; pp. 83-84)

(Peng et al, 2010) (Peng ZR, Zhong WH, Liu J, Xiao PT. Effects of the combination of hyperbaric oxygen and 5-fluorouracil on proliferation and metastasis of human nasopharyngeal carcinoma CNE-2Z cells. Undersea Hyperb Med. 2010;37:141–150)

(Perrins, 1966) (Perrins, J.D. Hyperbaric oxygenation of ischemic skin flaps and pedicles. In Brown, I.W. and Cox, B.G. (Eds): Proceedings of the Third International Congress on HBO Medicine. Durham, North Carolina: Duke University Press, 1966; pp. 613-620)

(Perrins, 1967) (Perrins, J.D. Influence of hyperbaric oxygen on the survival of split skin grafts. Lancet 1967; 1: 868-871)

(Perrins, 1970) (Perrins, J.D. Influence of hyperbaric oxygen on the survival of split skin grafts. In Wada, J. and Iwa, T. (Eds): Proceedings of the Fourth International Congress on HBO Medicine. London: Baillere, 1970; pp. 369-376)

(Perrins, Cantab, 1967) (Perrins DJD, Cantab MB. Influence of hyper-baric oxygen on the survival of split skin grafts. Lancet. 1967;II:868–871)

(Pinheiro et al, 2002) (Pinheiro AL, Carneiro NS, Vieira AL, Brugnera A Jr, Zanin FA, Barros RA, Silva PS. Effects of low-level laser therapy on ma-lignant cells: in vitro study. J Clin Laser Med Surg. 2002 Feb;20(1):23-6)

(Plafki et al, 2000) (Plafki C, Peters P, Almeling M, et al. Complications and side effects of hyperbaric oxygen therapy. Aviat. Space Environ. Med. 2000;71:119–124)

(Powell et al, 2005) (Powell TM, Paul JD, Hill JM, et al. Granulocyte colony-stimulating factor mobilizes functional endothelial progenitor cells in patients with coronary artery disease. Arter. Thromb. Vasc. Biol. 2005;25:296–301)

(Priestley, 1775) (Priestley, J. 1775. An account of further discoveries in air. Philos. Trans. 65: 384-94)

(Raa et al, 2007) (Raa A, Stansberg C, Steen VM, Bjerkvig R, Reed RK, Stuhr LE. Hyperoxia retards growth and induces apoptosis and loss of glands and blood vessels in DMBA-induced rat mammary tumors. BMC Cancer. 2007;7:23)

(Radi et al, 2002b) (Radi R, Cassina A, Hodara R, Quijano C, Castro L. Peroxynitrite reactions and formation in mitochondria. Free Radic Biol Med. 2002b;33:1451–1464)

(Reillo, 1997, 51) (Reillo, M. AIDS Under Pressure. Kirkland, Washington: Hogrefe & Huber, 1997; pp. 51-53)

(Reillo, 1997) (Reillo, M. AIDS Under Pressure. Kirkland, Washington: Hogrefe & Huber, 1997; pp. 39-45)

(Reillo, Altieri, 1996) (Reillo MR, Altieri RJ. HIV antiviral effects of hyper-baric oxygen therapy. J Assoc Nurses AIDS Care. 1996 Jan-Feb;7(1):43-5)

(Reiten et al, 1990) (Reiten, J.A., Kien, N.D., Thorup, S. et al. Hyperbric oxygen increases survival following carotid ligation in gerbils. Stroke 1990; 21: 119-123)

(Risers, Tyssebotn, 1986) (Risers, J. and Tyssebotn, I. Hyperbaric expo-sure to a 5 ATA He-$N_2$-$O_2$ atmosphere affects the cardiac function and organ blood flow distribution in awake trained rats. Undersea Biomed Res. 1986; 13: 77-90)

(Rockswold, Ford, 1985) (Rockswold, G.L. and Ford, S.E. Preliminary results of a prospective randomized trail for treatment of severely brain-injured patients with hyperbaric oxygen. Minn Med 1985; 68: 533-535)

(Roje et al, 2008) (Roje Z, Roje Z, Eterovic D, et al. Influence of adjuvant hyperbaric oxygen therapy on short-term complications during surgical reconstruction of upper and lower extremity war injuries: retrospective cohort study. Croat Med J.2008;49:224–232)

(Rosenthal, 1970) (Rosenthal, A.M. Treatment of patients with pressure sores in the hyperbaric chamber. Proceedings of the American Congress of Rehabilitation in Medicine. New York, 1970)

(Ross, McAllister, 1965) (Ross RM, McAllister TA. Protective action of hyperbaric oxygen in mice with pneumococcal sipticaemia. Lancet. 1965:579–581)

(Rothfuss, Radermacher, Speit, 2001) (Rothfuss A, Radermacher P, Speit G. Involvement of heme oxygenase-1 (HO-1) in the adaptive protection of human lymphocytes after hyperbaric oxygen (HBO) treatment. Carcinogenesis. 2001;22:1979–1985)

(Sayday et al, 2003) (Saydah SH, Platz EA, Rifai N, Pollak MN, Brancati FL, Helzlsouer KJ. Association of markers of insulin and glucose control with subsequent colorectal cancer risk. Cancer Epidemiol Biomarkers Prev. 2003;12:412–418)

(Scheele, 1777) (Scheele, C. W. 1777. Chemische abhandlung von der luft und dem feuer. Uppsala and Liepzig. Section 2. Chemical treatise on air and fire. In The Collected Papers of Carl Wilhelm Scheele. Trans!. L. Dobbs, 1931. London: G. Bell. Republished 1971, pp. 85-178. New York: Kraus Reprint)

(Schonmeyr et al, 2008) (Schonmeyr BH, Wong AK, Reid VJ, Gewalli F, Mehrara BJ. The effect of hyperbaric oxygen treatment on squamous cell cancer growth and tumor hypoxia. Ann Plast Surg.2008;60:81–88)

(Schreiner, 1974) (Schreiner, A. Hyperbaric oxygen therapy in bactericides infections. Acta Chir Scand 1974; 140: 73-76)

(Schroedl et al, 2002) (Schroedl C, McClintock DS, Budinger GR, et al. Hypoxic but not anoxic stabilization of HIF-1alpha requires mitochondrial reactive oxygen species. Am J Physiol Lung Cell Mol Physiol. 2002;283:L922–L931)

(Scibior-Bentkowska, Czeczot, 2009) (Scibior-Bentkowska D, Czeczot H. Cancer cells and oxidative stress. Postepy Hig Med Dosw (Online). 2009 Feb 23;63:58-72)

(Selvendiran et al, 2010) (Selvendiran K, Kuppusamy ML, Ahmed S, Bratasz A, Meenakshisundaram G, Rivera BK, Khan M, Kuppusamy P. Oxygenation inhibits ovarian tumor growth by downregulating STAT3 and cyclin-D1 expressions. Cancer Biol Ther. 2010;10:386–390)

(Semenza, 2000) (Semenza, G.L. HIF-1: Using two hands to flip the angiogenic switch. Cancer Metastasis Rev 2000; 19: 59-65)

(Semenza, 2001) (Semenza GL. HIF-1 and mechanisms of hypoxia sensing. Current Opinion in Cell Biology. 2001;13:167–171)

(Sethi et al, 1999) (Sethi, T., Rintoul, R.C., Moore, S.M., MacKinnon, A.C., Salter, D. and Choo, C., et al. Extracellular matrix proteins protect small cell lung cancer cells against apoptosis: A mechanism for small cell lung cancer growth and drug resistance in vivo. Nat Med 1999; 5: 662-668)

(Sheffield, 1984) (Sheffield, P.J. Tissue oxygen measurements with respect to soft-tissue wound healing with normobaric and hyperbaric oxygen treatments. In Gottlieb, S.F., Longmuir, I.S. and Totter, J.R. (Eds): Oxygen: An In-Depth Study of its Pathophysiology. Bethesda, Maryland: Undersea Medical Society, 1984; pp. 241-277)

(Sheffield, 1985) (Sheffield, P.J. Tissue oxygen measurements with respect to soft-tissue wound healing with normobaric and hyperbaric oxygen. HBO Review 1985; 6: 18-46)

(Sheffield, 1985) (Sheffield, P.J. Tissue oxygen measurements with respect to soft-tissue wound healing with normobaric and hyperbaric oxygen. HBO Review 1985; 6: 18-46)

(Sheffield, 1988) (Sheffield, P.J. Tissue oxygen measurements. In Davis, J.C. and Hunt, T.K. (eds): Problem Wounds: The Role of Oxygen. New York: Elsevier, 1988; pp. 17-51)

(Scheml et al, 2010) (Schreml S, Szeimies RM, Prantl L, Karrer S, Landthaler M, Babilas P. Oxygen in acute and chronic wound healing. Br J Dermatol. 2010 Aug;163(2):257-68)

(Schoemaker, 1964) (Schoemaker, G. Oxygen tension measurements under hyperbaric conditions. In Boerema, I., Brummelkamp, W.H. and Meijne, N.G. (Eds): Clinical Applications of Hyperbaric Oxygen.

Proceedings of the First International Congress on Hyperbaric Oxygen. Amsterdam: Elsevier, 1964; pp 330-335)

(Schwan, 1996) (Schwan, T.    National Institutes of Health, Rocky Mountain Laboratory.  Personal letter, 21 August 1996)

(Sen, 2009) (Sen CK (2009) Wound healing essentials: let there be oxygen. Wound Repair Reg 17:1–18)

(Sepnov, Uglova, 1979) (Sepnov, V.N. and Uglova, M.V. Features of sternum regeneration in autoplasty under conditions of hyperbaric oxygen. Orthop Traumatol Protex 1979; 5: 51-53)

(Shandling et al, 1997) (Shandling AH, Ellestad MH, Hart GB, et al. Hyperbaric oxygen and thrombolysis in myocardial infarction: The HOT MI pilot study. Am.Heart J.1997;134:544–550)

(Shannon et al, 2003) (Shannon AM, Bouchier-Hayes DJ, Condron CM, Toomey D. Tumour hypoxia, chemotherapeutic resistance and hypoxia-related therapies. Cancer Treat Rev.2003;29:297–307)

(Sharifi et al, 2002) (Sharifi M, Fares W, Abdel-Karim I, et al. Inhibition of restenosis by hyperbaric oxygen: a novel indication for an old modality. Cardiovasc Radiat Med. 2002;3:124–126)

(Sharifi et al, 2004) (Sharifi M, Fares W, Abdel-Karim I, et al. Usefulness of hyperbaric oxygen therapy to inhibit restenosis after percutaneous coronary intervention for acute myocardial infarction or unstable angina pectoris. Am J Cardiol.2004;93:1533–1535)

(Sheikh et al, 2000) (Sheikh AY, Gibson JJ, Rollins MD, et al. Effect of hyperoxia on vascular endothelial growth factor levels in a wound model. Arch Surg. 2000;135:1293–1297)

(Sheridan and Shank, 1999) (Sheridan R.L., Shank E.S. (1999) Hyperbaric oxygen treatment: A brief overview of a controversial topic. J Trauma 47: 426–435)

(Shewell, Thompson, 1980) (Shewell J, Thompson SC. The effect of hyperbaric oxygen treatment on pulmonary metastasis in the C3H mouse. Eur J Cancer. 1980;16:253–259. doi: 10.1016/0014-2964(80)90157-7)

(Shi et al, 2005) (Shi Y, Lee CS, Wu J, Koch CJ, Thom SR, Maity A, Bernhard EJ. Effects of hyperbaric oxygen exposure on experimental head and neck tumor growth, oxygenation, and vasculature. Head Neck. 2005;27:362–369)

(Shimizu et al, 1995) (Shimizu, S., Eguchi, Y., Kosaka, H., Kamiike, W., Matsuda, H. and Tsujimoto, Y. Prevention of hypoxia-induced cell death by Bel-2 and Bel-xL. Nature 1995; 374: 811-813)

(Shiokawa, D., Fujishima, M., Yanai, T. et al. Hyperbaric oxygen therapy in experimentally induced acute cerebral ischemia. Undersea Biomed Res 1986; 13: 337)

(Shyu et al, 2008) (Shyu KG, Hung HF, Wang BW, et al. Hyperbaric oxygen induces placental growth factor expression in bone marrow-derived mesenchymal stem cells. Life Sci. 2008;83:65–73)

(Shulman, Krohn, 1867) (Shulman, A.G. and Krohn, H.L. Influence of hyperbaric oxygen and multiple skin allografts on the healing of skin wounds. Surgery 1967; 62(6): 1051-1058)

(Shupak et al, 1987) (Shupak, A., Gozal, A.A. et al. Hyperbaric oxygenation in acute peripheral posttraumatic ischemia. J Hyper Med 1987; 2: 7-14)

(Sies, 1991) (Sies, H. 1991. Oxidative stress: from basic research to clinical application. Am. J. Med. 91:31S-38S)

(Silver, 1984) (Silver, I.A. Cellular microenvironment in healing and non-healing wounds. In Hunt, T.K., Heppenstall, R.B., Pines, E. et al. (Eds): Soft and Hard Tissue Repair, New York: Praeger, 1984; pp. 50-66)

(Simon, 1976) (Simon, L. The concept of threshold of ischemia in relation to brain structure and function. J Clin Path 1976; 11(suppl): 149-154)

(Sinclair, 2002) (Sinclair, D.A. Paradigms and pitfalls of yeast longevity research. Mech Aging Dev 2002; 123: 857-867)

(Sirsjo et al, 1993) (Sirsjo A, Lehr HA, Nolte D. Hyperbaric oxygen treatment enhances the recovery of blood flow and functional capillary density in postischemic striated muscle. Circ Shock 1993;40:9-13)

(Skyhar, M.J., Hargens, A.R., Strauss, M.B. et al. Hyperbaric oxygen reduces edema and necrosis of skeletal muscle in compartment syndromes associated with hemorrhagic hypotension J Bone Joint Surg 1986; 68A: 1218-1224)

(Smith et al, 1961) (Smith, G., Lawson, D.D., Renfrew, S. et al. Preservation of cerebral cortical activity by breathing oxygen at 2 ATA pressure during cerebral ischemia. Surg Gynecol Obstet 1961: 13:13)

(Soengas et al, 1999) (Soengas, M.S., Alarcon, R.M., Yoshida, H., Giaccia, A.J., Hakem, R. and Mak, T.W., et al. Apaf-1 and caspace-9 in p53-dependent apoptosis and tumor inhibition. Science 1999; 284: 156-159)

(Sohal, 1993) (Sohal, R. S.. The free radical hypothesis of aging: an appraisal of the current status. Aging Clin. Exp. Res. 5: 3-17, 1993)

(Soolsma, 1996) (Soolsma, S.J. (1996) The effect of intermittent hyperbaric oxygen on short term recovery from grade II medial collateral ligament injuries. Thesis, University of British Columbia, Vancouver)

(Staples and Clement, 1996) (Staples J., Clement D. (1996) Hyperbaric oxygen chambers and the treatment of sports injuries. Sports Med 22: 219–227)

(Stattin et al, 2007) (Stattin P, Björ O, Ferrari P, Lukanova A, Lenner P, Lindahl B, Hallmans G, Kaaks R. Prospective study of hyperglycemia and cancer risk. Diabetes Care. 2007;30:561–567)

(Stavitsky et al, 1998) (Stavitsky Y, Shandling AH, Ellestad MH, et al. Hyperbaric oxygen and thrombolysis in myocardial infarction: the "HOT MI" randomized multicenter study. Cardiology. 1998;90:131–136)

(Strauss et al, 1983) (Strauss, M.B., Hargens, A.R., Gershuni, D.H., Greensberg, D.A., Crenshaw, A.G., Hart, G.B. and Akeson, W.H. Reductions of skeletal muscle necrosis using intermittent hyperbaric oxygen in a model compartment syndrome. J Bone Joint Surg 1983; 65A: 656-662)

(Strauss, Malluche, Faugere, 1982) (Strauss, M.B., Malluche, H.H. and Faugere, M.C. Effect of hyperbaric oxygen on bone resorption in rabbits. Seventh Annual Conference on Clinical Application of HBO, Anaheim, California, 8-18 June 1982)

(Strauss et al, 1986) (Strauss, M.B., Hargens, A.R., Gershuni, D.H., Hart, G.B. and Akeson, W.H. Delayed use of hyperbaric oxygen for treatment of a model anterior compartment syndrome. J Ortho Res 1986; 4: 108-111)

(Strauss, Hart, 1984) (Strauss, M.B. and Hart, G.B. Crush injury and the role of hyperbaric oxygen. Top Emer Med 1984; 6: 9-24)

(Strauss, Hart, 1989) (Strauss, M.B. and Hart, G.B. Hyperbaric oxygen and the skeletal-muscle compartment syndrome. Contemp Ortho 1989; 18: 167-174)

(Sturh et al, 2007) (Stuhr LE, Raa A, Oyan AM, Kalland KH, Sakariassen PO, Petersen K, Bjerkvig R, Reed RK. Hyperoxia retards growth and induces apoptosis, changes in vascular density and gene expression in transplanted gliomas in nude rats. J Neurooncol. 2007;85:191–202)

(Suehiro et al, 2008) (Suehiro T, Shimura T, Okamura K, et al. The effect of hyperbaric oxygen treatment on postoperative morbidity of left lobe donor in living donor adult liver transplantation. Hepato. Gastroenterology. 2008;55:1014–1019)

(Suit, Maeda, 1967) (Suit HD, Maeda M. Hyperbaric oxygen and radiobiology of a C3H mouse mammary carcinoma. J Natl Cancer Inst. 1967;39:639–652)

(Sukoff, Ragatz, 1982) (Sukoff, M.H. and Ragatz, R.E. Hyperbric oxygenation for the treatment of acute cerebral edema. Neurosurgery 1982: 10: 29-38)

(Sukoff, Gottlieb, 1998) (Sukoff, M.H. and Gottlieb, S.F. Hyperbaric oxygen therapy. In Nussbaum E. (Ed): Pediatric Intensive Care 2nd ed. Mount Kisco, New York: Futura Publishing Inc. 1998; 483-507)

(Sun, Chen, Hsu, 2004) (Sun TB, Chen RL, Hsu YH. The effect of hyperbaric oxygen on human oral cancer cells. Undersea Hyperb Med. 2004;31:251–260)

(Takahashi et al, 2011) (Takahashi H, Mizuta T, Eguchi Y, Kawaguchi Y, Kuwashiro T, Oeda S, Isoda H, Oza N, Iwane S, Izumi K, et al. Post-challenge hyperglycemia is a significant risk factor for the development of hepatocellular carcinoma in patients with chronic hepatitis C. J Gastroenterol. 2011;46:790–798)

(Tally et al, 1975) (Tally, F.P., Stewart, P.R., Sutter, V.L. and Rosenblatt, J.E. Oxygen tolerance of fresh clinical anaerobic bacteria. J Clin Microbiol 1975; 1: 161-164)

(Tan et al, 1984) (Tan, C.M., Im, M.J., Myers, R.A.M., et al. Effects of hyperbaric oxygen and hyperbaric air on the survival of island skin flaps. Plast Reconstr Surg 1984; 73: 27-30)

(Tandara, Mistoe, 2003) (Tandara AA, Mustoe TA. Oxygen in wound healing--more than a nutrient. World J Surg. 2004 Mar;28(3):294-300)

(Tang et al, 2009) (Tang H, Zhang ZY, Ge JP, Zhou WQ, Gao JP. Effects of hyperbaric oxygen on tumor growth in the mouse model of LNCaP prostate cancer cell line. Zhonghua Nan Ke Xue.2009;15:713–716)

(Tang et al, 2009, uro) (Tang H, Sun Y, Xu C, Zhou T, Gao X, Wang L. Effects of hyperbaric oxygen therapy on tumor growth in murine model of PC-3 prostate cancer cell line. Urology.2009;73:205–208)

(Teicher et al, 1990) (Teicher, B.A, Holden, S.A., Al-Achi, A. and Herman, T.S. Classification of antineoplastic treatments by their differential toxicity toward putative oxygenated and hypoxic tumor subpopulations in vivo in the FSaII murine fibrosarcoma. Cancer Res 1990; 50: 3339-3344)

(Teicher, 1994) (Teicher BA. Hypoxia and drug resistance. Cancer Metastasis Rev. 1994;13:139–168)

(Telcher, 2001) (Telcher, B.A. Hypoxia and drug resistance. Cancer Metastasis Rev 2001; 155: 837-846)

(Tepper et al, 2005) (Tepper OM, Capla JM, Galiano RD, et al. Adult vasculogenesis occurs through in situ recruitment, proliferation, and tubulization of circulating bone marrow-derived cells. Blood. 2005;105:1068–1077)

(Thackham et al., 2007) (Thackham JA, McElwain DLS, Long RJ (2007) The use of hyperbaric oxygen therapy to treat chronic wounds: a review. Wound Repair Reg 16:321–330)

(Thiery, 2002) (Thiery JP. Epithelial–mesenchymal transitions in tumour progression. Nat Rev Cancer.2002;2:442–454)

(Thom, 1989) (Thom SR. Hyperbaric oxygen therapy. J. Intensive Care Med. 1989;4:58–74)

(Thom, 1993) (Thom SR. Leukocytes in carbon monoxide-mediated brain oxidative injury. Toxicol Appl Pharmacol. 1993;123:234–247)

(Thom, 2009) (Thom SR (2009) Oxidative stress is fundamental to hyperbaric oxygen therapy. J Appl Physiol 106:988–995)

(Thom, 2011) (Stephen R. Thom. Hyperbaric oxygen – its mechanisms and efficacy. Plast Reconstr Surg. 2011 Jan; 127(Suppl 1): 131S–141S)

(Thom, Bhopale, 2008) (Thom SR, Bhopale VM, Mancini JD, et al. Actin S-nitrosylation inhibits neutrophil beta-2 integrin function. J Biol Chem. 2008;283:10822–10834)

(Thom, Lauermann, Hart, 1986) (Thom SR, Lauermann MW, Hart GB. Intermittent hyperbaric oxygen therapy for reduction of mortality in experimental polymicrobial sepsis. J Infect Dis. 1986;154:504–510)

(Thom, Mendiguren, Hardy et al, 1997) (Thom SR, Mendiguren I, Hardy K, et al. Inhibition of human neutrophil beta2-integrin-dependent adherence by hyperbaric $O_2$. Am J Physiol.1997;272:C770–C777)

(Thom, Milovanova, 2008) (Thom S, Milovanova T. Hyperbaric oxygen therapy increases stem cell number and HIF-I content in diabetics. Undersea and Hyperbaric Med.2008;35:280)

(Tibbles, Edelsberg, 1996) (Tibbles PM and Edelsberg JS. Hyperbaric-oxygen therapy. N Engl J Med 334: 1642-1648, 1996)

(Tikhilow, Akimov, Lotovin, 1980) (Tikhilow, R.M., Akimov, G.C. and Lotovin,A.P. Effects of oxygen barotherapy on the regeneration of bone tissue. Orthop Traumatol Protez 1980; 12: 51-52)

(Tonomura, Granowitz, 2007) (Tonomura N, Granowitz EV. Hyperbaric oxygen: a potential new therapy for leukemia? Leuk Res. 2007;31:745–746)

(Torbati et al, 1992) (Torbati D, Church DF, Keller JM, and Pryor WA. Free radical generation in the brain precedes hyperbaric oxygen-induced convulsions. Free Radic Biol Med 13: 101-106, 1992)

(Torbati et al, 1989) (Torbati D, Mokashi A, and Lahiri S. Effects of acute hyperbaric oxygenation on respiratory control in cats. J Appl Physiol 67: 2351-2356, 1989)

(Torubarov et al, 1983) (Torubarov, F.S., Pakhomov,V.I., Krylova, I.V., et al. Changes in cerebral hemodynamics in patients with vascular pathology in the late stages of radiation sickness treated with hyperbaric oxygenation. Zh Neuropatol Psikhiatr 1983; 83:: 28-33)

(Toufekstian et al, 2001) (Toufektsian, M.C., Boucher, F.R., Tanguy, S., Morel, S. and de Leiris, J.G. Cardiac toxicity of singlet oxygen: implication in reperfusion injury. Antioxid Redox Signal 2001; 3: 63-69)

(Turrens et al, 1982) (Turrens JF, Freeman BA, Levitt JG, Crapo JD. The effect of hyperoxia on superoxide production by lung submitochondrial particles. Arch Biochem Biophys. 1982;217:401–410)

(Turrens et al, 1985) (Turrens JF, Alexandre A, Lehninger AL. Ubisemiquinone is the electron donor for superoxide formation by complex III of heart mitochondria. Arch Biochem Biophys. 1985;237:408–414)

(Turrens, 2003) (Julio F Turrens. Mitochondrial formation of reactive oxygen species. J Physiol. 2003 Oct 15; 552(Pt 2): 335–344)

(Tyler, 1992) (Tyler, D. D. 1992. The Mitochondrion in Health and Disease, Cambridge, UK: VCH)

(Ueno et al, 2014) (Ueno T, Omi T, Uchida E, Yokota H, Kawana S. Evaluation of hyperbaric oxygen therapy for chronic wounds. J Nippon Med Sch. 2014;81(1):4-1)

(Urschel et al, 1965) (Urschell, HC et al, Cardiac resuscitation with hydrogen peroxide. Circulation, Supplement II. October, 1965. Volumes XXXI and XXXII)

(Valko et al, 2007) (Valko M, Leibfritz D, Moncol J, et al. Free radicals and antioxidants in normal physiological functions and human disease. Int J Biochem Cell Biol.2007;39:44–84)

(Valois, Schade, 1967) (Valois, J.D. and Schade, J.P. An electrophysiological study of histotoxic anoxia under normal and hyperbaric conditions. In Bourg H. and Ledingham, I.M.C. (eds.) Carbon Monoxide Poisoning. New York: Elsevier, 1967; pp. 183-197)

(Van Meter et al, 1986) (Van Meter, K., Lasater, S., Whidden, S.J. et al. Hyperbaric oxygen therapy and wound healing. Curr Con Wound Care, 1986; Fall: 7-10)

(Van Unnik, 1965) (Van Unnik, A.J.M. Inhibition of toxin production in Clostridium perfringens in vitro by hyperbaric oxygen. Antonie Leeuwenhoek Microbiol 1965; 31: 181-186)

(Vaupel et al, 1987)(Vaupel, P., Kallinowski, F. and Okunieff, P. Blood flow, oxygen consumption and tissue oxygenation of human breast cancer engrafts in nude rats. Cancer Res 1987; 47: 3496-3503)

(Vaupel, Kellecher, 1995) (Vaupel, P.W. and Kellecher, D.K. Metabolic status and reaction to heat of normal and tumor tissue. In: Seegenschmiedt, M.H., Fessenden, P. and Vernon, C.C. editors. Medical radiology - diagnostic imaging and radiation oncology, thermo radiotherapy and thermo chemotherapy. Berlin and Heidelberg (Germany) and New York (NY): Springer; 1995:157-176)

(Vaupel, Kelleher, 1999) (Vaupel, P. and Kelleher, D.K. editors. Tumor hypoxia: Pathophysiology, clinical significance and therapeutic perspectives. Stuttgart (Germany): Wissenschaftliche Verlagsgesellschaft; 1999)

Prof Randolph M. Howes MD,PhD

(Vaupel, Mayer, 2007) (Vaupel P, Mayer A. Hypoxia in cancer: significance and impact on clinical outcome.Cancer Metastasis Rev. 2007;26:225–239)

(von Harsdorf et al, 1999) (von Harsdorf, R., Li, P.F. and Dietz, R. Signaling pathways in reactive oxygen species-induced cardiomyocyte apoptosis Circulation 1999; 99: 2934-2941)

(Wada et al, 1965) (Wada, J., Ikeda, T., Kamada, K., et al. Oxygen hyperbaric treatment for severe CO poisoning and severe burns in coal mines (Hokutan-Yubari) gas explosion. Igaku Jpn 1965; 54: 68)

(Warburg, Geissler, Lorenz, 1968) (Warburg, 0., Geissler, A. W., Lorenz, S. 1968. Oxygen the creator of differentiation. In Aspects of Yeast Metabolism, ed. A. K. Mills, H. A. Krebs, pp. 327-37. Oxford: Blackell. 345 pp)

(Waterhouse et al, 1993) (Waterhouse M, Zamboni W, Brown R, et al. The use of HBO in compromised free tissue transfer and replantation: a clinical review. Undersea and Hyperbaric Med. 1993;20 Suppl:64)

(Weaver, 1995) (Weaver LK. Hyperbaric medicine for the hospital-based physician. Hosp Pract (1995). 2012 Aug;40(3):88-101)

(Weaver et al, 2002) (Weaver LK, Hopkins RO, Chan KJ, et al. Hyperbaric oxygen for acute carbon monoxide poisoning. N Engl J Med. 2002;347:1057–1067)

(Weaver, 2011) (Weaver LK. Hyperbaric oxygen in the critically ill. Crit Care Med. 2011 Jul;39(7):1784-91)

(Webster et al. 2002) (Webster A., Syrotuik D., Bell G., Jones R., Hanstock C. (2002) Effects of hyperbaric oxygen on recovery from exercise-induced muscle damage in humans. Clin J Sports Med 12: 139–150)

(Weinstein et al, 1986) (Weinstein, P.R., Hameroff, S.R., Johnson, P. et al. Effect of hyperbaric oxygen therapy of dimethylsulfoxide on cerebral ischemia in unanesthetized gerbils. Neurosurgery 1986; 18: 528)

(Weiss, 1994) (Weiss EL: Connective tissue in wound healing, in McCulloch JM, Kloth LC, Feedar JA (eds): Wound Healing: Alternatives in Management, ed 2. Philadelphia, FA Davis Co, 1994, pp 16-31)

(Weiss, Neville, 1989) (Weiss, J.P. and Neville, E.C. Hyperbaric oxygen: primary treatment of radiation-induced hemorrhagic cystitis. J Urol 1989; 142: 43-45)

(Weisz et al, 1997) (Weisz G, Lavy A, Adir Y, et al. Modification of in vivo and in vitro TNF-alpha, IL-1, and IL-6 secretion by circulating monocytes during hyperbaric oxygen treatment in patients with perianal Crohn's disease. J Clin Immunol.1997;17:154–159)

(Wells et al, 1977) (Wells, C.H., Goodpasture, J.E., Horrigan, D.J. and Hart, G.B. Tissue gas measurements during hyperbaric oxygen exposure. In Smith, G. (ed): Proceedings of the Sixth International Congress on Hyperbaric Medicine. Aberdeen, Scotland: Aberdeen University Press, 1977; pp. 118-124)

(Wells, Hilton, 1977) (Wells, C.H. and Hilton, J.G. Effects of hyperbaric oxygenation on host burn plasma extravasation. In Davis, J.C. and Hunt T.K. (eds): Hyperbaric Oxygen Therapy. Bethesda, Maryland: Undersea Medical Society, 1977; pp. 259-265)

(Welsh et al, 2003) (Welsh, S.J., Williams, R.R., Birmingham, A., Newman, D.J., Kirkpatrick, D.L. and Powis, G. The thioredoxin redox inhibitors 1-methylpropyl 2-imidazolyl disulfide and pleurisy inhibit hypoxia-induced factor 1a and vascular endothelial growth factor formation. Molecular Cancer Therapeutics 2003; 2: 235-243)

(West, 1991) (West, J.B. Cardiac energetics and myocardial oxygen consumption. Physiologic basis of medical practice. 1991; Williams and Wilkins. Baltimore, MD 250-260)

(Whalen, Heyman, Saltzman, 1966) (Whalen, R., Heyman, A. and Saltzman, H. The protective effect of hyperbaric oxygen in cerebral ischemia. Arch Neurol 1966; 14: 15)

(Wheeler et al, 2014) (Wheeler KT, Payne V, D'Agostino RB Jr, Walb MC, Munley MT, Metheny-Barlow LJ, Robbins ME. Impact of breathing 100% oxygen on radiation-induced cognitive impairment. Radiat Res. 2014 Nov;182(5):580-5)

(Wike-Hooley et al, 1984) (Wike-Hooley, J.L., Haveman, J. and Reinhold, H.S. The relevance of tumor pH to the treatment of malignant disease. Radiol Oncol 1984; 47: 687-696)

(Wilkinson, et al, 1970)(Wilkinson, F.F., Rosasco, S.A., Calori, B.A., Equia, O.F. and Rubio, R.A. Conclusions preliminaries sobre el uso del oxygeno hiperbaro en lepr lepromatosa. {Preliminary conclusions on the use of hyperbaric oxygen in leprosy]. Revist de Leprologia 1970; 7: 459-471)

(Wilmeth, Gazau, 1982) (Wilmeth, J.B. and Gazau, A. Hyperbaric oxygen as an adjunct to the treatment of orthopedic injuries with full thickness grafts. Seventh Annual Conference on the Clinical Application of HBO, Anaheim, California, 9-11 June 1982)

(Winter, Perrins, 1969) (Winter, G.D. and Perrins, D.J.D. Effects of hyperbaric oxygen treatment on epidermal regeneration. In Wada, J. and Iwa, T. (Eds): Proceedings of the Forth International congress on Hyperbaric Medicine. Baltimore: Williams and Wilkins, 1969; pp. 363-368)

(Wlaschek and Scharffetter-Kochanek, 2005) (Wlaschek M, Scharffetter-Kochanek K (2005) Oxidative stress in chronic venous ulcers. Wound Repair Reg 13:452–461)

(Xu, Zhu, Shu, 2014) (Xu CX, Zhu HH, Zhu YM. Diabetes and cancer: Associations, mechanisms, and implications for medical practice. World J Diabetes. 2014 Jun 15;5(3):372-80)

(Yu et al, 2005) (Yu S, Chiu J, Yang S, et al. Preconditioned hyperbaric oxygenation protects the liver against ischemia-reperfusion injury in rats. J Surg Res.2005;128:28–36)

(Zamboni et al, 1993) (Zamboni WA, Roth AC, Russell RC, et al. Morphologic analysis of the microcirculation during reperfusion of ischemic skeletal muscle and the effect of hyperbaric oxygen. Plast. Reconstr. Surg. 1993:91)

(Zavesa, 1977) (Zavesa, P.X., Shavab, Y.Y. and Abduchudonov, S.S. Effects of local oxygen therapy on reparative regeneration of the bone. Orthop Traumatol Protez 1977; 1: 71-72)

(Zhang et al., 2005) (Zhang JH, Lo T, Mychaskiw G et al. (2005) Mechanisms of hyperbaric oxygen and neuroprotection in stroke. Pathophysiology 12:63–77)

(Zhang et al, 2008) (Zhang Q, Chang Q, Cox RA, et al. Hyperbaric oxygen attenuates apoptosis and decreases inflammation in an ischemic wound model. J Invest Dermatol.2008;128:2102–2112)

(Zhang, Gould, 2014) (Zhang Q and gould LJ. Hyperbaric Oxygen Reduces Matrix Metalloproteinases in Ischemic Wounds through a Redox-Dependent Mechanism. J Invest derbatol 2014 Jan;134(1):237-46)

(Zhang, Piston, Goodman, 2002) (Zhang Q, Piston DW, Goodman RH. Regulation of corepressor function by nuclear NADH. Science. 2002;295:1895–1897)

(Zijl et al, 2011) (Zijl F, Krupitza G, Mikulits W. Initial steps of metastasis: cell invasion and endothelial transmigration. Mutat Res. 2011;728:23–34)

# ABOUT THE AUTHOR

## Dr. Randolph M. Howes M.D., Ph.D.

**Biographical sketch:**

As a champion of the people, Dr. Howes anticipates and hopes for the active involvement of all connected parties (patients, caregivers, health-care professionals, etc.) as an integral approach to educating consumers and the public about the potential dangers of excessive antioxidant-containing supplements.

Some people are born with a silver spoon in their mouth but Dr. Howes had to earn his. Even as a child, Dr. Howes could think with adult clarity. He could envision his future but it would require "decades of dedication" to make it a reality.

From childhood, Dr. Howes was motivated to become a medical doctor and scientist. Assuredly, having been born on a small strawberry farm in rural Louisiana, his journey to the top has proved to be arduous and demanding.

However, he was fortunate to acquire the confidence of Sister Elizabeth Rose at St. Joseph's school and went on to gain the support of his high school speech teacher, Mrs. Iris Brann, who also had strong beliefs in his abilities and potential. Ultimately, with the help of his guitar and his singing ability, he defeated the star quarter back of the high school football team to become the president of the student body.

With the aid of a $25 dollar legislative scholarship, he went on to Southeastern Louisiana College (SLC). At SLC, he was selected for honors chemistry, made the Dean's list, worked at the Psychology Research Lab forty hours a week, maintained a premed study load, and was elected president of the Junior Class and the Interfraternity Council.

To earn badly needed funds, he played music on weekends in a small combo, The Three Blind Mice. Next, he matriculated to Tulane University School of Medicine.

His initial dream was to try to combine both medicine and science. In that regard, he began work as a technician with Dr. Andrew Schally at the Endocrine Polypeptide Lab in the isolation of thyrotropin releasing factor. This work led to a Nobel Prize for Dr. Schally.

Dr. Howes had been highly impressed with the enthusiasm of biochemist, Dr. Richard H. Steele, who accepted him as a doctoral candidate under his tutelage. Dr. Howes graduated in the top 10 of his class, won the Louisiana Pathology Association Award, was elected to the Sigma Xi honor fraternity and was the first in the history of Tulane to become a Doctor of Medicine and a Ph.D. in biochemistry concurrently.

Next, he was selected to pursue a career in surgery at the prestigious Johns Hopkins Hospital.

Unbelievably, at Dr. Howes' urging, he was allowed to operate his own research lab during his surgical internship and residency training while at Johns Hopkins Hospital. He worked hand in hand with the greats in American medicine and surgery.

Independently, he garnered grants, trained lab techs, wrote papers, slept on the cold floor, proudly served as a Captain in the U.S. Army Reserves Medical Corp and finished with board eligibility in both general and plastic surgery in an unheard of six year period.

In another first, he was appointed as an Adjunct Assistant Professor of Plastic Surgery at Johns Hopkins Hospital.

For decades, Dr. Howes gave unselfishly to pro bono medical missions in the Philippines and he holds the Ernesto Espaldon Chair as Professor of Plastic Surgery at the University of Santo Tomas.

Upon retirement from a career in cosmetic plastic surgery, he is living his dream of trying to revolutionize the treatment of cancer, heart disease, HIV/AIDS and malaria, with his in depth knowledge of the arcane biochemistry of oxygen metabolism. He is a work in progress! Dedicated and passionate, he is on a mission for mankind.

Dr. Howes invented the triple lumen venous catheter, which has been credited with helping save the lives of over 20 million critically ill patients worldwide. His catheter is the number one venous catheter in the world today and his name is well recognized in over 100 countries. He has been recognized as a humanitarian, visionary, entrepreneur, singer, songwriter, inventor and author.

He received the Harper Award for innovative research from the American College for Advancement in Medicine, served as their keynote speaker and his peers refer to him as "a walking encyclopedia on oxygen metabolism."

He is a Dr. Norman Vincent Peale Unsung Hero award winner, which recognized his awesome "versatility." Additionally, even though he is humble and does not like talking about it, he is a self made multi-millionaire.

He is currently doing extensive research on cures for cancer and heart disease and development of revolutionary treatment modalities. He has written 21 books over the past 5 years on the subject of oxygen metabolism, as it relates to protection from cancer, heart disease, diabetes, malaria, HIV/AIDS, Alzheimer's disease, aging and arthritis. He has written nine sci-fi novels, many scientific and medical papers and has lectured nationally and internationally. He has written over 500 medical letters to the editor on popular topics.

His research has shown that currently common antioxidant vitamins, such as vitamins A & E, (and vitamin C to a lesser extent) can be harmful and that oxygen free radicals protect us from bacterial, fungal and viral infections and they help to control cancer growth.

He has developed an effective, inexpensive singlet oxygen generating system, from orthomolecular agents, for the treatment of cancer and heart disease. He is passionate about his research and hopes to have his discoveries at the patient's bedside in his lifetime. Admittedly, this is an extremely ambitious goal.

There are over 12,000 pages in his magnum opus and at the Howes World Selective Library on Oxygen Metabolism. **Over 3,000 pages of his opus are available online in a searchable format www. iwillfindthecure.org.**

**Companion Books of Prof. R. Howes, MD, PhD:**

Howes, R. M. *U.T.O.P.I.A. - Unified Theory of Oxygen Participation in Aerobiosis.* © 2004. Free Radical Publishing Co. Kentwood, LA, available at www. iwillfindthecure.org.

Howes R. M. *The Medical and Scientific Significance of Oxygen Free Radical Metabolism.* © 2005. Free Radical Publishing Co. Kentwood, LA. USA. available at www.iwillfindthecure.org.

Prof Randolph M. Howes MD,PhD

Howes, R. M. *Hydrogen Peroxide Monograph 1: Scientific, Medical and Biochemical Overview.* © 2006; Free Radical Publishing Co. USA. 200 pages. available at www.iwillfindthecure.org.

Howes, R. M. Monograph 2: *Antioxidant vitamins A, C & E: Equivocal Scientific Studies,* © 2006; Free Radical Publishing Co. USA. 171 pages. available at www.iwillfindthecure.org.

Howes, R. M. *Cardiovascular Disease and Oxygen Free Radical Mythology,* © 2006;

Free Radical Publishing Co. USA. 308 pages. available at www.iwillfindthecure.org.

Howes, R. M. *Diabetes and Oxygen Free Radical Sophistry,* © 2006; Free Radical Publishing Co. USA. Free Radical Publishing Co. USA. 366 pages. available at www.iwillfindthecure.org.

Howes, R. M. *Reactive Oxygen Species Insufficiency (ROSI) as the Basis for Disease Allowance and Coexistence: Extraordinary Support for an Extraordinary Theory* Vol I, II & III. © 2008; 1564 pages. available at www.iwillfindthecure.org. Howes, R. M. Volume I 501 pages #7 © 2008. Free Radical Publishing Co. USA. Howes, R. M. Volume II 505 pages #8 © 2008. Free Radical Publishing Co. USA. Howes, R. M. Volume III 562 pages #9 © 2008. Free Radical Publishing Co. USA.

Howes, R. M. *THE HOWES PAPERS* © 2009; Free Radical Publishing Co. USA. 211 pages

Howes R.M. *"COFFEE TABLE MUSINGS of the Da Vinci in COWBOY BOOTS"* Pithy Prose and Perspicacious Aphorisms. © 2009; 103 pages

Howes, R. M. Reactive Oxygen Species vs. Antioxidants: *"The Oxypocalypse"* or *"The war that never was"* © 2010; Free Radical Publishing Co. USA. 550 pages. available at www.iwillfindthecure.org.

Howes R.M. *Death in Small Doses?:* Antioxidant Vitamins A, C & E in the 21st Century Book One: *A Health Impact Statement For The Layman* © 2010; Trafford Publishing. Indianapolis, USA. 90 pages

Howes R.M. *Antioxidant Vitamins are Making A Killing;*
Antioxidant Vitamins A, C & E in the 21st Century
Book Two: *A Health Impact Statement For The Medical Scientist*
© 2010; 184 pages

- **Death In Small Doses? Books 1 and 2. Trafford Publishing,** © **2010**

- **Antioxidant Overkill, CreateSpace and Free Radical Publishing,** © **2011**

- **Dangers of Excessive Antioxidants in Cancer Patients, CreateSpace and Free Radical Publishing,** © **2011**

- **Heart Disease and Antioxidant Failures, CreateSpace and Free Radical Publishing,** © **2011**

- **Antioxidant Failures and Dangers, CreateSpace and Free Radical Publishing,** © **2011**

- **Anti-Aging Anti-oxidant Scams, CreateSpace and Free Radical Publishing,** © **2011**

- **Sports, Athletes, Exercise Facts and Antioxidant Myths, CreateSpace and Free Radical Publishing,** © **2011**

- **Alzheimer's Disease: Forget Antioxidants and Supplements, CreateSpace and Free Radical Publishing,** © **2012**

- **Sex, Performance, Reproduction, Naked Radicals And Antioxidants, CreateSpace and Free Radical Publishing,** © **2012**

- **Antioxidants Linked To Deadly Unintended Consequences, CreateSpace and Free Radical Publishing,** © **2013**

- **U.T.O.P.I.A.: Unified Theory of Oxygen Participation In Aerobiosis, CreateSpace and Free Radical Publishing,** © **2014, revised**

- Hydrogen Peroxide: A Health, Homeostatic and Protective Essentiality, CreateSpace and Free Radical Publishing, © 2014

- Reactive Oxygen Species vs. Antioxidants: The Oxypocalypse or The War That Never Was, CreateSpace and Free Radical Publishing, © 2014

- Diabetes and Oxygen Free Radical Sophistry, CreateSpace and Free Radical Publishing, © 2014, revised

- FISH OIL (Omega3 fatty acids): Facts, Fantasies & Failures. CreateSpace and Free Radical Publishing, © 2014

-Vitamin D: Benefits & False claims. CreateSpace and Free Radical Publishing, © 2014

- Chocolate & Red Wine Antioxidants (Polyphenols, Flavonoids & Resveratrol): Facts vs. Falsehoods. CreateSpace and Free Radical Publishing, © 2015

- Blueberry, Tomato & CoQ10 Antioxidants (Anthocyanin, Lycopene & Ubiquinone): Claims vs. Facts. CreateSpace and Free Radical Publishing, © 2015

- Exercise and Reactive Oxygen Species. Likely the only health miracle out there. CreateSpace and Free Radical Publishing, © 2015

- Cancer and Longevity Answers: Naked Mole Rats, Exercise & EMODs (ROS). CreateSpace and Free Radical Publishing, © 2015

All books available at www.amazon.com; www.barnesandno-bles.com; www.booksamillion.com.

## Companion Papers of Prof. R. Howes, MD, PhD:

**Dr. Howes has authored over 500 medical publications in health related editorials.**

**Citation:** R. Howes: Mythology of Antioxidant Vitamins?. *The Journal of Evidence-Based Alternative and Complimentary Medicine*. April, 2011. 16(2): 149-189.

**Citation:** R. Howes: Cancer Therapy: A Review with Scientific Validation for the Role of Electronically Modified Oxygen Derivatives in Oncologic Treatment Modalities. *The Internet Journal of Alternative Medicine*. 2010 Volume 8 Number 1.

**Citation:** R. Howes: Hydrogen Peroxide: A review of a scientifically verifiable omnipresent ubiquitous essentiality of obligate, aerobic, carbon-based life forms. *The Internet Journal of Plastic Surgery*. 2010 Volume 7 Number 1.

Howes M.D., PhD., R. (2009). Dangers of Antioxidants in Cancer Patients: A Review. *PHILICA.COM Article number 153*. Published 7th February, 2009. (20 pages)

Howes M.D., PhD., R. (2008). Aging and anti-aging claims: a review on antioxidant vitamins A, C & E. *PHILICA.COM Article number 116*. Published on 12th January, 2008. (16 pages)

Howes M.D., PhD., R. (2007). Sleep: An original "radical" proposal. *PHILICA.COM Observation number 42*. Published on 5th October, 2007. (1 page)

Howes M.D., PhD., R. (2007). Antioxidant Vitamins A, C & E; Death in Small Doses and Legal Liability? *PHILICA.COM Article number 89*. Published on 5th April, 2007. (23 pages)

Howes M.D., PhD., R. (2007). Cancer, Apoptosis and Reactive Oxygen Species: A New Paradigm. *PHILICA.COM Article number 86*. Published on 26th February, 2007. (11 pages)

Howes M.D., PhD., R. (2007). Antioxidant Vitamins A, C and E: Assessing Potential for Harm. *PHILICA.COM Article number 83*. Published on 15th February, 2007. (14 pages)

Prof Randolph M. Howes MD,PhD

Howes M.D., PhD., R. (2007). The Consequent Downfall of the Free Radical Theory. *PHILICA.COM Article number 75.* Published on 22nd January, 2007. (9 pages)

Howes, R.M.: "The Free Radical Fantasy," The Annals of New York Academy of Sciences, 2006, Vol. 1067, pp. 22-26.

(Howes, 2005) (Howes, R.M. Tumoricidal Activity of An Injectable Singlet Oxygen System Generated From Physiological Agents: The Howes Singlet Oxygen Cancer Therapy System). In The Medical and Scientific Significance of Oxygen Free Radical Metabolism. © 2005. Free Radical Publishing Co. Kentwood, LA. pp. 893-912).

(Howes, Farber, 2005) (Howes, R.M. and Farber, G. Tumoricidal Activity of the Howes Singlet Oxygen Delivery System in Human Basal Cell Carcinoma. In The Medical and Scientific Significance of Oxygen Free Radical Metabolism. © 2005. Free Radical Publishing Co. Kentwood, LA. pp. 883-892).

(Howes et al, 1977) (Howes, R.M., Steele, R.H. and Hoopes, J.E., The role of Electronic excitation states in collagen biosynthesis, Persp. In Biol. And Med., Summer 1977, 20; 4:539-544).

(Howes, Steele, 1976) (Howes, R.M., Steele, R.H. and Hoopes, J.E., Peroxide induced Chemiluminescence in an in vitro proline hydroxylation system, 1976, 8; 1:77-84).

(Howes et al, 1976) (Howes, R. M., Allen, R.C., Su, C.T. and Hoopes, J.E., Altered polymorphonuclear leukocyte bioenergetics in patients with thermal injury, the Surgical Forum, 1976, 27:558-560).

(Howes, Steele, 1972) (Howes, R.M. and Steele, R.H., Microsomal chemiluminescence induced by NADPH and its relation to aryl-hydroxylations, Res Commun. Chem. Path. Pharmacol., March 1972, 3; 2:349-357).

(Howes, Steele, 1971) (Howes, R. M. and Steele, R. H., Microsomal chemiluminescence induced by NADPH and its relation to lipid peroxidation, Res. Commun. Chem. Path. Pharmacol., July-Sept. 1971, 2; 4 & 5:619-626).

**I despise precious time wasted,
for it alone, is the unfinished canvas
displaying the portrait of my life.
R. M. Howes, M.D., Ph.D.
9/7/09**

"We are what we repeatedly do. Excellence then, is not an act, but a habit." ~Aristotle

## OTHER BOOKS

**PUBLISHED: Partial list.** The Fire Eaters, Molding your own destiny more easily, Carnivore Press, © 1982

Uplift, The Answer Book to your plastic and cosmetic surgery questions, Carnivore Press, © 1986

The Pundit Speaks, vol. I. An Anthology of Neoclassical Poetic Philosophy, Carnivore Press, © 1990

The Pundit Speaks, Volume II, An Anthology of Neoclassical Poetic Philosophy, Free Radical Press, © 1994

The Pundit Speaks, Volume III, An Anthology of Neoclassical Poetic Philosophy, Free Radical Press, © 1996

The Pundit Speaks, Volume IV, An Anthology of Neoclassical Poetic Philosophy, Free Radical Press, © 2000

The Fable of the Chocolate Covered Strawberry Coloring Book, Free Radical Press, © 2001

The Pundit Speaks, Volume IV, An Anthology of Neoclassical Poetic Philosophy, Free Radical Press, © 2003

The Pundit Speaks, Volume V, An Anthology of Neoclassical Poetic Philosophy, Trafford Publishing, © 2009

Coffee Table Musings of The DaVinci In Cowboy Boots, Trafford Publishing, © 2010

Prof Randolph M. Howes MD,PhD

**Available at: www.philica.com**
**www.medi.philica.com**
**www.iwillfindthecure.org**
**www.amazon.com**

**DOC**
**R<sub>x</sub>ANDOLPH**
**HOWES**

**RAD!CAL**

**"Future's shape is sculpted by the**
**persistent kneading hands of**
**the impossible dreamer."**
R. M. Howes, M.D., Ph.D.
5/2/04